Japan's Wartime Medical Atrocities

Prior to and during the Second World War, the Japanese Army established programs of biological warfare throughout China and elsewhere. In these "factories of death," including the now-infamous Unit 731, Japanese doctors and scientists conducted large numbers of vivisections and experiments on human beings, mostly Chinese nationals. However, as a result of complex historical factors including an American cover-up of the atrocities, Japanese denials, and inadequate responses from successive Chinese governments, justice has never been fully served.

This volume brings together the contributions of a group of scholars from different countries and various academic disciplines. It examines Japan's wartime medical atrocities and their postwar aftermath from a comparative perspective and inquires into perennial issues of historical memory, science, politics, society and ethics elicited by these rebarbative events. The volume's central ethical claim is that the failure to bring justice to bear on the systematic abuse of medical research by Japanese military medical personnel more than six decades ago has had a profoundly retarding influence on the development and practice of medical and social ethics in all of East Asia. The book also includes an extensive annotated bibliography selected from relevant publications in Japanese, Chinese and English.

Jing-Bao Nie is an Associate Professor at the Bioethics Centre, University of Otago, New Zealand, and Furong Visiting Professor at the Centre for Moral Culture, Hunan Normal University, China.

Nanyan Guo is an Associate Professor at the International Research Center for Japanese Studies, Kyoto, Japan.

Mark Selden is a Research Associate in the East Asia Program at Cornell University, USA and a coordinator of *The Asia-Pacific Journal: Japan Focus*.

Arthur Kleinman is the Esther and Sidney Rabb Professor of Anthropology, Department of Anthropology, Faculty of Arts and Sciences and Professor of Medical Anthropology and Psychiatry at Harvard Medical School, USA.

Asia's Transformations
Edited by Mark Selden, Cornell University, USA

The books in this series explore the political, social, economic and cultural consequences of Asia's transformations in the twentieth and twenty-first centuries. The series emphasizes the tumultuous interplay of local, national, regional and global forces as Asia bids to become the hub of the world economy. While focusing on the contemporary, it also looks back to analyse the antecedents of Asia's contested rise.

This series comprises several strands:

Asia's Transformations
Titles include:

Debating Human Rights*
Critical essays from the United States and Asia
Edited by Peter Van Ness

Hong Kong's History*
State and society under colonial rule
Edited by Tak-Wing Ngo

Japan's Comfort Women*
Sexual slavery and prostitution during World War II and the US occupation
Yuki Tanaka

Opium, Empire and the Global Political Economy*
Carl A. Trocki

Chinese Society*
Change, conflict and resistance
Edited by Elizabeth J. Perry and Mark Selden

Mao's Children in the New China*
Voices from the Red Guard generation
Yarong Jiang and David Ashley

Remaking the Chinese State*
Strategies, society and security
Edited by Chien-min Chao and Bruce J. Dickson

Korean Society*
Civil society, democracy and the state
Edited by Charles K. Armstrong

The Making of Modern Korea*
Adrian Buzo

The Resurgence of East Asia*
500, 150 and 50 Year perspectives
Edited by Giovanni Arrighi, Takeshi Hamashita and Mark Selden

Chinese Society, second edition*
Change, conflict and resistance
Edited by Elizabeth J. Perry and Mark Selden

Ethnicity in Asia*
Edited by Colin Mackerras

The Battle for Asia*
From decolonization to globalization
Mark T. Berger

State and Society in 21st Century China*
Edited by Peter Hays Gries and Stanley Rosen

Japan's Quiet Transformation*
Social change and civil society in the 21st century
Jeff Kingston

Confronting the Bush Doctrine*
Critical views from the Asia-Pacific
Edited by Mel Gurtov and Peter Van Ness

China in War and Revolution, 1895–1949*
Peter Zarrow

The Future of US–Korean Relations*
The imbalance of power
Edited by John Feffer

Working in China*
Ethnographies of labor and workplace transformations
Edited by Ching Kwan Lee

Korean Society, 2nd Edition*
Civil society, democracy and the state
Edited by Charles K. Armstrong

Singapore*
The state and the culture of excess
Souchou Yao

Pan-Asianism in Modern Japanese History*
Colonialism, regionalism and borders
Edited by Sven Saaler and J. Victor Koschmann

The Making of Modern Korea, 2nd Edition*
Adrian Buzo

Re-writing Culture in Taiwan
Edited by Fang-long Shih, Stuart Thompson, and Paul-François Tremlett

Reclaiming Chinese Society*
The new social activism
Edited by You-tien Hsing and Ching Kwan Lee

Girl Reading Girl in Japan
Edited by Tomoko Aoyama and Barbara Hartley

Chinese Politics*
State, society and the market
Edited by Peter Hays Gries and Stanley Rosen

Chinese Society, 3rd Edition*
Change, conflict and resistance
Edited by Elizabeth J. Perry and Mark Selden

Mapping Modernity in Shanghai
Space, gender, and visual culture in the Sojourners' City, 1853–98
Samuel Y. Liang

Minorities and Multiculturalism in Japanese Education
An interactive perspective
Edited by Ryoko Tsuneyoshi, Kaori H. Okano and Sarane Boocock

Japan's Wartime Medical Atrocities
Comparative inquiries in science, history, and ethics
Edited by Jing-Bao Nie, Nanyan Guo, Mark Selden and Arthur Kleinman

Asia's Great Cities

Each volume aims to capture the heartbeat of the contemporary city from multiple perspectives emblematic of the authors' own deep familiarity with the distinctive faces of the city, its history, society, culture, politics and economics, and its evolving position in national, regional and global frameworks. While most volumes emphasize urban developments since the Second World War, some pay close attention to the legacy of the longue durée in shaping the contemporary. Thematic and comparative volumes address such themes as urbanization, economic and financial linkages, architecture and space, wealth and power, gendered relationships, planning and anarchy, and ethnographies in national and regional perspective. Titles include:

Bangkok*
Place, practice and representation
Marc Askew

Representing Calcutta*
Modernity, nationalism and the colonial uncanny
Swati Chattopadhyay

Singapore*
Wealth, power and the culture of control
Carl A. Trocki

The City in South Asia
James Heitzman

Global Shanghai, 1850–2010*
A history in fragments
Jeffrey N. Wasserstrom

Hong Kong*
Becoming a global city
Stephen Chiu and Tai-Lok Lui

Asia.com is a series which focuses on the ways in which new information and communication technologies are influencing politics, society and culture in Asia. Titles include:

Japanese Cybercultures*
Edited by Mark McLelland and Nanette Gottlieb

Asia.com*
Asia encounters the Internet
Edited by K. C. Ho, Randolph Kluver and Kenneth C. C. Yang

The Internet in Indonesia's New Democracy*
David T. Hill and Krishna Sen

Chinese Cyberspaces*
Technological changes and political effects
Edited by Jens Damm and Simona Thomas

Mobile Media in the Asia-Pacific
Gender and the art of being mobile
Larissa Hjorth

Literature and Society
Literature and Society is a series that seeks to demonstrate the ways in which Asian literature is influenced by the politics, society and culture in which it is produced. Titles include:

The Body in Postwar Japanese Fiction
Douglas N. Slaymaker

Chinese Women Writers and the Feminist Imagination, 1905–48*
Haiping Yan

Routledge Studies in Asia's Transformations
Routledge Studies in Asia's Transformations is a forum for innovative new research intended for a high-level specialist readership, and the titles will be available in hardback only. Titles include:

The American Occupation of Japan and Okinawa*
Literature and memory
Michael Molasky

Koreans in Japan*
Critical voices from the margin
Edited by Sonia Ryang

Internationalizing the Pacific
The United States, Japan and the Institute of Pacific Relations in war and peace, 1919–1945
Tomoko Akami

Imperialism in South East Asia*
'A fleeting, passing phase'
Nicholas Tarling

Chinese Media, Global Contexts*
Edited by Chin-Chuan Lee

Remaking Citizenship in Hong Kong*
Community, nation and the global city
Edited by Agnes S. Ku and Ngai Pun

Japanese Industrial Governance
Protectionism and the licensing state
Yul Sohn

Developmental Dilemmas*
Land reform and institutional change in China
Edited by Peter Ho

Critical Asian Scholarship

Critical Asian Scholarship is a series intended to showcase the most important individual contributions to scholarship in Asian Studies. Each of the volumes presents a leading Asian scholar addressing themes that are central to his or her most significant and lasting contribution to Asian studies. The series is committed to the rich variety of research and writing on Asia, and is not restricted to any particular discipline, theoretical approach or geographical expertise.

* Available in paperback

Japan's Wartime Medical Atrocities

Comparative inquiries in science, history, and ethics

Edited by Jing-Bao Nie, Nanyan Guo, Mark Selden and Arthur Kleinman

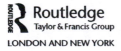

Routledge
Taylor & Francis Group

LONDON AND NEW YORK

First published 2010
by Routledge
2 Park Square, Milton Park, Abingdon, Oxon OX14 4RN

Simultaneously published in the USA and Canada
by Routledge
270 Madison Ave, New York, NY 10016

*Routledge is an imprint of the Taylor & Francis Group, an informa
business*

Typeset in Times New Roman
by Keystroke, Tettenhall, Wolverhampton
Printed and bound in Great Britain
by CPI Antony Rowe, Chippenham, Wiltshire

British Library Cataloguing in Publication Data
A catalogue record for this book is available
from the British Library

Library of Congress Cataloging-in-Publication Data
Japan's wartime medical atrocities: comparative inquiries in science, history,
and ethics / edited by Jing-Bao Nie . . . [et al.].
    p. cm.
    Includes bibliographical references and index.
    1. World War, 1939–45–Atrocities–Japan. 2. World War,
    1939–45–Biological warfare–Japan. 3. World War,
    1939–45–Atrocities–China. 4. Human experimentation in
    medicine–Japan–History–20th century. 5. Human experimentation
    in medicine–Moral and ethical aspects. 6. War crimes–History–
    20th century. 7. War crime trials–History–20th century. I. Nie,
    Jing-Bao, 1962–
    D804.J3J38 2010
    940.54'050952–dc22
    2009052329

ISBN10: 0-415-58377-2 (hbk)
ISBN10: 0-203-84904-3 (ebk)
ISBN13: 978-0-415-58377-0 (hbk)
ISBN13: 978-0-203-84904-0 (ebk)

To all victims of medical atrocities for whom justice has never been fully served

Contents

Notes on contributors

Till Bärnighausen is Assistant Professor of Global Health at the Harvard School of Public Health. Previously, he was Associate Professor of Health and Population Studies at the University of KwaZulu-Natal and senior epidemiologist at the Africa Centre for Population Studies in South Africa, prior to which he worked as senior associate at McKinsey & Company and as post-doc at the Centre for Health Care Administration at Tongji Medical University, Wuhan, China. Till Bärnighausen is a medical specialist in family medicine. He has published more than 30 articles in peer-reviewed journals, three books and multiple book chapters (on HIV epidemiology, population health, health systems, and history of medicine). He holds doctoral degrees in History of Medicine (University of Heidelberg, Institute for History of Medicine) and in International Health (Harvard School of Public Health, Department of Global Health and Population), and Master's degrees in Health Systems Management (London School of Hygiene and Tropical Medicine) and Financial Economics (University of London, School of Oriental and African Studies).

Peter A. Degen holds a Ph.D. in History of Science from Drew University in Madison, NJ. Before taking up his current position as an independent researcher at the Horst-Goertz Institute for Chinese Life Sciences at the Charite, Berlin, he was affiliated with the Institute for History of Science at the Goethe University in Frankfurt. He was postdoctoral Fellow at the Office for History of Science and Technology, University of California, Berkeley from 1989–93 and at the Center of Biomedical Ethics, Stanford University Hospital and Packard Children's Hospital in 1992. He has published in history of science and medicine, for example, in *Historical Studies in the Physical and Biological Sciences* and *Isis*. He is interested in the area of science and religion, particularly physics and religion; see, for example: "Albert Einstein. Ein deutsch-jüdischer Physiker zwischen Assimilation und Zionismus" in *Den Menschen zugewandt leben. Festschrift für Werner Licharz* (1999), ed. Ulrich Lilienthal und Lothar Stiehm (Innsbruck: secolo Verlag, pp. 147–63) and in the history of informed consent in medicine and the life sciences; see, for example: "Reflections of a Protestant Christian on the History of Informed Consent in Germany" in *Advances in Chinese Medical Ethics* (2001), ed. Ole Döring and R.B. Chen, pp. 73–84.

Ole Döring is a philosopher and sinologist with a special focus on bioethics in China and cross-cultural understanding. He holds a Magister Artium degree from Göttingen University and a Ph.D. from Bochum University. Since 1996, he has conducted several pioneering research projects, in Hamburg and Bochum, as part of a research program for culturally reflected bioethics, in a diversity of areas of application, including "Concepts of Humanity in Contemporary Chinese Bioethics" (DFG funded Research Group, Culture Transcending Bioethics, KBE). He teaches at different German and Chinese universities, has published widely and serves as a consultant in international bioethics for government, industry and stakeholder organizations. Currently, he is a core member of the European-Chinese FP6 consortium BIONET: "Ethical Governance of Biological & Biomedical Research: China–EU Co-operation," EC FP6. His numerous publications include the seminal monograph: *Chinas Bioethik verstehen* (Hamburg 2004).

Nanyan Guo was educated at Fudan University, Shanghai. She holds M.A. and Ph.D. degrees in Japanese literature from Ochanomizu University, Japan. She is Associate Professor at the International Research Center for Japanese Studies, Kyoto, Japan. Before taking up her current position, she taught at the University of Otago, New Zealand, from 1993 to 2008. Her research interest includes modern Japanese literature, environmental culture and China–Japan relations. Her recent publications include *Tsugaru and Otago: Periphery in Intellectuals' Consciousness* (Hirosaki University Press 2007), *The Environmental Culture of the Ogasawara Islands from the Perspective of the Asia-Pacific Region* (Hibonsha, Tokyo 2005), *Tsugaru: Regional Identity on Japan's Northern Periphery* (University of Otago Press 2005), and *The Formation of Tsugaru's Identity* (Iwata shoin, Tokyo 2004).

Tsuneishi Keiichi is a Professor at Kanagawa University in Japan. His major research field is history of science. He is a researcher in Unit 731 network's activities. He has published widely on Unit-related topics. His major books are *Epidemiology of Battle Field* (Kaimeisha, 2005), *Crimes by Chemical Weapons* (Kodansha, 2003), *The Crossroad of Conspiracy: The Investigation of the Empire Bank Incident and Unit 731* (Nihon hyoronsha, 2002), *The Organized Crimes of Medical Personnel: Unit 731 of the Kwangtong Army* (Asahi Shimbunsha, 1999), *Unit 731: Truth of Crimes by Biological Weapons* (Kodansha, 1995), and *The Disappeared Biological Warfare Unit* (Kaimeisha, 1981 and later from Chikuma shobo, 1993).

Arthur Kleinman, M.D., is one of the world's leading medical anthropologists. He is also a major figure in cultural psychiatry, global health, and social medicine. Kleinman is the Esther and Sidney Rabb Professor of Anthropology, Department of Anthropology, Faculty of Arts and Sciences, and Professor of Medical Anthropology and Psychiatry at Harvard Medical School. He is currently Victor and William Fung Director of Harvard University's Asia Center. His chief publications are *Patients and Healers in the Context of*

Culture; Social Origins of Distress and Disease: Neurasthenia, Depression and Pain in Modern China; The Illness Narratives; Rethinking Psychiatry; Culture and Depression (co-editor); *Social Suffering* (co-editor); and his most recent book, *What Really Matters*.

David B. MacDonald holds a Ph.D. in International Relations from the London School of Economics. He is currently Associate Professor of the Political Science Department at the University of Guelph. Prior to this he was Senior Lecturer at Otago University, and Assistant Visiting Professor at the Graduate School of Management, Paris. His first book, *Balkan Holocausts? Serbian and Croatian Victim Centred Propaganda and the War in Yugoslavia*, was published in 2002 by Manchester University Press. His second book *Identity Politics in the Age of Genocide*, was published in 2008 by Routledge. He is also co-editor of *The Ethics of Foreign Policy* (Ashgate Press, 2007) and is published widely in peer-reviewed journals and edited books. His third book, *Thinking History, Fighting Evil*, was published in 2009 by Lexington/Rowman & Littlefield.

Jing-Bao Nie, B.Med., M.Med., M.A., Ph.D., is an Associate Professor at the Bioethics Centre, University of Otago, New Zealand, and Furong Visiting Professor at the Centre for Moral Culture, Hunan Normal University, China. Growing up in a remote Southern Chinese village, he was trained in traditional Chinese medicine and medical history in China, and lectured at Hunan College of Chinese Medicine for several years. He also received training in sociology, medical humanities and bioethics in North America. He has published nearly 80 journal articles and book chapters including three chapters in *The Cambridge World History of Medical Ethics* (Cambridge University Press, 2009). He is the author of *Behind the Silence: Chinese Voices on Abortion* (Rowman & Littlefield, 2005) and *Medical Ethics in China: A Cross-cultural Study* (forthcoming). Currently, he is working on a research project entitled "Predicaments of Social Engineering: The Ideologies and Ethics of China's Birth Control Program."

Mark Selden is a Research Associate in the East Asia Program at Cornell University and a coordinator of *The Asia-Pacific Journal: Japan Focus* at http://www.japanfocus.org. A specialist in the modern and contemporary geopolitics and political economy of the Asia Pacific, his recent books include: *War and State Terrorism: The United States, Japan, and the Asia-Pacific in the Long Twentieth Century*; *Censoring History: Citizenship and Memory in Japan, China and the United States*; *China in Revolution: The Yenan Way Revisited*; *Chinese Society: Change, Conflict and Resistance*; and *Chinese Village: Socialist State*.

Suzy Wang holds two Master's degrees – one in International Relations and the other in International History. Born of German and Chinese descent, Suzy grew up learning about the history of the war (1931–45) from both the perspective of a victim (China) and the aggressor (Germany). Having encountered a "general amnesia" regarding Japan's actions during that period while studying for her

B.A. there, she began her research on Japan's medical atrocities. Spanning over a decade, Suzy's research has taken her to archives in Japan, China and the U.S. She is currently completing her doctorate degree in International History at the University of Chicago.

Boris G. Yudin holds a Ph.D. in Philosophical Sciences (since 1987) and since 1990 has been a Professor of Lomonosov's Moscow State University, and is Corresponding Member of the Russian Academy of Sciences (since 2000). He has served as editor-in-chief of the journal *Voprosy Istorii Estestvoznaniya I Tekhniki* (*Questions of History of Natural Sciences and Technology*) at the end of the 1980s, editor-in-chief of the scientific and popular journal *Chelovek* (*The Human Being*) since 1989, and as the Russian representative in the Steering Committee on Bioethics of Council of Europe since 1997, Director of Institute of Human Studies of Russian Academy of Sciences from 1998 to 2004, Head of Department of Comprehensive Problems of Human Studies of the Institute of Philosophy in Russian Academy of Sciences since 2005, Head of the Center of Bioethics in Moscow Humanitarian University since 2006, and Vice-Chairman of the Russian Bioethics Committee under the Commission of RF for UNESCO since 2006. His areas of research include philosophy and sociology of science, ethics of science and bioethics.

Acknowledgments

This volume would not have been possible without the generous support of many individuals and institutions. It is especially heart-warming to acknowledge our gratitude to them here, as the book's subject matter is so inherently dispiriting.

This volume is the first of two final products resulting from a research project supported by a grant (2003–5) from the Marsden Fund of the Royal Society of New Zealand, with Jing-Bao Nie as principal investigator, Nanyan Guo and Arthur Kleinman as associate investigators, and Mark Selden as advisor (the second product is a forthcoming volume by Nie). Two grants from the Bequest Fund of the Dunedin School of Medicine provided financial support for Nie to conduct a pilot study and for professional editing of the chapters written by scholars whose first language is not English.

We are grateful to all the contributors. Most of the chapters are based on material presented at three separate conference sessions: a panel (co-organized by Nie and Japanese bioethicist Takashi Tsuchiya) at the fourth annual meeting of the American Society for Bioethics and Humanities (Nashville, October 2001); a symposium (co-organized by Nie and Korean historian of science and bioethicist Sang-yong Song) at the 22nd International Congress of the History of Science (Beijing, July 2005); and a special session (organized by Nie) at the 8th World Congress of Bioethics (Beijing, August 2006). We highly appreciate the participation and inspiration of Takashi Tsuchiya and Sang-yong Song and greatly regret that they were unable to contribute to this volume due to extremely heavy workloads.

Along with all the contributors, we owe special thanks to Dunedin-based freelance writer and editor Dr Paul Sorrell, who has expertly exercised his professional skills on our research proposal and chapters 3, 5, 6, 7, 8 and 10; and to Dr Rachel Hall-Clifford in Boston, research assistant to Arthur Kleinman, for her marvelous editorial work on the whole manuscript.

We also thank Li Fujun, the Beijing science reporter for *Nanfang Zhoumo* (*Southern Weekend*) and Li Wenjing, currently a Ph.D. student in the philosophy of science at Beijing University, for their thoughtful reports to a Chinese audience on our project and research results presented at the 2005 Beijing International Conference on the History of Science.

Earlier versions of chapters 1 and 10 were published in *The Asia-Pacific Journal: Japan Focus* (available online at www.japanfocus.org) respectively on November 20, 2005 and April 15, 2008. Chapter 4 is based on materials published in W. Eckart (ed.) 2005, *Man, Medicine, and the State: The Human Body as an Object of Government Sponsored Research, 1920–1970* (Stuttgart: Franz Steiner Publishing House) and A. Frewer and U. Schmidt (eds) 2006, *History of Medical Ethics and Ethics of Human Experimentation* (Stuttgart: Franz Steiner Publishing House). We thank the editors and publishers for their permission to include the modified and revised versions of these articles and book chapters in this volume.

The reports by two anonymous reviewers of Routledge have been very helpful for revising the whole manuscript.

We hope that this book will serve as a material witness of our collegiality, friendship and the good times we – editors, contributors and associates – have spent together in different parts of our small planet as well as via enormous email communications.

Finally and most importantly, we hope that this volume will serve as a reminder of the medical atrocities for which justice has never been fully served. We would like our work to stand as a humble memorial to all those who were "sacrificed" in the course of the medical atrocities discussed here. Let us never forget, we dare not forget, the victims of all medical atrocities and of any kind of unethical medical research or practice.

Jing-Bao Nie (Dunedin)
Nanyan Guo (Kyoto)
Mark Selden (Ithaca)
Arthur Kleinman (Boston)
November 2009

Introduction

Medical atrocities, history and ethics

Arthur Kleinman, Jing-Bao Nie and Mark Selden

Facing Japanese wartime medical atrocities

If our age – the long twentieth century – has exhibited remarkable progress in areas of science, technology, and economic and social development, it has been equally notable for the scale of violence and destruction: including two World Wars, genocide, mass political violence, and terrorism. To this deplorable list, it is necessary to add Japanese wartime medical atrocities. From the early 1930s to the end of the Second World War, Japanese military doctors and scientists conducted a wide range of experiments with infectious disease agents and the vivisection of thousands of human guinea pigs in a quest to develop effective biological weapons. These horrific medical atrocities were carried out mainly in the biological warfare (BW) programs that the Japanese Imperial Army established throughout occupied China and Southeast Asia, among which those of Unit 731 were the most extensive and the best documented. Japanese researchers also actively participated in employing bacteriological and chemical weapons not only in military battles but in bombing entire city and village populations.

This was not just another serious if less well-known episode of human cruelty, one limited in its significance to Japan's war in Asia and the Pacific. This was the counterpart of Nazi medicine for East Asia. While significant political, social historical, and cultural differences exist between Nazi medicine and Japanese wartime medical atrocities, in both cases doctors and scientists participated in the state-sanctioned intentional killing and torture of human beings in the name of nation, science, and medicine, and other "sacred" causes (Bauman 2000). Like Nazi medicine, we aver, Japanese wartime medical atrocities constitute a paradigmatic case of how human lives and fundamental values such as justice, caregiving, medical ethics, and scientific integrity can all be sacrificed in the pursuit of winning wars and advancing ideology. Like Nazi medicine, Japanese wartime medical atrocities rank among the most egregious misuses of science and technology under state power. The enormity of this abuse raises the questions: How do we persist in resisting inhumanity and in advocating for humanity? And how do we do so not in an ideal world of ethical dreams, but in the gritty, gray, everyday world of contradictory, untoward, and inadequate moral realities? Indeed, as Nanyan Guo points out in Chapter 5 (this volume), the seeds of atrocities may be found in all of us, capable of surfacing under stressful conditions. If dictatorships are particularly prone to such abuses, Ole Döring observes in Chapter 7, it is important to reflect on "the different ways in which abuses can become embedded within 'normal' life and what they have to tell us about the structures of inhumane practices that begin with 'exceptions' and slippery slopes that start off ever so gently."

As in the case of Nazi medicine, and not only in the case of Nazi medicine, there are universal ethical lessons to be drawn from Japanese medical atrocities, in addition to the unique historical issues that we must also address.

These medicine-related war crimes, in Asia or in Europe, are not isolated events (for a comparative study on wartime science and politics, see Sachse and Walker 2005). War crimes such as slaughtering civilians have been practiced from the dawn of world history. During the Second World War, both the Axis powers and the Allies routinely bombed non-combatant areas and populations, and mistreated and abused captured prisoners. This was total war in which the commission of war crimes, specifically the slaughter of civilians and non-combatants, was not limited to one side. Indeed, some of the largest killing of civilians took place during the carpet bombing and the firebombing of Japanese and German cities in 1944 to 1945 (Selden and So 2004; Selden 2007). In assessing Japanese wartime medical atrocities, the authors of this volume seek to locate them within the structure of war-making during the Second World War and subsequent wars.

Along with wartime medical atrocities, the Japanese Imperial Army committed massacres of Chinese soldiers and civilians as exemplified by the Nanjing (Nanking) Massacre, carried out the Three All Policy (burn all, kill all, and loot all) across the Chinese countryside, created the "comfort women" (enslaving women as military prostitutes), and forced hundreds of thousands of civilians and captured prisoners into hard labor with inadequate food and minimal, if any, care. The subject of this book needs to be seen in the context of the 50 million deaths that took place during the Second World War.

Like many other events of mass violence in recent history, one of the most disturbing features of the case at hand is the international community's failure to pursue justice. Japanese wartime medical atrocities have been largely ignored by the world, with the partial exception of China, for nearly four decades. It was not until the 1980s that the Asian version of Nazi medicine started to become widely known to researchers and the public. The historical fate of those Japanese who engaged in medical atrocities has been very different from that of most Nazi doctors. The International Military Tribunal for the Far East (the Tokyo Trials) failed to recognize, address, or pursue Japanese microbiological and chemical warfare and the involvement of doctors in inhuman experimentation, a position that remained unchanged after Soviet prosecutors drew attention to these crimes and offered to present documentation (Boris Yudin, Chapter 3, this volume). The United States government instead struck a secret deal with the perpetrators immediately after the war, accepting "precious" scientific data in exchange for a cover-up and cash payments, and shielding the scientists from prosecution. No official inquiry has ever addressed this U.S.–Japanese devil's bargain. Moreover, neither Chinese Nationalist nor Communist governments have seriously sought justice for the victims, most of whom were Chinese civilians and soldiers. No Japanese government has officially admitted to or apologized for these atrocities, or provided compensation for victims.

Although the issues remain contentious, numerous historical and journalistic works on this subject have been published in Japan, China, and the West over the past three decades (see the comprehensive bibliography at the end of this book). This is one aspect of the emergence of worldwide concern about war crimes since the 1980s. Yet, in the case of Japanese wartime medical atrocities, the central theme of this work – namely, the ethical and human rights implications of human testing – remains largely unexplored. We have yet to fully gauge the nature and depth of the inhumanity of these wartime medical atrocities as a form of state violence committed in East Asia by the military and medical professions in the name of science. Nor have we located it in a broad global context as one of the signal ethical and scientific events of modern warfare. The experiments performed by Japanese perpetrators on human subjects as well as the employment of bacteriological and chemical weapons on Chinese troops and civilians raise crucial historical, political, cultural, and legal questions. Not least of these is the existential question of the relevance of these abuses for the contemporary moral experience of physicians, researchers, and patients in today's East Asian societies.

Through the contributions of scholars from China and Japan as well as from Europe and the United States, and from various academic disciplines, this volume examines Japanese wartime medical atrocities in multiple comparative perspectives: cross-national, cross-cultural, cross-disciplinary, and crossing local and global boundaries of politics, law, ethics, and lived experiences. The chapters present fresh studies of historical events and historical framings of what happened, new explorations of the moral responsibility of individuals and scientific communities, comparisons with Nazi Germany and with the Germany of today, reflections on U.S. wars and atrocities since the Second World War, and investigations of war and historical remembrance in East Asia, Europe, and the United States.

It is our aim to show how the silence over these and other wartime atrocities necessitates a more central place for ethics and the tenets of international law in considerations of medicine, science, ordinary social life, and history in East Asia and beyond. It is our belief that only by starting from the stark inhumanity of these terrible practices and the failure of politics, law and ethics that followed can the culture of silence and denial that has so frequently accompanied war crimes and atrocities in East Asia and beyond be transformed. In its place, we foresee possibilities for a more reflective, critical, and enabling culture of empathy and responsibility that replaces nationalism with justice, retribution, and reconciliation as a means toward pro-social policies and practices that build a more human world. The double failure – in the atrocities of war and in the subsequent state and societal responses – requires that ethics now be given a heightened place in global thinking.

In the aftermath of wartime atrocities, whether those of Japan, of Nazi Germany, of the United States, or others, human beings carry a grave responsibility to safeguard humanity and advance ethics. As the writer and conscience of the twentieth century's horrors, Albert Camus, once reminded us, we never know when the "plague" will return. Our ordinary lives must strip away silence and pretense to examine the past failure of our existential responsibility for moral practices in the face of catastrophe in order to create a more humane future.

Medical atrocities in East Asia

It is far from unusual for scientists in all countries to devote themselves to serving national power, especially in a time of war and cross-national conflict. Here we draw attention to the active role played by Japanese physicians and scientists in setting up biological warfare programs, including manufacturing biological agents in laboratories, testing them on unwilling participants, and employing microbiological weapons in the field to kill as well as to test and refine weapons of mass destruction. The 1925 Geneva Protocol, which was created in response to the horrors of the First World War, banned biological and chemical warfare. Signed by the great powers with the exception of Japan and the United States, it established an international milieu critical of its use (Geneva Protocol of 1925). The Japanese army invested heavily in creating a BW system, beginning in the early 1930s as it embarked on the conquest of Manchuria and continued research and testing throughout the war years. While other major powers created BW programs then and since, Japan alone appears to have systematically deployed BW warfare in the Second World War against both military and civilian targets. The heart of this system was an extensive network of programs centered in Northeast China (Manchuria), with additional facilities in other parts of China and Southeast Asia. Its most important components were Unit 731 in Pingfang (near Harbin) with branches in Mudanjiang, Hailar, and Dalian; Unit 100 in Changchun; Unit 1855 in Beijing; Unit 1644 in Nanjing; Unit 8604 in Guangzhou and Hong Kong; and Unit 9420 in Singapore.

General Ishii Shiro, a specialist in microbiology, a physician, and the major designer and leader of the BW program in the Japanese Army, described human experimentation as the system's "secret of secrets." To speed up the development of biological weapons, Japanese doctors and scientists experimented upon thousands of live human subjects. Their experiments involved:

- Intentionally infecting healthy men and women with the disease agents causing plague, anthrax, cholera, and typhoid by injection, by breathing in contaminated air, or by eating food and drinks laced with specific germs.
- Conducting vivisections and autopsies on these human subjects in order to study the natural progression of the infectious diseases created in them.
- Exposing research subjects to extreme cold for long periods of time to test physiological and psychological responses to frostbite, including use of anti-frostbite techniques.
- Experimenting with other responses to extreme conditions, such as deprivation of oxygen and high-voltage electric shocks.

- Exposing subjects to infectious agents released in explosions in order to evaluate the effects of biological weapons.
- Conducting experiments whose deadly consequences were predetermined, such as bleeding subjects to death, replacing human blood with horse blood, and injecting horse urine into the kidneys of human subjects.

(The Khabarovsk Trial 1950; Tsuneishi 1981; Chinese Central Archive 1989; Williams and Wallace 1989; Gold 1996; Fujii 1997; Harris 2002; Unit 731 Criminal Evidence Museum 2005; summarized in Nie et al. 2009).

Japanese doctors did not see the Chinese and other subjects of their gruesome experiments as human beings, but rather as "experimental materials." Those who tortured and murdered referred to their victims simply as *maruta*, a Japanese term for "logs of wood" or "lumber." People were sent to Unit 731 and other units by the Japanese military and their policy on "special consignment." Japanese doctors and scientists vivisected healthy people as well as patients in order to perfect their surgical skills and to teach human anatomy and pathology. Vivisection was also conducted to prepare medical specimens, and there is evidence that it was performed at times simply for fun (Chinese Central Archive 1989: 747–830).

The victims were mostly Chinese, but also included Russians and Koreans. Most of these human subjects were healthy men, women, and children. They included a three-day-old baby. Unit 731 alone, from 1939 through 1945, killed as many as 600 subjects each year (The Khabarovsk Trial 1950: 57).

Many more died as a result of the Japanese Army's BW program. In addition to the use of BW weapons in battle, notably in the attack on Soviet forces at Nomonhan in 1939, the Japanese Army carried out BW attacks on cities, towns, and villages throughout China. Ningbo in Zhejiang and Changde in Hunan were among the major aerial targets. Human experimentation, then, was not limited to the research facilities, the so-called "factories of death." Experimentation also took the form of the deployment of biological weapons in bombs.

Justice denied

In contrast to the punishment of some of the abuses of Nazi medicine in Europe, justice has never been served for the perpetrators and victims of Japanese military medical atrocities. While Japanese war crimes and atrocities were prosecuted at Tokyo, and in subsequent B and C class tribunals most of the perpetrators of Unit 731 were never prosecuted. Whereas many Nazi doctors were charged and sentenced or their careers ruined because of involvement with atrocities, most Japanese perpetrators got off scot-free. Ishii Shiro and his colleagues lived with impunity on generous pensions. The knowledge, skills, connections, and experience gained in the BW program fostered careers which made several of them pillars of the medical establishment in education, research, and administration (Williams and Wallace 1989: 286–304). Seven of the directors of Japan's postwar National Institute of Health, and five of the Institute's vice-directors, actively participated in these inhuman experiments during the 1930s and 1940s (Harris 2002: xiv,

336–344). Even today, their names and reputations are protected by the Japanese government.

How to face history has been and remains divisive in contemporary Japanese society, as the protracted controversies over colonial and war atrocities in textbooks, shrines, museums, monuments, and public statements demonstrate. Japanese courts have processed the lawsuits filed by Chinese victims supported by Japanese lawyers. In many instances the court accepted the fact of human experimentation and BW-related deaths, but did not award compensation to victims, citing statute of limitations (Chapter 2, this volume). As the bibliography here shows, numerous ground-breaking scholarly and journalistic reports have been published in Chinese, Japanese, and English, with quite a few translated into Chinese and other languages. As a result of the joint efforts of local governments in Tokyo and many volunteers, the traveling Unit 731 exhibition, a remarkable event, increased public awareness in Japan (Gold 1996). Japan's numerous private peace museums, as well as art exhibits and memorials have repeatedly brought other Japanese war atrocities to public attention (Lafleur et al. 2007; Nishino 2007; Xinhua 2009). However, the Japanese government, while apologizing repeatedly for various war atrocities, continues to adhere to a policy of no admission, no apology, and no compensation to victims or their heirs for BW crimes. It continues overall to refuse official compensation for victims of atrocities, claiming that its responsibilities have been fulfilled in postwar treaties re-establishing diplomatic relations with China, South Korea, and other nations.

This pattern contrasts strongly with that of the German government, for which the Nazi era with its crimes against humanity, most notably the Holocaust, eventually elicited strong official expressions of national responsibility accompanied by extensive programs of mass education, laws and ethical codes, public monuments consecrating apologies, a public attitude of regret, remorse and restitution, and large payments to victims and their heirs (Buruma 2002; Underwood 2006; Jager and Mitter 2007; Dudden 2008; Bazyler 2009). Denial of the Holocaust and other Nazi atrocities is in fact illegal in Germany. In Japan, despite heroic efforts by many individuals and organizations to face history squarely, official denial of war crimes and denial of official compensation for victims, supported by neo-nationalist individuals and non-governmental groups of "deniers," remain in place.

How did this come about?

In late 1949, the former Soviet Union conducted a public trial of eight Japanese physicians and research scientists and four other military servicemen in the eastern Siberian city of Khabarovsk on the Russian–Chinese border. In spite of its ideological framing and lack of international participation, as well as shortcomings in legal procedure, and despite the fact that the Soviets, who also had a BW program, were interested in obtaining the Japanese data, the trial established beyond reasonable doubt that the Japanese Army had prepared and deployed bacteriological weapons, and that Japanese researchers had conducted cruel and inhuman experiments on captive human subjects (the Khabarovsk Trial Materials 1950; Yudin, Chapter 3, this volume). In the geopolitical context of the Cold War, the trial, its evidence, and major findings were published in Russian, Japanese, Chinese, English, and other languages in 1950. Over time, its findings have proved remarkably accurate, but they were dismissed at the time in the West as communist propaganda and, until the 1980s, were largely ignored (Nie 2004).

The role of the U.S. was particularly troubling. With the aim of monopolizing the "scientific" data obtained by Japanese researchers and thereby advancing its own BW programs, notably those at Fort Detrick in Maryland, U.S. authorities immediately after the war secretly granted immunity from war crimes prosecution to those involved in the research. U.S. authorities also publicly denounced the findings of the Khabarovsk Trial and evidence from other sources (Powell 1981; Williams and Wallace 1989; Harris 2002). Recent research documents the fact that U.S. authorities paid Unit 731 researchers for information (Tsuneishi 2005). The American cover-up took place shortly after the U.S.-led Nuremberg and Tokyo trials. Privileging security concerns, the U.S. scientific and military authorities engaged in what the English Common Law tradition defines as "complicity after the fact" (Nie 2006). To this day, the U.S. has never formally admitted to or publicly apologized for covering up and exploiting the information generated by Japanese military medical atrocities.

The U.S. government also classified and systematically suppressed information on Japanese and American research on the medical effects of the atomic bombings in Hiroshima and Nagasaki, information that could have been used to alleviate the suffering of atomic survivors (Hein and Selden 1997). Moreover, at the height of the Cold War, a number of U.S. government-sponsored research projects exposed unknowing citizens to radiation (Advisory Committee on Human Radiation Experiments 1996), and radiation experimentation is but one of the cases of secret state-sponsored experiments which American scientists and research conducted upon human beings (Moreno 2001). Recently, U.S. medical professionals and psychologists participated in designing and implementing the abusive interrogation and torture of prisoners detained in Guantánamo Bay, Abu Ghraib, and other U.S.-maintained or supported torture sites scattered across the globe (McCoy 2006; Miles 2006). In the U.S., as in wartime Japan, medical and scientific ethics have frequently been sacrificed at the altar of the national security or the anti-terrorist state.

Chinese responses to the suppression of information about Japanese wartime medical atrocities have been puzzling. On the one hand, Japanese wartime atrocities are even today still publicly recalled by Chinese people with deep anguish. This should not be surprising given wartime devastation and Chinese death-tolls estimated at between 10 and 30 million. Yet neither the Republic of China on Taiwan nor the People's Republic of China has systematically pursued justice in the international community on behalf of victims. These ambiguous attitudes toward medical atrocities echo the silent stance of the Nationalist representatives at the Tokyo Trial and of communist authorities subsequently. Nevertheless, a number of high-profile efforts by Chinese victims and non-official organizations have been made since the 1990s to file suits in Japanese courts concerning war crimes, including exposure to biological and chemical warfare, forced labor, and coerced "comfort women" (Underwood 2006; Kingston 2008).

Remarkably, international bioethics, which has remained focused on Nazi crimes against humanity, has paid little attention to Japanese atrocities. In Japan and China, as well as in Europe and North America, the subject was long treated as if it held little relevance to contemporary science, medicine, or medical ethics. Only in the last decade have bioethicists, in small ways, begun to initiate ethically relevant analyses (e.g., Tsuchiya 2000; Döring 2001; Nie 2001, 2002, 2003, 2004, 2005, 2006; for a review see Nie et al. 2009). The questions that have been explored in this limited literature include the following: What historical, sociocultural and medical environments led to the establishment of factories of death and prevented doctors from resisting? What are the challenges of those atrocities for medical ethics today, notably for East Asian medical ethics? How can East Asia learn from the past in light of German experience? Why should we bring up past atrocities at all? Can the argument that "it was wartime" justify the atrocities and the failure to bring the doctors who perpetrated them to justice?

The studies included here document the fact that Japan's medicine-related war crimes during the Second World War and earlier "have been denied and marginalized" (Barenblatt 2004: xxii). Jing-Bao Nie has called the postwar response to Japanese wartime medical atrocities "the triumph of inhumanity" (Nie 2004: 32). This verdict can and should be reversed. This volume is an attempt to face up to the implications of these and other instances of inhumanity and the failure of ethics, and to assess responses to them.

Part I of this volume elucidates Japan's medical war crimes and examines the postwar trials of these crimes. In Chapter 1, Keiichi Tsuneishi, the leading authority on Unit 731 and Japan's wartime BW program, summarizes a scholarly lifetime of historical research. He describes in detail the origins and development of the Japanese Imperial Army's BW program. He outlines the human experimentation conducted in Unit 731, with an emphasis on large-scale BW field trials and the failure of a new type of biological bomb. Finally, he, together with Suzy Wang in Chapter 2, documents the American authorities' decision to shield 731 scientists from prosecution and to buy their research findings.

Historian Suzy Wang examines various war crimes trials and shows how Allied courts handled Japanese BW and medical atrocity cases. After noting how the International Military Tribunal for the Far East (IMTFE) declined to investigate the BW program despite having collected evidence, she examines the "B and C War Crimes Trials" on human experimentation involving American POWs. She also studies trials held by Soviet authorities, by Chinese Nationalist and communist governments, and, more recently, by Japanese courts. For Wang, while justice has never been fully served, the trials conducted in the course of six decades establish irrefutable evidence of Japan's medicine-related crimes.

In Chapter 3, Russian bioethicist Boris Yudin offers a historical analysis and ethical interpretation of the 1949 Khabarovsk Trial. Drawing on Russian primary and secondary materials, he emphasizes the extraordinary rapidity of the trial and the leniency in sentencing convicted war criminals. Interrogating the evidence uncovered in the trial, he inquires into the nature of the abusive wartime culture of coerced human experimentation.

Guilt and responsibility: individual, professional, state, and transnational

A vast international literature assesses the ethical implications of war atrocities and the responsibility of perpetrators. Shortly after the fall of the Third Reich, to address "the question of German guilt," one of the great twentieth-century philosophers Karl Jaspers (1948), who experienced what he called "internal exile" under the Nazis, distinguished four types of responsibility: criminal or legal guilt, political guilt, moral guilt, and metaphysical guilt. Although only a finite number of individuals are directly responsible for criminal actions, as citizens and human beings, all of us bear moral and metaphysical responsibility for the perpetration of atrocities by our government and the failure to bring the perpetrators to justice. Later, the influential political philosopher Hannah Arendt deliberated on the issue of responsibility from both societal and individual perspectives. While in *The Origins of Totalitarianism* (1951) she traced the social and historical roots of Nazism and Stalinism, in *Eichmann in Jerusalem: A Report on the Banality of Evil* (1963) she stressed that individuals are ultimately responsible for their judgments and actions. That is to say, in collective guilt – in this case that of the Nazi Party – the individual remains responsible for his or her specific acts, including acts of omission.

The Nuremberg and Tokyo trials established the responsibility of individuals from citizens to generals and presidents for the conduct of their states. Yet levels of responsibility require attention: What is the degree of responsibility of the soldier or bombardier who, following orders, carries out lethal medical tests or unleashes bombs on civilians? What is the responsibility of the generals or national leaders who went to war and command at the highest level? What are the ethical responsibilities of medical, research and other professionals in time of war? And what is the level of responsibility borne by later generations for war crimes or atrocities committed by their nations during previous wars? These are among the issues addressed by the authors of this volume.

Elsewhere, Arthur Kleinman (1995, 2006; Kleinman et al. 1997) has argued that a major obstacle to the development of a serviceable ethics for health care and health science professionals is the tendency to refrain from confronting ethical ideals and aspirations with on-the-ground moral realities. Genuine reality (as William James named it) constitutes the actual lived experience of ordinary people situated in a particular life world where serious issues are at stake – status, careers, resources, relationships, religious and cultural commitments, life itself. In this sense of lived values, we are always engaged in moral worlds, yet the moral may be, and often is, in opposition to the ethical, as in the case of murderous racism. That is to say, entire communities have acted on shared racist values to injure human targets of racial hatred. Here, racism is a shared moral practice – people are committed to it – that needs to be so described and then criticized in terms of ethical aspirations that transcend the local. Or indifference may implicate us through compliance with, conformity to, and collaboration with inhuman values and practices such as slavery, abuse of children, and murder of research subjects. Absent real cases that highlight the political, economic, cultural, institutional, and relational constraints on local worlds and people's lives that clarify real moral practices, statements of ethical requirements sound hollow, utopian, and irrelevant.

No progress in human values can be achieved unless there is *acknowledgment* of the actual limitations and abuses of the moral worlds we live in and the lives we lead. Acknowledgment of what is unacceptable requires *criticism* of real moral conditions (Jonas 1984; Kleinman 1986; Glover 1999). Where such criticism does not exist locally, it is the responsibility of outsiders to help inform it.

It may at first seem ludicrous and even dangerous to classify the abuses by Japanese perpetrators as "moral practices," but doing so enables us to understand how these inhuman acts were sustained in an actual world by real people. For what was at stake for (and deeply valued by) Japanese physicians and scientists were not only careers, technological goals, institutional commitments, and close relationships, but a political and cultural orientation that privileged the survival and flourishing of an expansive nation predicated on the subordination of China to Japanese power. The same value orientation that stripped the humanity from Chinese and other research subjects viewed the construction of Japan's Asian imperium as a force for overcoming the baneful effects of European colonialism and creating a Greater East Asia Co-Prosperity Sphere that would bring salvation to Asian people.

Below we consider examples of some Japanese researchers and military physicians who were reluctant to participate in the program, or who even resisted. Most, however, assiduously carried out their terrible responsibilities and many expressed commitment to, even passion for, their work in private and public communications. We know this was the case with many Nazi perpetrators, too, who believed in killing Jews, felt good in doing so, and committed themselves passionately to the worst atrocities. Even when ordinary Nazis felt their religious or family backgrounds to be in conflict with their professional and institutional commitments to eliminationist anti-Semitism, many struggled to be "responsible" Nazis by killing Jews. In contrast to the eliminationist goals of many Nazi researchers, Japanese physicians and researchers of Unit 731 bore no such animus toward the Chinese people. They nevertheless likewise bear ethical and legal responsibility for conducting wartime medical atrocities.

Noda Masaaki's *War, Crime and Responsibility* (1998) examines the unwillingness of many Japanese to accept responsibility for crimes they committed in the Second World War. He claims Japanese culture has a tendency to suppress consciousness of guilt. Japan's postwar peace movements are mainly based on the consciousness of being victims. Thus Noda and others have pointed out that participants in anti-nuclear movements in response to Hiroshima and Nagasaki or the bombing of other cities, as well as those Japanese who experienced the war as soldiers, frequently privilege their experience as victims of war. Yet it is also the case, as Selden argues in this volume, that significant elements of Japanese anti-war and peace movements have recognized Japanese war responsibility. Important examples include the Beheiren movement (Japan Peace for Vietnam) of the 1960s and 1970s which recognized the position of Japanese in the Asia-Pacific War as both assailants and victims – aggressors in war, but also victims both of the Japanese military and the bombing that destroyed almost every Japanese city and took more than half a million lives (Tanaka 2007).

Noda interviewed military doctors, military police, and ordinary soldiers in order to understand their perceptions of the Chinese. He draws on the analysis by psychologist Stanley Milgram who conducted a series of famous experiments from 1960 to 1963 on obedience to authority, in which, with rare exceptions, participants followed orders and showed no sympathy toward their "victims." Noda points out a similarity among Japanese interviewees to those analyzed by Milgram. In both cases, people suppressed their sensitivity or their ability to make moral adjustments when obeying immoral orders. They tried to justify their obedience retrospectively, frequently blaming their superiors for any moral lapses. Noda is surely correct that most Japanese followed orders even where they were led to commit horrific crimes, but does this require an understanding of a unique Japanese pathology? Comparative studies of, for example, German or U.S. military and civilian wartime behavior does not result in substantially different findings: whether our point of reference is Auschwitz or the bombing of German or Japanese cities, or the napalming of Vietnamese. We need to understand the powerful positive and negative incentives that lead many people under wartime conditions to obey orders whose consequences may cross both legal and ethical lines, just as we need to understand the conditions under which some break with such behavior and challenge the legitimacy of such orders.

In spite of pressures to conform, Noda notes situations in which other outcomes are sometimes possible: among those who look to a higher authority such as religion, those who refuse military service, and those who critically examined their own actions.

Although rare, some did refuse to obey illegitimate authority due to their religious values. Buddhism, particularly Zen, actively promoted the Japanese war effort and trained its disciples for war (Victoria 2006). Yet some Japanese monks had refused to kill Chinese on the basis of Buddhist beliefs on the sanctity of life; others refused to follow orders to raid civilian homes, and a few refused to accept a military pension after the war. Some Japanese soldiers, following detention in China, returned to Japan and publicly criticized the atrocities they had themselves committed. Some Americans became conscientious objectors during the Second World War and in all subsequent wars; others chose draft resistance, desertion, or anti-war activities during the Vietnam and Iraq Wars. Nevertheless, in all societies that we have studied, including Japan, Germany, and the United States, organized religions – Buddhist, Protestant, Catholic, and Jewish – worked with the military in support of the war effort, and the great majority of citizens obeyed orders to fight, apparently without feeling any sense of personal wrongdoing, even in ethically compromised situations involving committing atrocities such as those outlined above and discussed in other chapters in this volume.

Among 2000 patients in the Konodai Army Hospital in Chiba prefecture, a research center for mental illness in the years 1937 to 1945, Noda found that only two were overcome by memories of slaughtering victims. Both repeatedly saw the faces of the Chinese in their dreams. Noda uses several examples to show that recalling victims' faces is usually the beginning of recognizing the victims' humanity, and the start of regretting war crimes. This is also a healing process of regaining the perpetrators' humanity that was lost in the war, and of reconciling with victims. Noda emphasizes the importance of each individual accepting moral responsibility as a means to reduce obedience to immoral orders. In contrast to the findings of Noda and others, Janice Matsumura challenges statistics indicating the exceptionally low incidence of Japanese soldier trauma, noting that there were severe pressures on military psychiatrists and hospital staff to suppress such information and to send traumatized soldiers back to the front as quickly as possible (Matsumura 2004).

Part II of this book explores the responsibility of nation-states, scientific communities, and individuals from the perspective of human ethics. Chapter 4 by physician and public health expert Till Bärnighausen focuses on scientific data obtained under inhumane conditions. He addresses two key questions: Are the bestial human experiments conducted by Japanese military scientists of any scientific value, and should data that were thus obtained be used for scientific and medical purposes today? Bärnighausen, through examining the Japanese experiments for their reliability and validity as well as considering research alternatives from the scientific angle, concludes that, contrary to the assumptions of the U.S. investigators who struck a deal with the perpetrators, they were of virtually no scientific value. Further, he argues that unethically obtained data, even those that are scientifically relevant and reliable, should never be used except for historical documentation and ethical condemnation.

Nanyan Guo (Chapter 5) examines the moral life and ethics of Japanese who perpetrated atrocities. Drawing from primary Japanese accounts (e.g., participants' confessions and testimonies of witnesses) she presents examples of those who refused to directly participate in atrocities and those who experienced a sense of remorse over their participation in causing the suffering and death of others. Even in the midst of this dark account of barbarity, criticism and aspiration for something more human, though limited and fragile, was not entirely absent. Indeed, these examples of going against the grain in the face of powerful impulses of careerism, nationalism, perverse scientism, and pressures to conform reveal that some had the strength to resist the most inhumane practices in the face of intense pressures to conform.

For ethicist and historian of medicine Jing-Bao Nie (Chapter 6), Japanese wartime medical atrocities constitute a paradigmatic case of how human lives and fundamental values such as morality, justice, professional ethics, and scientific integrity can be sacrificed on the altar of the nation-state and its nationalistic ideology. He explores the role of the nation in this two-sided ethical failure: both the abdication of human and professional ethics on the part of Japanese scientists who participated in the Unit 731 experiments, and the United States in covering up Japanese atrocities on the basis of a national security calculation. Nie goes on to observe that nationalism has also dominated China's retrospective responses to the war, including Japanese medical atrocities. Drawing on the major East Asian moral tradition of Confucianism, he argues that, in the face of the increasing power of the state and nationalistic ideology, it is urgent to uphold the ethical core of Chinese and East Asia medical ethics. Here, in common with the highest international ethics, medicine is defined as an art of humanity (*yi nai renshu*), rather than a political tool of the nation.

Lessons from Germany and historical memory

We have repeatedly referred to Nazi medicine as a point of reference in our discussion of Japanese medical atrocities. Not only is it the archetype of the dark side of modern medicine and science, but Nazi medicine is also the most thoroughly studied case. There are far more important historical, psychological, sociological, legal, and ethical studies on Nazi medicine than on Japanese medical war crimes (see Lifton 1986; Annas and Grodin 1992; Caplan 1992; Nicosia and Huener 2002). Some significant similarities exist in these two major cases of medical atrocities, notably the fact that both involve systematic torture and killing of human beings in the name of science and medicine. At the same time, while it is crucial to highlight shared aspects of the two cases, one should not ignore their unique features. For instance, Nazi medicine was integral to the Final Solution to eliminate the "unfit" (the Jewish people and other targeted victims including homosexuals and Roma) through eugenics, euthanasia, and inhuman experimentation. Japanese medical war crimes, while founded on racist assumptions concerning the superiority of Japanese in contrast with Chinese, never sought to eradicate an entire people. Rather, Japan sought to conquer and colonize China. Nonetheless, the killing of tens of millions of Chinese during the 15-year China–Japan War underscores the seriousness of the case and provides a benchmark for comparison with the Holocaust.

Part III includes two chapters that draw parallels with the German case and two chapters that grapple with the ethical implications of the construction of Japanese wartime medical atrocities, both for the past and the future. Sinologist and bioethicist Ole Döring (Chapter 7) examines Nazi medicine in the setting of the German concentration camp at Ravensbrück. He draws from poetic and philosophical traditions to provide an account of individual moral integrity. Rejecting ethical relativism and local exceptionalism, Döring insists that accounts of moral life transcend particularly situated worlds. Only by advancing universal values, he argues, can we make sense of Japanese wartime medical atrocities and inhuman practices in general, and that critical sense is crucial for preventing similar abuses from happening again. For Döring, it is critical to continuously *remember* the social and individual suffering caused by crimes against humanity as a way of living a moral life. Historical remembrance concerns not only what happened in the past, but provides a guide to what should be done now. In this sense, historical remembrance is always about the future.

Historian of science Peter Degen (Chapter 8) examines the influence of racial eugenicist Otmar von Vershuer on his infamous Nazi student, Josef Mengele. His focus is on facing up to the denial of historical truths that challenge our deeply held moral biases. In contrast to Nanyan Guo's account of religion as a source of inner resistance to participation in atrocities, Degen offers a cautionary tale of how religious institutions and commitments can serve to protect perpetrators from public scrutiny and just punishment, even (and most troubling) from awakening a genuine sense of responsibility and guilt.

The remaining two chapters concern the historical remembrance of Japanese wartime medical atrocities and the postwar failure of justice in East Asia, Europe and, in particular, the United States. David MacDonald (Chapter 9) explores the implications of U.S. suppression of information about Japanese war crimes. Seen not as an isolated event, but rather as part of a larger social amnesia that kept Americans "innocent" of genocide and mass political murders, particularly those committed by Americans, MacDonald argues that American responsibility for the cover-up of Japanese wartime medical crimes should be viewed in light of their own suppressed crimes. From the ethnocide of American Indians to radiation experiments without informed consent and the Tuskegee syphilis study supported by the U.S. Public Health Service, Americans have not drawn historical lessons that might help to prevent future abuses. MacDonald emphasizes the failure of the U.S. government to acknowledge either atrocities committed by its military or its own central role in the cover-up.

Mark Selden (Chapter 10) concludes this book by offering comparative reflections on historical memories of Japanese and American war atrocities and possibilities for reconciliation. He considers wartime medical atrocities in light of other war crimes committed by the Japanese Imperial Army, including the Nanjing Massacre, enslavement of the military comfort women and the killing of prisoners, locating the activities of Unit 731 within the wider structure of violence in the Asia-Pacific War. Selden points to an often ignored dimension of war crimes, the United States bombardment of more than 60 Japanese cities prior to dropping the atomic bombs in both Hiroshima and Nagasaki, initiating a pattern of civilian bombing that the U.S. would relentlessly pursue in subsequent wars in Korea, Vietnam, Iraq, and Afghanistan. He concludes that not only Japanese medical experiments but also American bombing practices systematically violate both international laws and ethical norms that mandate protection of civilians during warfare. Selden breaks with analyses that highlight exclusively the failures of Japanese and Americans to come to terms with their nations' war atrocities, noting in particular the strengths of postwar Japanese pacifism, and the contributions of Japanese scholars to unearthing the truth about the Nanjing Massacre, the coercion of the comfort women as well as of Chinese and Korean forced laborers, and the activities of Unit 731. Perhaps most important, he links the citizen response to the defeat and destruction that the Asia-Pacific War brought to Japan to the fact that for 60 years since its surrender in 1945, Japan has not gone to war, though it has faithfully provided support for successive U.S. wars. Nevertheless, much remains to be done by the Japanese and U.S. governments and their citizens. Ultimately, reconciliation and peace in the Asia-Pacific region and beyond require that Japan and the United States, as well as others, reassess the historical record and, where appropriate, apologize and provide compensation to victims of their abuses. Such actions make it possible to bring to closure unresolved war legacies and create a moral climate conducive to the prevention of future conflicts and wars.

Defending humanity and ethics in East Asia and globally

The bibliography compiled and annotated by Nanyan Guo and Jing-Bao Nie offers a survey of the major available primary sources, important historical studies, journalistic investigations, and ethical inquiries in Chinese, Japanese, and English on Japan's wartime medical atrocities. This provides a guide to the development and current status of studies conducted in China, Japan, and internationally that constitute a new field of scholarly inquiry. Together with the chapters in this book, these works represent a quest for discovering historical truth, creating cross-national understanding, finding justice, and commencing restitution that merits the attention of those who seek to repair and rebuild the world and to enhance human ethics.

We recognize that the failure to pursue justice with respect to perpetrators of war crimes and atrocities in the Asia-Pacific War and subsequent wars seriously impedes the development of medical ethics and ethics more generally. That delayed development continues to be challenged by powerful cultural and political forces associated with nationalism in Japan, China, the U.S. and beyond that make serious engagement with the devastating moral reality depicted in this volume difficult. Other forces at work in East Asia suggest more hopeful possibilities, at least in the case of Japanese atrocities: after years of official resistance to reparations for victims by both the Japanese government and corporations that profited from forced labor, there are preliminary signs of willingness by both to accept responsibility and provide compensation (Underwood 2009). The changing outlook is a product not only of the deepening economic bonds among East Asian nations of China, Japan, and Korea, but also of the findings by Japanese courts that the Japanese government is not *legally* liable for war compensation. As in the case of Germany, this could open the way for a new Japan Democratic Party government that has prioritized its relations with East Asia to take creative and ethical steps to resolve the issues. Nevertheless, it will require bold efforts by the governments concerned to bring the issues to closure through apology and reparations for victims, steps that seem far more likely in the case of Japan than of the United States.

To prevent recurrence of the war crimes that we describe in this volume, together with the contributors, we call on nations, communities, and individuals to face facts, criticize moral premises that their forebears took for granted and valued, and acknowledge the dark aspects of their histories so that ethical alternatives may be articulated and practiced. We note some encouraging achievements in addressing historical injustice, including the German government's apology and compensation to Nazi victims and U.S. government apology and compensation to Japanese Americans interned during the Second World War. The Japanese government has also issued a number of apologies for its wartime conduct. It has, for example, apologized and provided compensation to the comfort women, albeit it has thus far chosen to do so through an ostensibly private fund that shields the government from assuming full responsibility. These are promising, albeit limited developments, which point to a way forward.

We contend that it is both necessary and possible to confront history in the service of ethical aspirations for justice and a better world. On both societal and individual levels, we see such ethical analysis and reframing as the basis not only for resisting collaboration with unethical practices, but for preventing future medical atrocities and promoting human rights. Ethics, understood in these terms, is essential for our professions, our institutions, ourselves, and above all for international peace and harmony.

Core unresolved political, ethical, and professional questions remain: What kind of justice can be served for these crimes against humanity? What should and can be done to remake the value structure of medicine and science? In general, how do we defend humanity, ethics, human dignity, fundamental human rights, and the professional integrity of medicine and science in the face of a variety of yet-to-be-healed historical wounds and new challenges that are rooted in the human condition? The response to these catastrophes must simultaneously address both what is culturally distinctive and also universal in our worlds and lives.

References

Advisory Committee on Human Radiation Experiments. 1996. *Final Report of the Advisory Committee on Human Radiation Experiments*. New York: Oxford University Press.

Annas, G.J. and Grodin, M.A. 1992. *The Nazi Doctors and the Nuremberg Code: Human Rights in Experimentation*. New York: Oxford University Press.

Arendt, H. 1973 (first edition 1951). *The Origins of Totalitarianism*. New York: Harvest Books.

Arendt, H. 2006 (first edition 1963). *Eichmann in Jerusalem: A Report on the Banality of Evil*. London: Penguin Books.

Barenblatt, D. 2004. *A Plague upon Humanity: The Secret Genocide of Axis Japan's Germ Warfare Operation*. New York: HarperCollins.

Bauman, Z. 2000 [1989]. *Modernity and the Holocaust*. Ithaca, NY: Cornell University Press.

Bazyler, M. 2009. *Japan Should Follow the International Trend and Face Its History of World War II Forced Labor*. http://japanfocus.org/-Michael-Bazyler/3030.

Buruma, I. 2002 (first edition 1994). *The Wages of Guilt: Memories of War in Germany and Japan*. London: Phoenix.

Caplan, A.L. 1992. *When Medicine Went Mad: Bioethics and the Holocaust*. Totowa, NJ: Humana Press.

Chinese Central Archive (Zhongyang danganguan), eds. 1989. *Xijunzhan he Duqizhan* ([Japanese] Biological and Chemical Warfare). Beijing: Chinese Bookstore.

Döring, O. 2001. Comments on Inhumanity in the Name of Medicine: Old Cases and New Voices for Responsible Medical Ethics from Japan and China. *Eubios Journal of Asian and International Bioethics*, 11: 44–47. http://www2.unescobkk.org/eubios/EJ112/ej112e.htm.

Dudden, A. 2008. *Troubled Apologies Among Japan, Korea and the United States*. New York: Columbia University Press.

Fujii, S. 1997. *Qisanyi Budui* (Unit 731: Horrors of Japanese Devilish Biological Warfare Campaign). Taipei: Wenyintang.

Geneva Protocol of 1925. Protocol for the Prohibition of the Use in War of Asphyxiating, Poisonous or Other Gases, and of Bacteriological Methods of Warfare. http://www.fas.org/nuke/control/geneva/text/geneva1.htm.

Glover, J. 1999. *Humanity: A Moral History of the Twentieth Century*. London: Pimlico.

Gold, H. 1996. *Unit 731: Testimony*. Tokyo: Charles E Tuttle.

Harris, S. 2002 (revised edition; first edition 1994). *Factories of Death: Japanese Biological Warfare, 1932–1945 and the American Cover-up*. New York: Routledge.

Hein, L. and Selden, M. 1997. Commemoration and Silence; Fifty Years of Remembering the Bomb in America and Japan. In L. Hein and M. Selden, eds, *Living With the Bomb: American and Japanese Cultural Conflicts in the Nuclear Age*. Armonk: M.E. Sharpe, 1997, pp. 3–36.

Jager, S.M. and Mitter, R. eds (2007). *Ruptured Histories. War, Memory, and the Post-Cold War in Asia*. Cambridge, MA: Harvard University Press.

Jaspers, K. 2001 (first edition 1948). *The Question of German Guilt*, trans. E. B. Ashton. New York: Fordham University Press.

Jonas, H. 1984. *The Imperative of Responsibility: In Search of an Ethics for the Technological Age*. Chicago, IL: University of Chicago Press.

The Khabarovsk Trial. 1950. *Materials on the Trial of Former Servicemen of the Japanese Army Charged with Manufacturing and Employing Bacteriological Weapons*. Moscow: Foreign Language Publishing House.

Kingston, J. 2008. Nanjing's Massacre Memorial: Renovating War Memory in Nanjing and Tokyo. http://japanfocus.org/-Jeff-Kingston/2859.

Kleinman, A. 1986. *Social Origins of Distress and Disease: Depression, Neurasthenia, and Pain in Modern China*. New Haven, CT: Yale University Press.

Kleinman, A. 1995. *Writing at the Margin: Discourse between Anthropology and Medicine*. Berkeley: University of California Press.

Kleinman, A. 2006. *What Really Matters: Living a Moral Life Amidst Uncertainty and Danger*. New York: Oxford University Press.

Kleinman, A., Das, V. and Lock, M., eds. 1997. *Social Suffering*. Berkeley: University of California Press.

Lafleur, W.R., Böhme, G. and Shimozono, S., eds. 2007. *Dark Medicine: Rationalizing Unethical Medical Research*. Bloomington: Indiana University Press.

Lifton, R.J. 1986. *The Nazi Doctors: Medical Killing and the Psychology of Genocide*. New York: Basic Books.

Matsumura, J. 2004. State Propaganda and Mental Disorders: The Issue of Psychiatric Casualties among Japanese Soldiers During the Asia-Pacific War. *Bulletin of the History of Medicine*, 78: 804–835.

McCoy, A. 2006. *A Question of Torture: CIA Interrogation, From the Cold War to the War on Terror*. New York: Metropolitan Books.

Miles, S.H. 2006. *Oath Betrayed: Torture, Medical Complicity, and the War on Terror*. New York: Random House.

Moreno, J.D. 2001. *Undue Risk: Secret State Experiments on Humans*. New York: Routledge.

Nicosia, F.R. and Huener, J. 2002. *Medicine and Medical Ethics in Nazi Germany: Origins, Practices, and Legacies*. New York: Berghahn Books.

Nie, J.B. 2001. Challenges of Japanese Doctors' Human Experimentation in China for East-Asian and Chinese Bioethics. *Eubios Journal of Asian and International Bioethics*, 11: 3–7. http://www2.unescobkk.org/eubios/EJ111/ej111d.htm.

Nie, J.B. 2002. Japanese Doctors' Experimentation in Wartime China. *The Lancet*, 360: s5–s6.

Nie, J.B. 2003. Let's Never Stop Bashing Inhumanity: A Reply to Frank Leavitt and a Call for Further Ethical Studies on Japanese Doctors' Wartime Experimentation. *Eubios Journal of Asian and International Bioethics*, 13: 106–107. http://www2.unescobkk.org/eubios/EJ135/ej135b.htm.

Nie, J.B. 2004. The West's Dismissal of the Khabarovsk Trial: Ideology, Evidence and International Bioethics. *Journal of Bioethics Inquiry*, 1: 32–42.

Nie, J.B. 2005. State Violence in Twentieth-century China: Some Shared Features of Japanese Army's Atrocities and the Cultural Revolution's Terror. In L. Kühnhardt and M. Takayama, eds, *Menchenrechte, Kulturen und Gewalt: Ansaetze einer Interkulturellen Ethik* (Human Rights, Cultures, and Violence: Perspectives of Intercultural Ethics). Baden-Baden: Nomos, pp. 161–176.

Nie, J.B. 2006. The United States Cover-up of Japanese Wartime Medical Atrocities: Complicity Committed in the National Interest and Two Proposals for Contemporary Action. *American Journal of Bioethics*, 6: W21–W33.

Nie, J.B., Tsuchiya, T. and Li, L. 2009. Japanese Doctors' Experimentation in China, 1932–1945, and Medical Ethics. In R. Baker and L. McCullough, eds, *The Cambridge World History of Medical Ethics*. New York and London: Cambridge University Press, pp. 589–594.

Nishino, R. 2007. The Women's Active Museum on War and Peace: Its Role in Public Education. http://japanfocus.org/-Rumiko-NISHINO/2604.

Noda, M. 1998. *War, Crime and Responsibility*. Tokyo: Iwanami shoten. [In Japanese]. A Chinese version, translated by C.L. Zhu and Y. Liu, was published by Guangxi Normal University Press in 2000.

Powell, J.W. 1981. Japan's Biological Weapons: 1930–1945, A Hidden Chapter in History. *Bulletin of the Atomic Scientists*, 37: 44–52.

Sachse, C. and Walker, M. 2005. *Politics and Science in Wartime: Comparative International Perspectives on Kaiser Wilhelm Institutes*. *Osiris*, Vol. 20. Chicago, IL: University of Chicago Press.

Selden, M. 2007. A Forgotten Holocaust: US Bombing Strategy, the Destruction of Japanese Cities and American Way of War from World War II to Iraq. *The Asia-Pacific Journal: Japan Focus*, May 27, 2007. http://japanfocus.org/-Mark-Selden/2414.

Selden, M. and So, A.Y. 2004. *War and State Terrorism: The United States, Japan, & the Asia-Pacific in the Long Twentieth Century*. Lanham and Oxford: Rowman & Littlefield.

Tanaka, Y. 2007. Oda Makoto, Beheiren and 14 August 1945: Humanitarian Wrath against Indiscriminate Bombing. *The Asia-Pacific Journal: Japan Focus*. http://japanfocus.org/-Yuki-TANAKA/2532.

Tsuchiya, T. 2000. Why Japanese Doctors Performed Human Experiments in China 1933–1945. *Eubios Journal of Asian and International Bioethics*, 10: 179–280. http://www2.unescobkk.org/eubios/EJ106/ej106c.htm.

Tsuneishi, K. 1981. *The Germ Warfare Troops that Vanished: Unit 731 of the Kwantung Army.* Tokyo: Kaimeisha.

Tsuneishi, K. 2005. New Facts about US Payoff to Japan's Biological Warfare Unit 731. *Japan Focus. The Asia-Pacific Journal.* http://japanfocus.org/-Tsuneishi-Kei_ichi/2209.

Underwood, W. 2006. Names, Bones and Unpaid Wages (1): Reparations for Korean Forced Labor in Japan. *The Asia-Pacific Journal.* http://japanfocus.org/-William-Underwood/2219, http://japanfocus.org/-William-Underwood/2225.

Underwood, W. 2009. New Era for Japan-Korea History Issues: Forced Labor Redress Efforts Begin to Bear Fruit. *The Asia-Pacific Journal.* http://japanfocus.org/-William-Underwood/2689.

The Unit 731 Criminal Evidence Museum (Qinhua rijun 731 budui zuizheng chenlieguan), ed. 2005. *Unit 731: Japanese Germ Warfare Unit in China.* Beijing: China Intercontinental Press.

Victoria, B. 2006. *Zen at War*, 2nd edition. Lanham, MD: Rowman & Littlefield.

Williams, P. and Wallace, D. 1989. *Unit 731: The Japanese Army's Secret of Secrets.* London: Hodder & Stoughton.

Xinhua. 2009. August 10, Japan Holds Memorial Service for Wartime Chinese Forced Laborers. http://www.chinadaily.com.cn/world/2009-08/10/content_8547791.htm.

Part I

Japan's medical war crimes and post-war trials

1 Unit 731 and the Japanese Imperial Army's biological warfare program

Tsuneishi Keiichi, translated by John Junkerman

The Ishii Network

Unit 731 was the common name of a secret unit of Japan's Manchuria-based Kwantung Army whose official name was the Epidemic Prevention and Water Supply Department. The leader of the unit was Ishii Shiro (1892–1959), who held the rank of lieutenant general at the end of World War II. The unit epitomized the extensive organization for the development of biological weapons within the Imperial Army, which was referred to, beginning in the late 1930s, as the Ishii Network.

The Network itself was based at the Epidemic Prevention Research Laboratory, established in 1932 at the Japanese Army Military Medical School in Tokyo. Unit 731 was the first of several secret, detached units created as extensions of the research lab; the units served as field laboratories and test sites for developing biological weapons, culminating in the experimental use of biological weapons on Chinese cities. The trial use of these weapons on urban populations was a direct violation of the 1925 Geneva Protocol, which outlawed the use of biological and chemical weapons in war. It was also understood by those involved that the use of human subjects in laboratory and test site experiments was inhumane. This was why it was deemed necessary to establish Unit 731 and the other secret units.

Lt. General Ishii Shiro

The Epidemic Prevention Research Laboratory was created under the initiative of Ishii Shiro after he returned from two years of field study of American and European research facilities. It was set up, with the approval of top-level army authorities, as a facility to develop biological weapons. It is said that Ishii first became convinced of the need to develop biological weapons with the signing of the Geneva Protocol in 1925.

The biological weapons Ishii sought to develop had humans as their target, and Unit 731 was established with this goal in mind. In order to produce biological weapons as quickly as possible, Ishii considered it essential to have a human experimentation site at the disposal of his research laboratory. Japan had occupied northeastern China, and in 1932, the puppet state of Manchukuo was established.

Within this "safe zone," Ishii set up what was called the Togo Unit, based in the village of Beiyinhe, about 100 kilometers south of Harbin. Human experimentation began there in the fall of 1933. The Togo Unit was a secret unit under the vice-chief of staff of the Kwantung Army. It was set up to determine whether it was possible to conduct human experiments in northeastern China and, if it was possible, whether the experiments would produce useful results. The launching of this feasibility study reflects the deliberate nature of Ishii as the organizer of the research. All of those involved in this research and development were military doctors, but they all used false names. At this stage, the scale of the project involved about ten doctors, along with a staff of about 100.

The inauguration of Unit 731

Unit 731 was officially established in 1936. Its establishment is reflected in a memo dated April 23, 1936, entitled "Opinion Regarding the Reinforcement of Military Forces in Manchuria," from the chief of staff of the Kwantung Army to the vice-minister of the Ministry of War (contained in the Ministry of War Journal for the army in Manchuria, Rikuman Mitsu-dainikki). Under the heading "Establishment and Expansion of the Kwantung Army Epidemic Prevention Department," the memo states that the department will be "newly established" in 1936, and "one part of the department will be expanded in fiscal 1938." This is the oldest official document concerning Unit 731 that has been found to date.

In addition to inaugurating Unit 731, this memo also laid the foundation for establishing two other units. It called for the establishment of an additional biological weapons development unit, independent of Ishii's unit, which was called the Kwantung Army Military Horse Epidemic Prevention Workshop (later referred to as Manchuria Unit 100), and for preparations to set up a chemical weapons development unit called the Kwantung Army Technical Testing Department (later referred to as Manchuria Unit 516).

Several months later, the memo's recommendations were approved by Emperor Hirohito, the two units were established, and preparations began for creating the Testing Department. The Ministry of War Journal for May 21, 1936, recorded this development under the heading "Imperial Hearing on Military Force Improvement Consequent upon Budget Approval." The journal noted, "Units concerned with epidemic prevention: One unit each is established for epidemic prevention among humans and horses."

Having been officially established, Unit 731 moved its facilities from Beiyinhe to a newly established laboratory at a hospital in Harbin. This laboratory served as a front-line headquarters while the unit's permanent facilities were being built in Pingfan, outside of the city of Harbin. These facilities were completed and capable of conducting research in the fall of 1939, after the hostilities at Nomonhan (on the border between Manchuria and Mongolia) had ended.

With the construction of the Pingfan facilities, the primary research staff changed in composition from the military doctors of the Togo Unit to private-sector medical researchers affiliated with universities and other institutions. The first group to be posted to the unit was a team of eight assistant professors and instructors from Kyoto Imperial University in the spring of 1938. The group consisted of two bacteriologists, three pathologists, two physiologists, and one researcher specializing in experiments using animals. Within a year, a second group had arrived at the facility, and the research staff had expanded considerably. The prominence of researchers in pathology and physiology in the development of biological weapons reflected the need for specialized judgment in assessing the results of human experimentation.

With the expansion of the war front throughout China after 1937, sister units affiliated with Unit 731 were established in major Chinese cities. These units were also called Epidemic Prevention and Water Supply Departments. Then Unit 1855 was established in Beijing on February 9, 1938; Unit 1644 in Nanjing on April 18, 1939; and Unit 8604 in Guangzhou on April 8, 1939. Later, after Japan occupied Singapore, a similar unit (Unit 9420) was established there on March 26, 1942. These affiliates comprised the scope of the Ishii network through the end of the war. As of the end of 1939 (that is, before the establishment of the Singapore unit), the network had a total staff of 10,045, of which 4,898 were assigned to the core units in Tokyo and Pingfan.

Human experimentation

Human experimentation took place at all the units of the Ishii network, but it was conducted systematically by Unit 731 and Unit 1644. Of these two, there are extant reports from a U.S. Army survey of human experimentation by Unit 731, so the general outline of its program is known.

Table 1.1 was compiled from two sources: a report to U.S. occupation authorities dated December 12, 1947 by Edwin Hill and Joseph Victor, concerning human experimentation by Unit 731 and related facilities; and a list of specimens brought back to Japan by a Unit 731 pathologist in July 1943. Aside from Ishii and another unit leader, Kitano Masaji, the names of individual researchers do not appear; they are identified as military personnel: (M), primarily military doctors, (C), civilian technicians conducting research within the military, and (PT), part-time researchers working outside of the military.

The number of specimens reflects the number of subjects who died as a result of human experimentation as of July 1943. Consequently, the total number of victims of human experimentation at the time of Japan's surrender two years later would be higher than these figures. The figures also do not include victims of germ bomb tests at the Anda field test site or from other experiments.

Technicians who were civilian employees of the army were treated as officers. The status of civilian employees ranged from infantry class to general class, but technicians were treated as lieutenants and above. Ranking below the technicians were operators, clerks, and staff. For the most part, the Ishii Network took on university researchers as technicians. The part-time researchers were part-time employees of the Military Medical School Epidemic Prevention Research

Table 1.1 The number of specimens in human experimentation by July 1943

Subject	Researcher	Total specimens	Medically usable specimens
Anthrax	M	36	31
Botulinus	Ishii	2	0
Brucellosis	Ishii, M, C, M	3	1
CO	poisoning	1	0
Cholera	C, C	135	50
Dysentery	M, M, PT, PT, M	21	12
Glanders	Ishii, C	22	20
Meningitis	Ishii, C	5	1
Mustard gas		16	16
Plague	Ishii, C, M, C	180	42
Plague (from the Shinkyo [Changchun] epidemic)		66	64
Poison		2	0
Salmonella	M, C	14	11
Songo (epidemic hemorrhagic fever) C, Kitano, C		101	52
Smallpox	Ishii, C	4	2
Streptococcus		3	1
Suicide		30	11
Tetanus	Ishii, PT, C	32	14
Tick encephalitis	C, Kitano	2	1
Tsutsugamushi (scrub typhus) C		2	0
Tuberculosis	C, Ishii	82	41
Typhoid	C, C	63	22
Typhus	C, M, C, Kitano, C	26	9
Vaccine		2	2
Total		850	403

Laboratory; they were professors at Tokyo and Kyoto imperial universities who were contracted to perform research in their own laboratories. In short, a large number of civilian researchers were mobilized.

Biological warfare trials

For the most part, the use of the biological weapons developed by the Ishii Network amounted to field trials. The first of these trials took place during the Nomonhan Incident in 1939. In August, toward the end of the hostilities, pathogens that cause gastrointestinal disease were placed in the Holsten River, a tributary of the Halha River that the Soviet Army used as its source of water. It is not clear how many Soviet soldiers suffered from this attack, but it is thought that casualties were not widespread. This was because the typhoid bacillus and the other pathogens that were used lose their infectivity when placed in water. This fact was known to Ishii's group. It is thought that they nonetheless carried out the attack because they wanted to conduct a field test of biological weapons in combat. While there were likely few Soviet casualties, at least one Japanese soldier became infected when he spilled liquid from a drum filled with contaminated water while dumping it into the river. He died of typhoid fever at an army hospital in Hailar.

During the following year, 1940, larger-scale field trials were conducted in central China, using biological weapons dropped from airplanes. The pathogens were cultivated by Unit 731 and shipped to Unit 1644 in Nanjing, which served as the forward base for the attacks through 1942. During the first two years, these attacks were carried out in cities along the Yangzi River. Of these, the large-scale attack on the city of Ningbo on October 27, 1940 is well documented and has also been thoroughly investigated by the Chinese.

The attack took place at 7 a.m. from heavy bombers flying a low-altitude run at 200 meters. The bombers dropped fleas, grain, and strips of cotton on the streets in the center of the city. The fleas were infected with the plague. They had ingested blood from plague-infected rats and were called "plague fleas." The plague bacteria were not dissipated directly, as it was considered more effective to infect the carrier fleas and release them, in order to target a specific area with a focused attack. It was also expected that the bacteria would live longer in the bodies of the fleas. The fleas were dropped with grain and cotton to ensure that they reached the target area, and it was also thought that the cotton would absorb some of the shock of impact on the ground.

The first death was recorded on the fourth day, October 30, and casualties increased rapidly in the days that followed. By November 2, it was clear that the disease was an epidemic, and the area was sealed off as disease-contaminated. The following day, it was determined that the disease was the plague. By then 37 deaths had been reported. The quarantine imposed on the area slowed down the spread of the epidemic.

The plague epidemic ended on December 2, with the death of the last two victims. Deaths totaled 106 people. These figures were reported in a survey, conducted by two Ningbo researchers and published in March 1994 by Dongnan University Press. This historical account of the epidemic tracked down all of the victims and listed them by name, and it is thus a very valuable document. This attack, killing more than 100 people, was the most lethal in this series of attacks on Chinese cities. However, when one considers that the attack was carried out by heavy bombers on a risky low-altitude run, these results have to be considered a military failure.

There were two primary reasons for this failure. First, the bacteria used was so infectious that it immediately set off alarms among its victims. Second, there were exaggerated expectations of the ability to artificially spark an epidemic. In February 1941, Ishii reported to his superior officer, Lt. Gen. Kajitsuka Ryuji, chief of the medical department of the Kwantung Army, "plague epidemics arose easily under natural conditions, but that it was not easy to induce them artificially. A study of the reasons for this showed . . . that it was not enough to have the pathogenic agents to start an epidemic; it was necessary to have a good knowledge of physiological conditions and the physiological properties of human beings." (The Khabarovsk Trial 1950: 299) It was expected that pathogens dropped in a densely populated area like Ningbo would quickly spread from person to person, but these expectations were unfulfilled.

Great failures

In November 1940, the month after the attack on Ningbo, the Chinese began to take countermeasures in response to biological warfare attacks on urban populations. On November 28, the central Chinese city of Jinhua was the target of a failed attack. According to a Chinese Ministry of Health document

> At the time that the plague epidemics were continuing in Ningbo and its vicinity, three Japanese airplanes flew over Jinhua and dropped a large number of small granules the size of small shrimp eggs. These strange objects were gathered and examined at a local hospital. . . . They showed the physical characteristics of the bacteria that cause the plague. In any case, the plague did not break out in Jinhua and as far as this town was concerned the Japanese experiment in germ warfare ended in failure.

No effort was made to collect the material dropped from the airplanes on Ningbo, but one month later the objects dropped on Jinhua were gathered and analyzed. There had been rapid progress in securing evidence in response to the attacks. It is also likely that townspeople were warned to stay inside their houses. As a result, the Japanese experiment was deemed a failure.

Biological weapons are not only useful as potent instruments of war. Their use can also be accompanied by an important element of strategic disinformation, if it is claimed that the enemy itself used them, or if it is implied that they were used in retaliation. In this sense, when biological weapons are used, one tactic is to cause confusion as to whether they were used or not, but if the enemy deems the trial use a failure, the tactic itself fails decisively.

Nonetheless, the trial use of biological weapons on central Chinese cities continued in the fall of 1941. One of the targets was the city of Changde, about 1000 kilometers west of Shanghai in the Chinese interior. The Chinese applied the lessons they learned the previous year and were able to keep casualties in the single digits. Thus the results of the trials through the end of 1941 indicated that dropping plague fleas from airplanes as a means of attacking urban areas was some what ineffective.

Beginning in 1942, Japan began dropping pathogens from airplanes into battlefield zones, on a scale that amounted to a combat operation. In April, Japan launched the Zhejiang campaign. During this campaign, Ishii and company carried out massive biological weapons attacks. Cholera bacteria was the main pathogen employed, and the attacks resulted in more than 10,000 casualties. It has also been reported that some victims contracted dysentery and the plague. More than 1700 soldiers died, mostly from cholera. This would have been considered a great success for the Ishii group, save for the fact that all of the victims were Japanese soldiers.

A Japanese medic captured by American forces at the end of 1944 described the casualties among the Japanese Army during his interrogation:

> When Japanese troops overran an area in which a [biological weapons] attack had been made during the Chekiang [Zhejiang] campaign in 1942, casualties upward from 10,000 resulted within a very brief period of time. The Diseases were particularly cholera, but also dysentery and pest [bubonic plague]. Victims were usually rushed to hospitals in rear. . . . Statistics which POW saw at Water Supply and Purification Dept Headquarters at Nanking showed more than 1,700 dead, chiefly from cholera; POW believes that actual deaths were considerably higher, "it being a common practice to pare down unpleasant figures."

A new type of bomb

Following the 1942 failure, the Japanese army general staff lost all confidence in the efficacy of biological weapons. The pressure was on to find a new approach that would ensure the safety of friendly troops and deliver a more reliable, more devastating blow to the enemy.

The new approach developed was to pack the pathogens in bombs or shells, which would be dropped from airplanes or delivered by artillery. This would satisfy both of the requirements to deliver massive carnage while maintaining the safety of the attacking troops. At the same time, the only way to prevent disasters like that of the Zhejiang campaign was to improve communication among the troops.

Two hurdles confronted the effort to load bombs with pathogens. The first was the need to keep the pathogens alive for long periods of time. The second was the need to develop a bomb made of materials that would break apart upon impact using little or no explosives; this would prevent the pathogen from being destroyed by heat. Alternatively, if a bombshell could not be made of fragile material, a pathogen that could withstand the heat of an explosion would have to be selected. When a bomb or a shell lands, people do not immediately gather at the point of impact, so it was necessary to convey the pathogen from that spot to wherever people were located. Again a live host like a plague flea that would physically carry the pathogen and infect people was considered the best solution to this problem.

A bacteria bomb using the plague bacteria was developed to satisfy most of these requirements. The bomb used plague fleas packed in a shell casing of unglazed pottery made from diatomaceous earth (a soft, sedimentary rock containing the shells of microscopic algae). This same material was used in a water filter that Ishii had developed and patented. Since this bomb would break apart using minimal explosive, it was expected that the plague fleas inside would survive the heat and scatter in all directions, to bite people and spread the disease. This bomb, called the Ishii bacterial bomb, was perfected by the end of 1944. At the beginning of 1945, the collection of rats went into high gear, and Unit 731 went to work cultivating fleas to be infected with the plague.

Japan's defeat

The main force of Unit 731 left the unit headquarters by train soon after the Japanese surrender and returned to Japan between the end of August and early September 1945. Some members of the unit and officers of the Kwantung Army were captured by the Soviet military. Twelve of these POWs were tried by the Soviet Union at a war crimes trial in Khabarovsk in December 1949. In addition to members of Unit 731, officers of the Kwantung Army and the Army's chief medical officer were also charged as responsible parties. All of those charged were given prison sentences ranging from two to 25 years, but aside from one man who committed suicide just before returning to Japan, all had been repatriated by 1956. The record of the Khabarovsk trial was published in 1950 as Materials on the Trial of Former Servicemen of the Japanese Army Charged with Manufacturing and Employing Bacteriological Weapons (Foreign Languages Publishing House, Moscow).

On the other hand, not one of the members of Unit 731 who safely returned to Japan immediately after the defeat was tried as a war criminal. Instead, the American military began investigating the Unit in September 1945, and Unit officers were asked to provide information about their wartime research, not as evidence of war crimes, but for the purpose of scientific data gathering. In other words, they were granted immunity from prosecution in exchange for supplying their research data. The American investigation continued through the end of 1947, and resulted in four separate reports. The investigation took place in two phases.

The first phase resulted in the Sanders Report (dated November 1, 1945) and the Thompson Report (dated May 31, 1946). These two reports contained information on the Unit's bacteria bombs, but did not address the subject of human experimentation or the trial use of biological weapons. Kitano Masaji, who was in Shanghai at the time of Japan's surrender, was interrogated in January 1946. However, he was instructed by Lt. Gen. Arisue Seizo, the Japanese chief of intelligence, that he should not talk about "human experimentation and biological weapons trials," Kitano later told the author of this chapter. In other words, until that time, these two subjects had been effectively concealed.

Body disposal at Unit 731

However, at the end of 1946, American authorities received notice from the Soviets that they intended to try cases involving human experimentation and biological warfare. Ishii and others were interrogated again, and they confirmed the general content of the Soviet claims. The American investigation began anew, headed by new investigators. Two additional reports were produced: the Fell Report (dated June 20, 1947) and the Hill and Victor Report (dated December 12, 1947). These documents described the human experiments conducted by Unit 731 and its related units, based primarily on the interrogation of researchers involved in the experiments.

The Hill and Victor Report concludes with the following evaluation:

> Evidence gathered in this investigation has greatly supplemented and amplified previous aspects of this field. It represents data which have been obtained by Japanese scientists at the expenditure of many millions of dollars and years of work. Information had accrued with respect to human susceptibility to those diseases as indicated by specific infectious doses of bacteria. Such information could not be obtained in our own laboratories because of scruples attached to human experimentation.

The above account makes clear the nature of the crimes committed by the Ishii Unit. At the same time, it is necessary to question the responsibility of the American forces who provided immunity from prosecution in exchange for the product of these crimes.

Acknowledgment

This chapter was originally written by Tsuneishi Keiichi for publication in *Sekai senso hanzai jiten* (Encyclopedia of War Crimes in Modern History) (Tokyo: Bungei Shunju, 2002), edited by Hata Ikuhiko, Sase Masamori, and Tsuneishi. This English version was first posted at the online journal *Japan Focus* on November 20, 2005.

References

The Khabarovsk Trial 1950, *Materials on the Trial of Former Servicemen of the Japanese Army Charged with Manufacturing and Employing Bacteriological Weapons*. Moscow: Foreign Language Publishing House.

Kobayashi, Hideo 小林英夫 & Kojima Toshiro 児嶋俊郎 1995, ed. *Germ Troops of Unit 731: New Material from China* 七三一細菌戦部隊・中国新資料, Tokyo: Fuji shuppan.

Tanaka, Akira and Matsumura Takao 田中明, 松村高夫 1991, ed. *Documents from Unit 731* 七三一部隊作成資料, Tokyo: Fuji shuppan.

Tsuneishi, Keiichi 常石敬一1984, *Targeting Ishii: Unit 731 and the American Army's Intelligence Service* 標的・イシイ：七三一部隊と米軍諜報活動, Tokyo: Otsuki shoten.

—— 1994, 1999 *Organized Crimes by Medical Researchers: Unit 731 of the Kwantung Army* 医学者たちの組織犯罪：関東軍第七三一部隊, Tokyo: Asahi shimbunsha.

—— 1995, *Unit 731: The Truth about Biological Weapons and Crimes* 七三一部隊：生物兵器犯罪の真実, Tokyo: Kodansha.

2 Medicine-related war crimes trials and post-war politics and ethics

The unresolved case of Unit 731, Japan's bio-warfare program

Suzy Wang

Introduction

The International Military Tribunal (IMT) held in Nuremberg, and the International Military Tribunal for the Far East (IMTFE) held in Tokyo, were meant to be, as their titles suggest, *international* in nature, and in both cases they included judges, investigators, and prosecutors from multiple nations (four in the German case and 11 in the Japanese case). Military, civilian, and economic leaders charged primarily with Crimes against Peace, but also including Crimes against Humanity and Conventional War Crimes, made up the list of defendants: 24 in the German case and 25 in the Japanese case.

In addition to these international tribunals, provisions were made with Control Council Law No. 10 which also allowed occupying authorities to prosecute war criminals who committed conventional crimes. The official website for the Museum of Tolerance provides a postwar estimate of 80,000 Germans and tens of thousands of local collaborators convicted for their crimes in Europe during World War II. Between 1945 and 1949, over 500 Nazi criminals were convicted in the American, British, and French zones alone. Similarly, between October 1945 and April 1956, over 2200 trials were held in 49 locations in Asia and the Pacific simultaneously with and subsequently to the IMTFE by various authorities, including those of the U.S., China, Australia, and Britain. According to a 2002 report by the Interagency Working Group of the United States National Archives, of the 5700 war criminals charged,[1] 4300 were convicted, with 984 sentenced to death and 475 sentenced to life imprisonment. Investigations into war crimes were conducted on a wide range of issues over a vast territory occupied by Japanese forces.[2] Politics also dictated which crimes would be tried and by whom. These were known as B and C class trials, as opposed to the IMT and IMTFE trials, and they received far less international attention. A review of these trials permits a better understanding of issues surrounding contemporary trials and controversies taking place in Japan.

International Tribunal for the Far East (Tokyo Tribunal)

By the time the IMTFE (May 3, 1946 to November 12, 1948) was created as the Asian counterpart to the IMT, Cold War tensions had begun and politics played a much larger role in how the tribunal was run.[3] Although the number of participating nations at the Tokyo Tribunal was 11 compared to the four in the German case, General Douglas MacArthur, the central figure in the U.S. occupation, controlled many decisions pertaining to the legal proceedings, much to the exasperation of investigators from other nations.[4] The goal of the United States to contain communism and quickly rebuild Japan governed many of the decisions made by SCAP even before the tribunal convened in early May 1946.

Various declassified archival materials and testimonies reveal that Japan's BW program, headed by Ishii Shiro, had conducted inhumane experiments – including vivisections, freezing experiments, BW, and chemical warfare (CW) experiments as well as aerial tests and bombing of Chinese, Korean, Manchurian, Mongolian, and Soviet subjects (which were conducted in a controlled environment at Unit 100) from as early as 1932 to the end of the War.[5] While most of the victims were Chinese, some testimonies have also claimed that U.S. prisoners of war were subjects of such human experimentation (The Khabarovsk Trial 1950).

The numerous declassified government documents lay to rest any doubts about the U.S. government's postwar cover-up of Japan's BW program. Not only did the Japanese scientists receive 250,000 yen in payments in exchange for their data, but immunity from prosecution of war crimes was also granted to all those associated with the program.[6] The deal was struck with full knowledge that the data collected were from human subjects, almost all of whom were killed in the experiments. Although internal memos indicate otherwise, the United States government continues to maintain that no U.S. prisoners of war were victims of the experiments conducted under the BW program.[7]

The issue of the Japanese BW program was virtually excluded from the IMTFE with the exception of comments made on record by an American Associate Prosecutor of the International Prosecution Section (IPS) assigned to the China case, David Nelson Sutton. This, together with the Khabarovsk Trial conducted by the Soviet Union, would become the starting point for international research on the issue.

Significance of the IPS documents

While discussing the Nanjing Massacre on August 29, 1946, Sutton shocked the IMTFE court when he mentioned the Tama Detachment of Nanjing (also known under the designation of Unit 1644) and the human medical experiments conducted by their detachment during the Japanese occupation of the city.

> Mr. [David Nelson] Sutton: The enemy's TAMA Detachment carried off their civilian captives to the medical laboratory, where the reactions to poisonous serums were tested. This detachment was one of the most secret organizations. The number of persons slaughtered by this detachment cannot be ascertained. . . .

> The President [Australian Chief Judge William Flood Webb]: Are you going to give us any further evidence of these alleged laboratory tests for reactions to poisonous serums? This is something entirely new, we haven't heard before. Are you going to leave it at that?
>
> Mr. [David Nelson] Sutton: We do not at this time anticipate introducing additional evidence on that subject.[8]
>
> (IMTFE 1946, 4546–4547)

The prosecution case remained firmly on the Nanjing Massacre, and thus the opportunity to include the issue of Japan's BW experiments was lost and never brought up again in the IMTFE proceedings. This exchange between Sutton and Webb is nevertheless significant, as it left a written record of early U.S. awareness of the program.[9]

Sutton's comments during the IMTFE proceedings are all the more surprising since Sutton, on April 25, had recommended to Chief of Counsel Joseph B. Keenan that "no attempt be made to establish the use of bacteria warfare by the Japanese against China" due to lack of evidence.[10]

Interestingly, a month before the group's departure to China in April 1946 for collecting evidence, Colonel Thomas H. Morrow, Sutton's colleague at the IPS, had written a series of reports concerning the BW and chemical warfare (CW) issues for Keenan. His recommendations indicated that the responsibility lies in "the Tokyo Government and not field commanders," thus implying the inclusion of this issue within the scope of war crimes to be raised in the IMTFE. Sutton's interest in collecting evidence of individual atrocity and Morrow's search up the chain of command for culpability led to their different recommendations. In his final report, handed to Keenan on the same day as Sutton's report on BW, Morrow concluded that there is enough evidence to charge Japan with the use of poison gas in China (Williams and Wallace 1989, 173).

The possibility of a Nanjing trial?

The difficulties of collecting evidence in China in the midst of a civil war became evident to the IPS. Sutton's mention of the Tama Detachment alerted researchers to the fact that the IPS may have known more than they were willing (or allowed) to let on. John W. Powell points out that "the Chinese procurator at Nanking [had] sent a report on the TAMA Detachment's activities to the IMTFE, in Tokyo, asking that it be included in the war crimes charges against the Japanese" (1980, 5). Perhaps the new evidence compelled Sutton to mention the use of poison gas by the Japanese.

A search into the materials held in Nanjing does reveal the existence of three indictments against 14 former members of the Tama Detachment dated October 22, 1946.[11] Xie Fusheng of the Nanking Central Hospital charged Nagayama (長山) with using Chinese Nationalist prisoners as subjects for experimentation, injecting them with various germs and drugs. The second indictment charged Senior Captain Hiromoto (広本) and First Lieutenant Morita[12] (森田) with choosing 100 prisoners of the Laohuqiao Camp in October 1942, to be sent to the Tama Detachment for experimentation, causing the death of all prisoners. The third indictment was based on the testimony of Xie Jinlong, a former laborer recruited from Taiwan, which charged First Lieutenant Morita with ordering Xie in January 1942 to transport over 100 prisoners to the Tama Detachment, where no one survived (Fujii 1997, 432–433). According to Zhang Lianghong, the historian and Director of the Nanjing Massacre Study Center at Nanjing Normal University (email correspondence, February 10, 2007), in addition to Xie's testimony, two others regarding human experiments committed by the Tama Detachment may be found in the Nanjing archives. Among them, the one by Chimba Osamu 榛叶修 (榛葉修) is especially significant, its being a rare testimony provided by a former member of the Tama Detachment who defected to China during the War.

Williams and Wallace (1989), in their archival research, also found the Chimba testimony among the IPS documents,[13] but under a slightly different name: Hataba Osamu (hereafter referred to as Chimba). Taken on April 17, 1946, Chimba describes the 1942 Zhejiang Campaign in which Ishii had solicited the support of the Tama Detachment. After reading reports of the spread of epidemics during 1942 and 1943 in the areas that had been targeted, Ishii was known to have touted the campaign as a major success (Harris 1994, 111). Chimba, however, insisted that the winds had changed course during the summer maneuvers and poisoned soldiers from the Tama Detachment were hospitalized well into September of the following year. Chimba's testimony corroborates previously gathered intelligence reports,[14] and Sutton's claim in court that poison was used by the Tama Detachment may have come from Chimba's statement in the affidavit that Japan's research was not confined to BW but to poisons as well (Williams and Wallace 1989, 176–177).

These materials, collected for the IMTFE or a subsequent trial, provide the first material evidence of the activities of the Tama Detachment as well as partial data indicating the specific number and location of Chinese prisoners taken from one camp to be killed by experimentation. More importantly, the materials serve as an early indication that Japan's BW program extended at least as far south as Nanjing and was not confined to Manchuria (present-day Northeast China).

Beginning in December 1945, military tribunals in postwar China ended in late 1947 due to "heavy court costs," while "mounting Communist rebellion diverted attention" away from the tribunals (Cady 1980, 172). According to John F. Cady, charges were brought against 41,000 Japanese war criminals; however, a Chinese source indicated that only 2435 were tried (of which 110 were executed) (*Zhongguowang* 2005). Currently available materials do not confirm whether those of the Tama Detachment charged with war crimes were ever brought to trial in China. As we will see later, U.S. investigators, hindered in their search for truth by SCAP directives protecting the Japanese scientists, missed opportunities to put the BW researcher under scrutiny. Investigators were stonewalled.

Subsequent U.S. Army and Navy trials –
USA vs. Karl Brandt et al.

Among the more infamous cases tried in Europe after the end of World War II was that of *United States of America vs. Karl Brandt et al.* Held between October 1946 and November 1947, "the Doctor's Trial," as it was commonly known, was the first of 12 cases to be brought before the Nuremberg Military Tribunal (NMT). The defendants included senior doctors and administrators in the armed forces and SS, charged with conducting a series of medical experiments (see Appendix A) during the course of the War within the context of genocide and the systematic elimination of those deemed "life unworthy" (United States Holocaust Memorial Museum).

PostWar discourse of medical atrocities committed by Imperial Japan often refers to the Doctor's Trial – citing it as an example of justice served in Europe but "denied" in the Asian case. Indeed, no case was filed against Japan comparable to that of *USA vs. Karl Brandt et al.* given the decision to protect the Japanese BW scientists from prosecution in exchange for their data.

Subsequent Japanese trials

Initial regulations governing the scope and procedures of trials to be conducted by the U.S. military commissions in the Asian Theater were set by General Douglas MacArthur on September 24, 1945, with subsequent changes implemented through SCAP. Japanese war criminals (including Koreans and Formosans serving the Japanese military) were tried by the US military commissions in Army and Navy courts.[15] The Army courts were held in China, Japan, and the Philippines and generally followed more relaxed SCAP regulations on evidence. However, according to Glazier (2003), the Navy, while recognizing the relaxed SCAP regulations, adhered to the stricter regulations found in the *Naval Courts and Boards*[16] and brought in Japanese lawyers as part of their defense team (p. 2070). Since this would be the Navy's first experience holding war crime tribunals, great efforts were made to ensure fair trials. The Navy also wanted to distinguish its trials from those of the IMTFE and the Army trials, which were being criticized for displaying "victor's justice."

Imperial Japan was not the only nation to have conducted research on BW. Others include Germany and the United States (For a list of U.S. experiments, see Appendix A). What stands out in the Japanese research, as in the case of Germany, is the extensive use of humans as experimental subjects with death as the prescribed outcome of the experiments. Given the extent of the cover-up by the U.S. government during and after the IMTFE proceedings, it is interesting that trial-related materials reveal at least three cases of human experimentation.

USA vs. Iwanami Hiroshi et al. and
USA vs. Asano Shimpei et al.

There was much postwar destruction of evidence and elaborate cover-ups designed to hide crimes by the Imperial Japanese Navy stationed at Dublon Island, Truk

Atoll, Caroline Islands. In the following case, it took an undercover operation to eventually reveal what had occurred during the War on this military installation.

The case file records of *United States of America vs. Iwanami, Hiroshi et al.* indicate that the atrocities committed went beyond the starvation and beatings of POWs and locals,[17] and included shocking details of experiments conducted on American airmen. On June 10, 1947, charges were brought against 19 Japanese defendants for murdering eight American POWs. According to William H. Stewart (1986), a Japanese defendant named Nakamura whose job was to take notes during the various experiments provides the fullest account.[18] Nakamura explained that Iwanami Hiroshi, the Commanding Officer of Fourth Naval Hospital on Dublon Island, Truk, requested eight American POWs from the Commanding Officer of the Naval Guard Unit, where the prisoners were kept, for use in experimentation. Details of the experiments were as follows:

> On 30 January 1944, two doctors, now deceased, and Iwanami performed shock experiments on four of the POWs by placing tourniquets on their arms and legs for long periods. The tourniquets were taken off of two POWs at the end of about two hours and off the other two at the end of seven hours, the latter died immediately from shock, the former survived. The four other POWs were injected with streptococcus bacteria to cause septicemia (blood poisoning). These four developed a high fever and soon died.
>
> *(USA vs. Iwanami, Hiroshi et al.)*

The two POWs who had survived the shock experiments were strangled to death the following day. This was after explosions of dynamite intentionally placed in shallow holes in proximity to the bound, naked POWs injured their legs but still left conscious and in pain. These, along with the bodies of the other two POWs, were taken to the hospital and all were dissected. The hearts and organs of the four POWs who were victims of the shock experiments were said to have been removed and placed in specimen bottles. Iwanami's files further indicate that he confessed to cutting off the heads of the shock experiment subjects and boiling them for specimens to be sent to Tokyo (*USA vs. Iwanami, Hiroshi et al.*).

During this trial, testimonies were given by two defendants in another case, *United States of America vs. Asano, Shimpei et al.* Ueno Chisato was the acting head medical officer of the Forty-first Naval Guard Unit and Nakase Shoichi was the acting executive officer of the same unit where Iwanami conducted his experiments. Five months after the experiments were conducted by Iwanami, a separate request for POWs came from Ueno Chisato.

Within the case file, a 1948 review of the trial by John D. Murphy[19] shows that the six Japanese defendants of *United States vs. Asano Shimpei et al.* were variously charged with cutting and wounding, beheading, and stabbing two American POWs. Among them, former Rear Admiral Asano Shimpei was charged with failing to control his subordinates and not protecting prisoners under his jurisdiction, while Ueno was charged with illegally mistreating and torturing one American POW (the other was spared vivisection but was killed as a target for bayonet practices).

The prosecution charged that Ueno had informed a surgeon lieutenant at the Naval Guard Unit that he was going to operate on the prisoners and that the operations would be of educational value for younger surgeons. According to the postwar review by Murphy, "The right toe nail was removed . . . the right thigh was incised and the femoral artery exposed . . . the right testicle was incised . . . and removed . . . an incision was made in the abdomen . . . and an incision was made in the right breast." Ueno, however, objected to the charges and claimed that the operation was to correct a paronychial (nail bed infection) condition and other incisions were made to check for internal bleeding *(USA vs. Asano, Shimpei et al.)*. Although not found in Murphy's review, Stewart, in his 1986 publication, stated that Ueno had killed "one prisoner by chloroforming him and dissecting him alive on the operating table" (p. 104). Iwanami, Asano, and Ueno were all sentenced to death by hanging and their sentences were carried out as part of a series of executions which began in 1949 (Stewart 1986). A point which warrants further scrutiny is the fact that while these individual cases brought to trial under the U.S. military ended up in the death of the perpetrators, the IMTFE failed to bring the Unit 731 scientists to trial – indeed, they received immunity and payments in exchange for their data.

The fact that two different naval doctors could at different times have access to POWs for use in experimentation indicates that these were not isolated acts. While Ueno's surgery may have been an isolated case of a medical surgeon seeing POWs as better utilized in experimental surgeries for "educational purposes," Iwanami's experiments point to a possible connection with the larger network under which Japan's BW program operates. It remains curious that the heads of the POWs were processed as skull specimens to be sent to Tokyo. What the review and memoranda do not indicate is where in Tokyo Iwanami sent the specimens.

Perhaps further investigation into related material would reveal whether the legal team pushed further for information regarding a possible connection between the Navy experiments in the Caroline Islands and Tokyo. So far, all indications are that the investigative style of the Navy investigators was similar to that of Sutton's, with the focus on the specific crimes rather than placing it within the larger context of the networks within the scientific community.

The Army trial: *USA vs. Kajuro, Aihara et al.*

In contrast to the two Navy trials that took place far from Japan, the case of *United States of America vs. Kajuro, Aihara et al.* was part of several that took place in Yokohama on the mainland and collectively referred to as the "Yokohama Trials" or the "B and C War Crimes Trials." The media on this case was short-lived and while there was almost disbelief that human experiments on POWs were conducted on Japanese soil, the headlines quickly moved on to other news. Over the early months of the occupation, SCAP received many anonymous and named tips asking the investigators to look into certain doctors connected to Unit 731 and to include their crimes in the IMTFE.[20] This, combined with the near exposure of Japan's BW program by Sutton during IMTFE proceedings and the continued Russian insistence on interrogating Ishii, resulted in the transfer of much effort from the prosecution of criminals to cover-up.

On May 5, 1945, on their return flight to Guam, after having completed their mission to attack the Tachiarai Air Base in southwestern Japan, Captain Marvin S. Watkins and the rest of his B-29 bomber crew were attacked and had to abandon their airplane. Watkins, who was sent to Tokyo owing to his rank and possible knowledge of intelligence, was thus spared the same fate as that of his crew members. According to Fukubayashi Toru, a co-founder of the POW Research Network Japan, in May 1945, Army District Headquarters were ordered from Tokyo "to dispose of" the bodies of crew members and interpreted this as execution without trial. In fact,

> in or about June 1945, Japanese Kempeitai commander Lt. Gen. Sanji Okido secretly ordered each Army District Kempeitai commander that they should make contact with the Army District commander and strictly dispose [sic] of all the captured fliers. This order substantially meant to execute the captured fliers secretly without trial.[21]

Between May 17 and June 2, 1945, a series of experiments was conducted on eight American fliers who were held in detention barracks near and under the jurisdiction of the Western Army Headquarters. The first experiments were performed to explore respiratory conditions; the second series of two operations was on the brain and the stomach; the third series of operations was on the liver, artery, stomach, and heart; and the fourth and final series was on the lung and the brain. Aside from one crewman, who was injured in a scuffle with locals when he landed, the other seven "all appeared to be in good health and did not need medical or surgical treatment and the organs removed did not appear diseased" – all were noted to have been able to walk into the autopsy room, believing that they were there to receive medical care (*USA vs. Kajuro, Aihara et al.*).

Kamisaka (1979) and Landas (2004), in their postwar study of the Kyushu Imperial Medical University experiments, both question the use of a less experienced prosecution team for this case. Moreover, in his research of SCAP Legal Section case files, Landas (2004) found Kyushu Imperial Medical University to be one of three main research centers experimenting with artificial blood substitutes. The other two were Nagoya Imperial University and Niigata Medical College. Landas explained that:

> each research facility conducted its own experiments and pursued different types of substitutes. They only needed to report their data and conclusions to the Densenbyo Kenkyusho. In that sense, each university and research laboratory functioned semi autonomously.

(Landas 2004, 146)

If the connection to Ishii's research had been pursued by the prosecutors, the larger network of the medical community, pharmaceutical companies, and the military government would have been exposed. Ultimately, on March 25, 1950, "the Office of the Judge Advocate General (JAG) ruled that due to severe judicial errors on the part of the presiding commission members, the rulings were deemed questionable" and that "the president-law member 'exhibited a decided lack of judicial temperament and control' " (Landas 2004, 253–54). Finally, a rehearing was ordered but was never carried out due to the changing political environment at the start of the Korean War and the official reduction of most of the sentences in September 1950 by General Douglas MacArthur. None of the 30 defendants in this case were executed for their crimes (Easton 1995), and by 1958, all had been freed following reversion to the Japanese government of responsibility for Japanese war criminals (Landas 2004, 255).

Significance of the trials

In the early 1990s, when atrocities committed by former members of the Imperial Army came to be widely debated, there were those who, in order to separate themselves from negative media attention, proudly emphasized that they had served in the Imperial Navy during the War and not in the Imperial Army. It has long been argued that the Imperial Army and the Imperial Navy largely operated separately and oftentimes disagreed with the military maneuvers of the other – yet again adding to the distancing between the two. Within this context, the Navy trials were significant because, though they were not of the large-scale organized nature of those of Unit 731, they left a record that proved human experimentation was not confined to the Imperial Army and the medical facilities attached to them. Furthermore, both the Army and Navy trials ask us to reconsider what was previously only thought of as a hierarchical relationship between the military and the medical community.

The fact that Iwanami admitted to preparing the skull specimens to be sent to Tokyo provides a likely link between the medical communities in both places. Understood in the context of Landas' (2004) allegations of a relationship between Kyushu Imperial University and Tokyo's Densenbyo Kenkyusho (Center for Infectious Diseases), it is quite probable that Iwanami's experiments were not simply isolated cases conducted in the Caroline Islands.

On July 22, 1989, over 100 human remains (including complete skulls) were found at a construction site in the vicinity of the former Tokyo Imperial Army Medical University and Ishii's wartime research laboratory. Seventeen years later, on June 24, 2006, *Asahi Shimbun* published an article that confirmed the connection between the remains and the Japanese Army Military Medical School ("What is the Problem of Human Remains?" 2003). A former nurse who worked there disclosed that she knew of at least three locations where human remains were buried and, furthermore, that these remains – both Japanese and foreign (including Chinese) – had been dissected, made into specimens, and stored at that location. In one location she had helped to remove specimens from their glass containers and bury them after the War to prevent discovery by the occupying forces.

This dispels any doubts that Japan's BW program was operating solely under the Imperial Army – more specifically, the Kwantung Army located in Manchuria. The larger question that certainly warrants further research should then be which governmental or military organization controlled the medical research networks within the scientific community.

United States vs. Kajuro, Aihara et al. is significant because it provides material evidence that human experimentation was conducted on the Japanese mainland – against the long-held belief that the rush of Japanese doctors to fill jobs in the colonies was because human experimentation was not allowed on the Japanese mainland. Both trials indicate that doctors were able to procure human subjects through the military.

Whether Watkins's postwar effort to locate his missing crew members led to prosecution in the Faculty of Medicine of Kyushu Imperial Medical University case and not in the case of the Tama Detachment experiments is not clear. What *is* clear, however, is that the United States placed national interests over justice.

Frustrated by the stonewalling and non-disclosure of the Americans at every turn when it came to trying members of Japan's BW program at the IMTFE, the Russians decided to hold their own trial in December 1949. Although officially known as the Military Tribunal of the Primorye Military Area, the trial has since commonly been referred to as the "Khabarovsk Trial."

Military tribunal of the Primorye military area, "Khabarovsk Trial"[22]

According to Georgy Permyakov, the tribunal was rushed because Stalin was to re-introduce the death penalty early in 1950 (Working and Chernyakova 2001). Unfortunately, the rushed nature of the tribunal lent itself to the image of a "show trial." Postwar comments made by MacArthur's camp jumped at the opportunity to reinforce that image of Stalin's Russia, dismissing the short five-day trial as "just another show trial" reminiscent of those reported by the media in 1938, and discrediting it as "communist propaganda" (Working and Chernyakova 2001; Powell 1981, 48–49).

Since the 1990s, the works of Sheldon H. Harris (1994) and Jingbao Nie (2004) have given the 1950 Russian publication and the proceedings of the tribunal greater credence. Harris reiterated his belief that "the evidence presented at the trial was reasonably faithful to the facts" seven years after the publication of his book (Working and Chernyakova 2001). Further research by authors such as Kondo Shoji (personal communication, November 17–18, 2006) indicates the existence of interrogation records of at least 100 other members of Japan's BW program within the 18-volume trial record. Thus despite accusations that the trial was merely a "show trial," evidence shows that the Russian prosecutors as well as scientists conducted thorough investigations before the five-day tribunal in December 1949 and indeed, that they had captured many more than the 12 who stood trial.

The Russian charges suggested that Emperor Hirohito as well as other members of the imperial family knew about the BW program and allowed the experiments.

It is the only primary material we have that specifically places the BW program within a larger context, one that includes the scientific community, the military, the government, and the emperor (The Khabarovsk Trial 1950).

Of the approximately 600,000 Japanese captured by the Russians at the end of the War, only a minority were prosecuted, while many more did forced labor at various railroad construction sites, during which 10 percent died and the final prisoners returned to Japan in 1956. About 3000 were deemed to be war criminals, and 2000 of them were indicted in Soviet military court. Some 969 were deemed to have committed crimes in China and were not tried by the Soviets (Zhang et al. 2005, 6).

Despite long being out of print, *Materials on the Trial of Former Servicemen of the Japanese Army Charged with Manufacturing and Employing Bacteriological Weapons*, published in 1950 in Chinese, English, and Japanese, survived the years in various libraries and countries. The Chinese version served later as a reference to the tribunal held in China in 1956.

Superior people's court special military tribunal (Shenyang and Taiyuan trials)

On February 14, 1950 the leaders of the Soviet Union and the People's Republic of China (PRC) signed the Sino–Soviet Treaty of Friendship, Alliance and Mutual Assistance. As a token of goodwill, the Russians transferred to the newly formed Communist government in July of the same year the 969 Japanese war criminals believed to have committed crimes against the Chinese during the War. Camp records (Zhang et al. 2005) and trial records (Wang 1991) indicate that at least nine prisoners admitted to either being part of the Unit 731 network or to having conducted vivisections on patients in hospitals. These prisoners were taken to Fushun Prison in Changchun, the former Japanese stronghold in the Northeast. Together with the 140 Japanese prisoners already held in the Taiyuan Prison in Shanxi,[23] these prisoners were to wait six years before any of them saw prosecution.

There were several reasons for the six-year interval between initial incarceration and the eventual trial of the Special Military Tribunal of the People's Supreme Court. The main reason was obvious. This would be the first major war crimes trial for the newly created Communist government. The sheer responsibility of the new nation to allocate[24] and train people in the legalities pertaining to these cases necessitated the assembly of a new team, which came to be known as the Northeast Working Group on the Processing of Japanese Prisoners (NEWG). The legal significance did not go unnoticed by members of the young regime, and exhaustive preparations were made to ensure that this trial would place China, if not within the international community, then at least within the international legal community. To help achieve this goal, Chinese delegates who had returned from the IMTFE were called to assist in training this team in international law.

Zhou Enlai, then PRC Premier and Foreign Minister, had taken part in the Soviet transfer of the prisoners and had on previous public occasions repeatedly instructed that they be treated humanely.[25] With those instructions, members of NEWG went about the difficult task of locating witnesses and collecting testimonies. As a result, in 1954, a series of simultaneous archiving of materials throughout the Northeast took place. After three years of substantial progress, the camp administrators were still faced with one of the biggest obstacles – despite repeated interviews, none of the prisoners had admitted to any wartime atrocities. In the beginning and well into the third year, most continued to deny personal responsibility for any crimes (Zhang et al. 2005, 32–37).

In late 1955, as the trials approached, Zhou again publicly stressed the government's policy regarding the Japanese prisoners.

> there will be no death penalty or life sentences given, and those who are sentenced should be few in number. The indictment should clearly state and verify the basic crimes [committed by the defendant] before it can be brought to court. There will be no charges brought against general crimes. This is the decision of the Central [government].[26]
>
> (Zhang et al. 2005, 227, Translated by author)

Zhou's statements were made available to the Japanese prisoners as reassurance from China's Premier. Emotions ran high during the trials (June to July 1956), and much publicity surrounded its proceedings and re-emphasized the humane treatment given to those who remained within the Fushun camp.[27] In a post-trial interview in the *People's Daily*, former IMTFE judge Mei Juao stressed the legality and fairness of the trial, stressing its legitimacy within the realm of international law.[28]

Collaboration between the military, medical universities and the pharmaceutical companies

Like other commanders stationed near the Russian border, Major Kamihara Toshio was given instructions to destroy all evidence of BW at his Unit 162 (an auxiliary of Unit 731) and evacuate before Russian troops entered Manchuria on August 8, 1945 (Zhang et al. 2005, 35). The immediate postwar destruction of evidence was so thorough that it was difficult to gauge the specific kinds of work conducted in any of the Units. The Chinese trial records, however, provide valuable information on the area of research as well as scale of production of the little known Unit 162, also known as the Linkou Unit, and the Chinese experts came to the same conclusion as the Russians – the fact that these BW units calculated the fleas in kilograms and bacteria culture in tons confirms that these materials could not be used for anything other than massive BW use (The Khabarovsk Trial 1950; Wang 1991, 466–85).

Moreover, Chinese trial records substantiate the Russian claim that the *Kempeitai* or military police supplied Japan's BW program with human experimental subjects, a claim documented at the Khabarovsk Trial proceedings. In Chinese custody were three former *Kempeitai* commanders who admitted to their connection with Unit 731. Major Horiguchi Masao (堀口正雄) admitted in his testimony that during his time in Jinzhou, he sent nine people to Unit 731 (Wang 1991, 179–80), while Lieutenant Colonel Kamitsubo Tetsuichi (上坪鉄一) admitted to sending 22 people to Unit 731 during his time in Siping (Wang 1991, 181–85). Unlike the Khabarovsk Tribunal, we are not given the full picture of Japan's BW program due mainly to the fact that former unit members in custody were very few in number and low in rank. Nevertheless, by sifting through the trial records and contextualizing the relevant testimonies, we are able to better understand the vast networks between the military and medical community under the umbrella of science, of which Japan's BW program was an intricate part. This is an important contribution to the discourse of wartime medical ethics. Not only does it widen the scope to include non-military experiments, it also clarifies the relationships between hospitals, the military, and pharmaceutical companies both in Japan and overseas.

Some of the more disturbing information revealed in the trial records may be found in the testimony of Major Kobayashi Kiichi (小林喜一). Kobayashi had worked at *Kempeitai* headquarters for five years but stated that he could not specify how many people he had sent to Unit 731 and to various hospitals for vivisection. Kobayashi testified that they were simply too many to recall. This testimony not only hints at the sheer volume of human experimentation victims who passed through *Kempeitai* hands, but undercuts any argument that Unit 731 had exclusive rights to request prisoners from the *Kempeitai*. The fact that the *Kempeitai* provided human subjects for various organizations makes clear that use of human experimental subjects within China was far from limited to the BW program. The testimonies of two other prisoners, Tamura Yoshio (田村良雄) and Yuasa Ken (湯浅謙), who continued to speak out against the atrocities following their return to Japan, add credence to this argument. Tamura admitted, in a 1954 testimony, to amputating the legs of a young Chinese patient in the Manchuria Medical University (now the China Medical University located in Shenyang, northeast China) without anesthetics, leading to blood-loss-related death (Eda et al. 1991, 25).

Indeed, the medical community in Manchuria was equally guilty of conducting human experimentation. Yuasa was a medical doctor and Associate Director at the Luan Army Hospital in Shanxi province, China from 1942 until the end of the War. He had studied medicine under Kitano Masaji, who taught at the Manchuria Medical University and for a time headed Unit 731 in Harbin. Although not for use in bacteriological experiments, Yuasa admitted that during the three years and six months he was at the Luan Army Hospital, he "practiced vivisections for the purpose of practicing surgery and other methods seven times on fourteen conscious Chinese victims'" (Kokoro 1994, 44).

Yuasa recalls the time when the five hospitals assembled 40 medics for group training.

> We all had to go to the Epidemic Prevention Center in Taiyuan for lectures. The next day we were brought to the Taiyuan Jail. They took four Chinese

men out, shot them each twice and told us to dissect them. I didn't want to do it, but the other medics told me, "Every military unit does it, you don't have to make such a big deal out of it."[29]

(Kokoro 1994, 48; translated by author)

We received requests from a Japanese pharmaceutical company for brain-cortex tissue. They were making adrenocortical hormones. We cut tissue from the brains and sent it along. We sent one bottle. Then a second request came from the company for ten bottles, which we filled. This was a "private route." Everybody was involved.

(Cook and Cook 1992, 150)

This testimony provides a picture of the far-reaching scope of this network within the Japanese scientific community,[30] which included not only units within Japan's BW program and medical universities/hospitals, but pharmaceutical companies as well.

In addition to research on chronic adrenocortical insufficiency (also known as Addison's disease), pharmaceutical companies in Japan were also interested in studying the effects of steroid hormones on asthma and rheumatism (Kokoro 1994, 48). According to Matsumura Takao, a professor emeritus at Keio University, medical universities in China were not the only ones seeking the "private route." Knowing that human experimentation was not allowed in Japan, "many doctors put in requests to Unit 731 so as to obtain accurate results" (Kokoro 1994, 21). To make sense of the seamless collaboration between these industries, one must take into account the hierarchical nature of the Japanese university and medical system, within which fraternity between classmates was especially binding. Ishii astutely involved the medical community within Japan as a source of financial and technical support, buying their allegiance and their silence about the atrocities by concealing their tacit participation in experiments which allowed them to obtain and use materials gathered through inhumane means. Unfortunately for researchers interested in exploring this connection, while numerous captured military documents may now be obtained through archival research, those of the pharmaceutical companies remain locked up in private archives. Even retired pharmaceutical company employees are tight-lipped about their companies and their personal involvement in medical research during the War.

Political significance of the trials

The political significance of the Shenyang and Taiyuan trials was not overlooked by Chinese leaders. When the prisoners were handed over to the Chinese in 1950, both China and the Soviet Union were at war with the Americans in Korea and, while pressure mounted for it to remilitarize, Japanese industry supported the U.S. war, thereby jump-starting its postwar economy. By June 1956, China's leaders were actively seeking to establish diplomatic relations with Japan. At the Third National People's Congress, Premier Zhou Enlai commented that

> even though both countries are still in a state of war, the Chinese government is taking its own initiative to adhere to the policy of leniency while processing the imprisonment and examination of Japanese war criminals. . . . The Chinese government has continued to make such efforts because of its correct appraisal that the people of both China and Japan not only want peaceful coexistence and friendly relations, but also the normalization of relations between the two countries.[31]
>
> (Zhang et al. 2005, 318; translated by author)

That same month, the Shenyang and Taiyuan trials took place. Of the 1108 prisoners, only 45 were charged in a series of tribunals that lasted two months. In the end, five of the nine who had ties with Unit 731 were sentenced to 12 to 15 years in prison. The other four were returned home on one of three repatriations of the remaining Japanese prisoners that took place in 1956.[32] As China and Japan had no formal relations at the time, the logistics for repatriation were handled by organizations including the Red Cross and the Sino-Japanese Friendship Association.

In 1957, former prisoners of the Fushun camp who had been returned to Japan formed the organization "Chukiren."[33] Members of the group published memoirs and books on wartime atrocities. They also criticized the remilitarization of Japan despite numerous threats to their lives by right-wing organizations. However, most of postwar Japan was eager to leave the War behind, and thus many of these publications as well as other discussions of the War were marginalized by the mainstream public discourse until the 1970s.

Recent trials in Japan

Zhou Enlai's 1956 speech at the National People's Congress foreshadowed the normalization of the Sino–Japanese relationship which was finally achieved in a series of communiqués and treaties in 1972 in the wake of the US-China opening.[34] These treaties would later be used by Japanese courts as proof that China had given up its claims for compensation for wartime atrocities. By 2007, at least 27 cases in Japan (Kang 2007),[35] 15 cases (including appeals) in the U.S., and one each in Korea and China sought compensation for victims for various wartime atrocities including those of forced labor, comfort women, and abandoned chemical weapons, as well as the BW case. The majority of the cases were filed on behalf of Korean and Chinese victims.

While most of the above-mentioned cases were not filed until after the death of Emperor Hirohito in 1989, a 1965 textbook screening lawsuit against the Japanese Ministry of Education brought by Ienaga Saburo, a Japanese historian, would lay the foundation for future World War II-related lawsuits. However, in a 1997 verdict, Ienaga was ordered to delete all descriptions related to Military Unit 731 "on the ground that no reliable academic study, paper or publication was available for reference by then, therefore it was too early to address this issue in a textbook" (Judgments of the Supreme Court 1997).

Ienaga's lawsuit spurred scholarly research into issues concerning Japanese wartime atrocities including the BW program. Ienaga enlisted the help of Japanese scholars to collaborate with Chinese scholars in order to collect victim testimonies and visit local Chinese archives for primary documents. The collaborations resulted in the publication of scholarly works that were later entered into evidence for the case.[36]

The Ienaga case and the 1989 discovery of buried human remains sparked the interest of citizen activist groups, Japanese lawyers, and scholars, who began recording the testimonies of former members of Japan's BW programs. According to Gold (1996), while the national government continued to deny wartime atrocities, some Japanese local governments were more responsive. Between 1994 and 1995, the efforts of various local governments and citizen activists resulted in a 61-location "Unit 731 Exhibition." A subsequent book by Gold contained the testimonies given by former Unit 731 members at the exhibit, many of whom were speaking out for the first time.

Two years after the first lawsuit of Chinese war victims was filed, a group of Japanese lawyers[37] sued the Japanese government on August 11, 1997 on behalf of 180 Chinese plaintiffs – all victims of Japan's bacteriological warfare. *Chinese Sufferers and Bereaved of the Victims by Bacterio-weapons of the 731 Corps of Japan Army v. Japan* or the "Unit 731 Lawsuit" was the first lawsuit specifically targeting Japan's wartime BW program filed in Japan.[38] Due largely to the scope of Japan's BW program and given the lack of Chinese primary materials and testimonies, the lawyers decided to limit their case to certain localities rather than filing a general lawsuit. The decision was made to focus on Changde (Hunan) and Yiwu (Zhejiang), two areas that were described in detail in the IPS documents submitted by Sutton to Keenan as well as submitted to IPS by the Chinese procurator in Nanking in 1946. Those documents as well as local newspaper reports during the 1941 and 1942 attacks corroborated that the two areas would yield the highest possible number of witness testimonies.

The Japanese courts, however, ignoring the evidence of atrocities, have repeatedly invoked the "statute of limitations" or "state immunity" to dismiss the cases. Nevertheless, five years after the Unit 731 trial was filed on June 12, 2001, in a case brought by Liu Lianren, a former Chinese forced laborer, the Tokyo District Court rejected the "statute of limitations" defense (Kang 2007).

In August 2002, the Tokyo District Court recognized for the first time that Japanese Army units had engaged in bacteriological warfare. Moreover, it recognized the responsibility of the State for its actions. However, the court dismissed demands for compensation on the ground that foreign individuals do not have the right to sue for war damages. With courts rejecting former defense arguments, in 2001 the Japanese government began using the argument of "abandonment of the right to claim" as its main defense. This argument maintains that the San Francisco Peace Treaty, the 1952 Sino–Japanese Peace Treaty (or

Treaty of Taipei),[39] and the 1972 Joint Communiqué of the Government of Japan and the Government of the People's Republic of China had already resolved the issues regarding war compensation (Kang 2007). In refutation of the Court's decision, the Chinese plaintiff's legal team cited a March 1995 statement made by China's Vice-premier Jiang Chunyun during the National People's Congress: "What China gave up was not compensation between individuals and nations, but only between nations. The government should not interfere with compensation matters, since each individual has a right to claim it" (Anti-Saikinsen Website 2002).

On July 19, 2005, the final verdict of the High Court was read by presiding Judge Ota Yukio who acknowledged that the Imperial Army had violated the Geneva protocol of 1925, which explicitly prohibits the use in war of asphyxiating, poisonous gases, and of bacteriological methods of warfare. Judge Ota also acknowledged that the use of bacteriological weapons ultimately caused the deaths in the two provinces that the cases covered. However, the judge affirmed the District Court's ruling of August 27, 2002 to dismiss the demand for direct compensation and apology from the Japanese government.

While it may still be too soon to determine the overall implications the trials will have for Japan and its neighbors, lasting legacies have already been made. Because of the trials, first- and second-hand witness testimonies of the remaining few living victims are being recorded in multiple areas in China for use in future court cases. Former Unit 731 members, mostly in their late eighties and nineties, now have a forum to leave behind a record of truth. Finally, the cases prompted the research and production of scholarly work on BW and Unit 731 within China, Japan, and internationally.

Conclusion

These court cases have proven that in the face of Japanese government intransigence, there are lawyers, citizen activists, and former imperial soldiers within Japan who are interested in seeing their government acknowledge its past atrocities and compensate its victims.

China has, on a number of occasions, brought up war issues in the context of criticizing official Yasukuni Shrine visits by successive Japanese Prime Ministers. Moreover, Chinese anger culminated in massive, simultaneous anti-Japanese demonstrations that occurred within various provinces in 2005. The focus of reparation efforts, according to Underwood (2007), may well shift to China. Chinese leaders announced in 2006 that they will not only permit non-profit organizations and the Non-governmental Fund to Support Lawsuits by Victims of the Japanese Army's War of Invasion, but also that they may allow lawsuits of former forced laborers to take place in Chinese courts. The significance of the latter has not gone unnoticed by major Japanese corporations with investments in China.

On January 15, 2007, Japan's Supreme Court decided to hold back on all decisions regarding wartime atrocity lawsuits – including the Unit 731 lawsuit –

and instead scheduled a March 16 debate on the "abandonment of the right to claim" issue. This historical debate is part of the forced laborer lawsuit that resulted in a 2004 victory for the plaintiffs in the Hiroshima High Court and was being appealed by the company sued, namely Nishimatsu Construction Company.

However, celebrating the road to legal justice, and the prospect for a sincere, official apology from the Japanese government to the victims of their wartime atrocities, may still be premature. Touted by the Chinese Embassy as a historic "ice-thawing" visit by Chinese Premier Wen Jiabao (the last visit to Japan by a Chinese premier was in 2000) to promote "political trust and expand reciprocal cooperation and friendly exchanges so as to push forward Sino–Japanese relations to develop in a long-term, healthy and stable way," Wen's public relations campaign followed Japan's Prime Minister Abe Shinzo's denial that there was any evidence that the military coerced women into sexual slavery.

On April 27, less than three weeks after Wen's visit, the Japanese Supreme Court deliberated on two landmark hearings – the Nishimatsu Forced Labor Case[40] and the Comfort Women Case – both of which resulted in defeat for the plaintiffs. The Supreme Court's debate ended with the ruling that the 1972 Joint Communiqué signed by Japan and China had settled all compensation issues, including those of individual claims (Kim 2009).

In a meeting called by lawyers of the plaintiffs of the two cases (and other pending cases) later that same day, citizen activists learned that lawyers of five other pending cases had been notified by telephone that their cases had been dropped by the Supreme Court. There was outrage expressed when no representatives from the Nishimatsu Corporation (or their lawyers) showed up for the verdict, while one of the plaintiffs, blind, hard of hearing, and in his nineties, had traveled all the way from rural China. During the meeting, the irony of the Comfort Women verdict was also emphasized. It was given on the same day as Abe Shinzo's apology to the United States president – not the victims – for his public remarks on the comfort women issue. Abe's goal was to weaken support for House of Representative Resolution H-121 calling on Japan to formally apologize and compensate the women,[41] which passed three months after his trip on July 10, 2007.

To say that we have a full understanding of Imperial Japan's wartime BW program and all its implications may still be premature, and a shift in focus from that of the International Tribunals to local trials may reveal a different perspective on events as well as offer new revelations of postwar politics. Furthermore, rather than understanding the most recent (2007) verdict of dismissal of the Unit 731 trial as just another failed lawsuit, the focus should be the Tokyo Supreme Court's first recognition that Japan's Unit 731 did indeed engage in bacteriological warfare and that the victims' testimonies and legal proofs given by the Japanese lawyers representing the plaintiffs prove that these were victims of Japan's bacteriological warfare program. Given the non-prosecution in the IMTFE, the marginalization of the Khabarovsk Trial by the West, and the relatively understudied other trials, this is no small feat. Most importantly for historians, the records of the testimonies should be collected and kept for future research.

Acknowledgment

Suzy Wang would like to dedicate this chapter to the memory of Attorney Tsuchiya Koken, former President of the Japan Federation of Bar Associations, and Chairperson of the Japan Committee of the International Solidarity Council for Redress of World War II Victims by Japan who passed away on September 25, 2009. Attorney Tsuchiya and his team of lawyers were very generous in supporting interested researchers by providing opportunities as well as primary sources. Despite battling kidney cancer for the last four years of his life, he continued his work in seeking compensation for the victims of Japan's wartime crimes until the end.

Notes

1 Of the defendants, five were sentenced to death by hanging, while 16 were sentenced to life imprisonment and two were given lesser jail terms. Other than those who were hanged and the six who died in prison, all were released by April 1958 (Interagency Working Group 2002).
2 According to Stratford, the British alone conducted investigations and trials in Burma, British North Borneo, the Netherlands East Indies, French Indo-China, Singapore, Hong Kong, Tianjin, Shanghai . . . etc., and by early 1948, 931 Japanese war criminals had already been tried by the British (Stratford 2007).
3 For an excellent article comparing the rules of evidence and procedure applied in the International Military Tribunal and the International Military Tribunal for the Far East, see Wallach 1999.
4 There were similar criticisms made concerning the IMT: critics, including some judges, charged that the trials exemplified victor's justice due to the ex-post facto nature of the trials, and that the U.S. "ran the show." The fact that the legal procedures protected Japan's imperial family from prosecution for war crimes was another issue raised by a number of the judges.
5 According to Guo (Anqing City 2005), Japan's BW program consisted of seven main units and 63 subunits, employing up to 20,000 personnel, and which claimed to have successfully employed BW 36 times.
6 A December 12, 1947 report written by Dr. Edwin V. Hill, Chief of Basic Sciences at Camp Detrick, Maryland, pointed out that 250,000 yen was "a mere pittance by comparison with the actual costs of the data" which the U.S. government was to purchase. These data, according to Hill, "have been obtained by Japanese scientists at the expenditure of many millions of dollars and years of work" (Powell 1981, 47). It has also been established that those involved in the cover-up included top leaders of the United States government and SCAP (Powell 1980, 1981; Harris 1994).
7 In a declassified May 23, 1995 memo titled "DOD Q's &A's Regarding Unit 731," the U.S. Department of Defense stated that "no documentary evidence could be found to support the claims that American POWs were used for Japanese BW experimentation and research." Provided by Wang Ao, President of the Mukden Prisoner of War Remembrance Society (MPOWRS) on August 25, 2009.
8 Copy of the Record of the Proceedings for August 29, 1946 provided by the Hoover Institution on War, Revolution and Peace.
9 The IMTFE was in session for 404 days and its more than 3000 court exhibits and 40,000 pages of the records of trial proceedings cover crimes committed between 1928 and 1945 (Liu 1948, 168). In his article, written before the verdict of the IMTFE was delivered, Liu stressed the importance of the IMTFE materials as offering a complete overview of Japan's history and urged the preservation of these materials. A year later, Delmer A. Brown wrote that within the IPS alone, 2200 of the 4336 exhibits were

submitted by the prosecution, but the numbering system indicated that there were at least 8279 documents within the IPS (Brown 1949, 1013). This material, which was published in the early 1990s (Awaya and Yoshida 1993), revealed further the extent of IPS knowledge of Japan's BW program in China (Williams and Wallace 1989, 176).

10 Sutton's 36-page report to Keenan included expert testimonies by Chinese and foreign observers such as Dr. P.Z. King, Director General of the National Health Administration of China, and Dr. Robert Pollitzer, who has been involved in public health and plague prevention work in China for 25 years. Their testimonies included autopsy reports on plague outbreaks in the cities of Chongqing (Sichuan), Ningbo (Zhejiang), and Changde (Hunan) – cities reportedly bombed with BW in the early 1940s. While reports of the plague outbreaks coincided with sightings of Japanese planes flying at low altitudes dropping globules and other matters, Sutton concluded that no direct correlation could be made without further investigation into the matter (Sutton 1946).

11 Author Fujii Shizue dates the handover of the report to Sutton as October 22, 1946, "to be presented at the IMTFE. But, because the Americans had already decided to cover up the issue, it was not taken up as evidence in the IMTFE" (1997, 43). The discrepancy between the dates may, however, be due to the fact that several of the reports sent to members of the Chinese prosecution team in Tokyo required follow-ups with the addition of new information.

12 First names not available in the document.

13 "Affidavit of Osamu Hataba, on Bacterial Warfare carried on by Ei 1644 Force in China, 1943" cited as IPS Evidentiary Document 1896, Files Unit of IPS Document Division (Williams and Wallace 1998, 176).

14 A December 18, 1944 U.S. Army G-2 intelligence report entitled "Japanese Chemical & Bacteriological Warfare in China," by the Sino-translations and Interrogation Center (SINTIC), noted that a Japanese captive revealed that "a BW attack . . . made during the Chekiang campaign in 1942, [Japanese] casualties upward from 10,000 resulted within a very brief . . . time. Diseases were particularly cholera, but also dysentery and [plague]. Statistics which POW saw at Water Supply and Purification Dept. Hq. at Nanking [TAMA Detachment headquarters] showed more than 1700 dead" (Powell 1980, 6).

15 Most trials were held to try war criminals for atrocities against Americans, but there were also cases where U.S. military tribunals tried war criminals for atrocities against the British or other local natives. There were also regulations for specific areas such as the China Theater which allowed for the "creation of mixed inter-Allied military tribunals" (Bradsher 2007, 186).

16 Timothy Maga's (2001) research showed that Rear Admiral John D. Murphy, the Navy's Director of War Crimes, "sought to protect the Navy's 'good name' against the backdrop of criticisms regarding IMTFE and Army trials, by emphasizing fairness and avoiding what he saw as Army and international tribunal mistakes." The Navy followed standard court martial procedures, allowed for Japanese counsel, and obtained live witnesses and physical evidence whenever possible (Glazier 2003, 2069–2070; Navy Department 1937).

17 According to Stewart (1986), "evidence was collected on war crimes committed against ten Americans, twelve Nauruans, five Australians, one British, one French, one Swiss, four Trukese and thirteen white victims whose nationality could not be established" (p. 103).

18 Nakamura committed suicide after having testified and thus his name was not included among the 19 charged.

19 A retired Rear Admiral of the U.S. Navy and Director of the War Crimes Commission, Pacific Fleet to the Commander in Chief of the Pacific, the United States Pacific Fleet, and the Commander of the Marianas Area.

20 For example, Nishimura Takeshi, in his 1946 letter to SCAP, accused three named veterinary surgeons of being connected with Unit 100 where Nishimura claimed that Allied POWs were dissected (Nishimura 1946). In the same year, Ueki Hiroshi, a former army doctor, also wrote to SCAP and specifically to General MacArthur that

52   Suzy Wang

Ishii had established in Harbin a laboratory where Allied POWs were executed through human experimentation (Ueki 1946). The major concern of Washington at the time was whether American POWs were used as human experimentation subjects of Japan's BW program. Despite various indications and charges to the contrary, it was officially concluded that no Americans were experimented on, thus paving the way for a deal. As a response to the postwar pleas by former U.S. POWs of Camp Hoten in Mukden, Manchuria, for medical care for illnesses related to experiments by the Japanese, the U.S. House Committee on Veterans' Affairs, Subcommittee on Compensation, Pension and Insurance held a hearing on September 17, 1986 and continued to officially state that no experiments were conducted on American POWs of Camp Hoten (Yang 2007).

21 Private email correspondence with Sasamoto Taeko, co-founder of the POW Research Network Japan, on August 10, 2007.

22 See Boris Yudin (Chapter 3, this volume) for an in-depth analysis of the Khabarovsk trial and its ethical implications.

23 Many of the prisoners in the Taiyuan Prison were either captured after the 15-year war as holdouts waiting for the remilitarization of Japan or those who had gone underground and mixed with the Nationalist troops during the civil war between the Nationalist (KMT) and Communist (CCP) forces. Because of this, many of them were regarded by the Communist government as having committed "double atrocities."

24 In 1949 a large number of professionals trained in law and government administration fled to Taiwan with Chiang Kai-shek.

25 Because many of the Chinese within NEWG suffered directly at the hands of the Japanese, there was repeated emphasis from government leaders that "though there may be personal hatred, the Party's enterprise may not be violated" and that "individual sentiment cannot replace the Party's policy" ("个人仇恨不能违背党的事业, 个人感情不能代替党的政策," Zhang et al. 2005, 19). Their goal was to make sure that these prisoners would move from their previous ideology of militarism to that of peace.

26 Original quote cited in pp. 432–433 of Liu and Tie (1993).

27 The conditions were designed as a model among Chinese prison camps – the Japanese prisoners were not forced to work and were well fed. They were treated promptly for illness and given expensive medical care to which the locals did not have access. These factors convinced the prisoners that execution may not be the only sentence in their future and that there was hope that they would eventually see their families in Japan. After confessions among the prisoners were completed and before sentencing began in 1956, the prisoners were taken on group trips around the Northeast to interact with their former victims as well as witness Chinese economic progress. Even after the trial, those who were sentenced were allowed visits with family members who had traveled from Japan (Zhang et al. 2005).

28 Judge Mei Juao stated in the article that "not only did we provide witness testimony and documentary evidence, each defendant was given the opportunity to defend themselves. This was completely in line with international regulations and international law. [The trials] were in the spirit of humanity and at the same time fulfilled the requirement of legal justice" (Wang 1991, 756; translated by author).

29 Yuasa recalls his first experience with vivisection:

> I was trembling with fear the first time, but the second time, the third time, I got more daring and I just did as if it were a normal procedure. During that time, I was trained as a soldier. I even remember calling the *Kempeitai* myself once to ask for a victim. I gave the Chinese victim anesthesia, opened him up and showed the younger soldiers, "this is the liver, this is the kidney, and this is the heart."
>
> (Kokoro 1994, 48)

30 Collaboration between pharmaceutical companies and the military is not particular to the Japanese case. Although the circumstances under which American experiments

were conducted differed, ethical questions surround both cases. See Appendix B for a preliminary list of experiments conducted by the U.S. military in conjunction with pharmaceutical companies and state prisons.

31 Original quote found in Central Chinese Archives, File Record 119–1, Record 584.

32 The first repatriation took place on June 21, 1956; the second on July 15, 1956, and the last on August 21, 1956 (Zhang et al. 2005). All Japanese prisoners held in China were repatriated to Japan by 1965.

33 中國歸還者連絡會 (Network of Returnees from China). The group, made up of former prisoners of the Fushun camp, is now officially run by younger support members due to the passing of most of its original members. <http://www.ne.jp/asahi/tyuukiren/web-site/index.htm> (February 15, 2007).

34 The Joint Communiqué of the Government of Japan and the Government of the People's Republic of China signed on September 29, 1972 and the Treaty of Peace and Friendship between Japan and the People's Republic of China signed on August 12, 1978.

35 The Center for Research and Documentation on Japan's War Responsibility numbered the trials taking place in Japan as 61, but that number includes appeals. According to Kang (2007), Chinese war victims have filed lawsuits in Japanese courts not only in Tokyo, but in "Sapporo, Kyoto, Nagano, Fukuoka, Niigata, Gunma, Yamagata, Miyazaki and Kanazawa."

36 For an example, see Matsumura et al. 1997.

37 The number of sponsoring lawyers listed in the most recent court document is 175. Court records, case number 4815 regarding appeals for case numbers 16684 and 27579. Final verdict from the High Court delivered on July 19, 2005.

38 An August 1995 lawsuit filed by a separate group of Japanese lawyers on behalf of the victims of the Nanjing Massacre included eight victims of Unit 731. This lawsuit was dismissed in September 1999 (Center for Research and Documentation on Japan's War Responsibility 2003).

39 Although most of the cases involved plaintiffs from the People's Republic of China and not Taiwan, the Court had on occasion used the Sino–Japanese Peace Treaty or Treaty of Taipei signed in 1952 between Japan and Taiwan as grounds to dismiss claims made by Chinese plaintiffs. Kang (2007) and other lawyers claim that the Japanese courts, by invoking this treaty, violated the 1972 Peace Treaty signed between the People's Republic of China and Japan, which recognizes one China. The actions of the Court, while trying to maintain the attitude of denial of wartime atrocities by the government, have contributed to more tension between the two nations.

40 Two years after the Court ruling, an illegal donations scandal related to bid-rigging involving the former Nishimatsu president Kunisawa Mikio and former Democratic Party leader Ozawa Ichiro led to a change in the company's top management. Along with this change came the voice of social responsibility, and the company's representatives began talks of a settlement for the former Chinese forced laborers (Kim 2009). On October 23 2009, Nishimatsu Construction Company agreed to 250 million yen (2.74 million U.S. dollars) to its Chinese victims as well as issuing an apology and building a memorial for them (Xiong 2009). This news brought about renewed hopes that while legal routes may have been effectively cut off, there may be other routes available to seeking compensation for the victims.

41 The resolution stipulated

> that the Government of Japan should formally acknowledge, apologize, and accept historical responsibility in a clear and unequivocal manner for its Imperial Armed Force's coercion of young women into sexual slavery, known to the world as "comfort women," during its colonial and wartime occupation of Asia and the Pacific Islands from the 1930s through the duration of World War II.
>
> (U.S. House 2007)

References and further reading

Annas, George J. and Michael A. Grodin (eds) (1992) *The Nazi Doctors and the Nuremberg Code: Human Rights in Human Experimentation*. New York: Oxford University Press.

安庆市疾病预防控制中心网站。*揭开[被隐瞒的一章] – 郭成周教授谈侵华日军细菌战历史真相* (2005) 健康报 [Anqing City Disease Prevention Center Website. *Exposing "A hidden chapter" – Professor Guo Chengzhou speaks on the historical truth of Japan's Bacteriological Warfare*. (2005) Health Newspaper] [online]. <http://www.aqcdc.org/newsout.asp?ID=611> (Accessed March 10, 2007).

Anti-Saikinsen Website (2002) *Statement of the Chinese Plaintiffs Legal Team* [online]. <http://www.anti731saikinsen.net/en/seimei-en.html> (Accessed on February 11, 2007).

栗屋憲太郎　吉田裕　編集・解説 (1993) 国際検察局 *<IPS>* 尋問調書 東京：日本図書センター現代資料出版事業部　第 1–27 巻 [Awaya, Kentaro and Yoshida Yutaka (compilation/explanation) (1993) *International Prosecution Section <IPS> Written Interrogation Records*. Tokyo: Nihon Tosho Center Modern Documents Publication Division, Vols 1–27].

Bradsher, Greg (compiled) (2007) "Japanese War Crimes and Related Topics: A Guide to Records at the National Archives." Maryland: Interagency Working Group (IWG), The U.S. National Archives and Records Administration (NARA).

Brown, Delmer A. (1949) "Instruction and Research: Recent Japanese Political and Historical Materials." *The American Political Science Review* 43 (5), pp. 1010–17.

Cady, John F. (1980) Review of *The Japanese on Trial: Allied War Crimes Operations in the East, 1945–1951. The Annals of the American Academy of Political and Social Science* 451, pp. 171–72.

Center for Research and Documentation on Japan's War Responsibility (2003) *Postwar Compensation Cases in Japan* [online]. <http://space.geocities.jp/japanwarres/center/hodo/hodo07.htm> (Accessed February 4, 2007).

Cook, Haruko Taya and Theodore F. Cook (1992) *Japan at War: An Oral History*. New York: The New Press.

Dower, John W. (1987) *War Without Mercy: Race and Power in the Pacific War*. New York: Random House.

Easton, Thomas (1995) "A Quiet Honesty Records a World War II Atrocity." *The Baltimore Sun*, May 28.

江田憲治、児島俊郎、古川万太郎（編訳）(1991)『生体解剖-旧日本軍の戦争犯罪』東京：同文館. [Eda Kenji, Kojima Toshio, and Furukawa Mantaro (compilation/translation) (1991) *Vivisection – the Crimes of former Japanese Soldiers*. Tokyo: Dobunkan.

Embassy of the People's Republic of China in the United States of America Website (2007) *Chinese Premier Begins "Ice-thawing" Visit to Japan* [online]. <http://www.china-embassy.org/eng/xw/t310544.htm> (Accessed August 15, 2007).

籐井志津枝. (1997)『 731 部隊：日本魔鬼生化的恐怖』台北：文英堂 [Fujii Shizue]. *Unit 731: The Horror of Japan's Monstrous Biological Weapon*. Taipei: Weningtang]

Glazier, David (2003) "Kangaroo Court or Competent Tribunal? Judging the 21st Century Military Commission." *Virginia Law Review* 89(8), pp. 2005–2093.

Gold, Hal (1996) *Unit 731 Testimony*. Tokyo: Yenbooks.

Harris, Sheldon H. (1994) *Factories of Death: Japanese Biological Warfare 1932–1945 and the American cover-up*. New York: Routledge.

"人骨「別にも埋めた」" (2006) 朝日新聞 ["Human Remains: Also Buried Elsewhere." *Asahi Shimbun*, June 24, 2006.

Interagency Working Group (IWG) (2002) "Implementation of the Japanese Imperial Government Disclosure Act and the Japanese War Crimes Provisions of the Nazi War

Crimes Disclosure Act: An Interim Report to Congress." The U.S. National Archives and Records Administration (NARA) [online]. <http://www.archives.gov/iwg/reports/japanese-interim-report-march-2002-1.html> (Accessed March 13, 2007).

International Military Tribunal for the Far East, Record of the Proceedings for August 29, 1946, pp. 4546–52.

姜力（編）《1949 伯力大审判 – 侵华日军使用细菌武器案庭审实录》解放军文艺出版社 (2006) [Jiang, Li (2006) *1949 Khabarovsk Trial – Trial Record of the Case of the Use of Bacteriological Warfare Weapons by the Japanese Military during the Invasion of China*. People's Liberation Army Literary Arts Publication Co.].

裁かれる細菌戦 (2002) 資料集シリーズ No. 8: "特集 7 3 1 部隊細菌戦裁判 第一審判決." 東京: 7 3 1 部隊細菌戦被害国家賠償請求訴訟弁護団、7 3 1 菌戦裁判キャンペーン委員会、ABC 企画委員会 [*Judged: Germ Warfare* (2002) Material Series No. 8: "Special Edition – First Judgment Decision of the Unit 731 Germ Warfare Case" Tokyo: Published jointly by Lawyers Group for Japan's Compensation for Victims of Unit 731 Germ Warfare, the Unit 731 Lawsuit Campaign Organization and the ABC Planning Organization].

Judgments of the Supreme Court (1997) *Case Number 1994(O) No.1119* [online]. <http://courtdomino2.courts.go.jp/promjudg.nsf/0/85ca688815fae0f649256c60002e13a1?OpenDocument> (Accessed February 11, 2007).

The Khabarovsk Trial 1950, *Materials on the Trial of Former Servicemen of the Japanese Army Charged with Manufacturing and Employing Bacteriological Weapons*. Moscow: Foreign Language Publishing House.

上坂冬子 (1979) 人体解剖：九州大学医学部事件. 東京：毎日新聞社. [Kamisaka, Fuyuko (1979) *Vivisection: The Incident at Kyushu University Medical Department*. Tokyo: The Mainichi Newspaper Co.].

Kang, Jian (2007) "The Basis of the 'Abandonment of the Right to Claim' Argument and the Reason for the Japan Supreme Court's Special March 16 Hearing." *The Asia-Pacific Journal* [online]. <http://www.japanfocus.org/products/details2369> (Accessed March 12, 2007).

Kim, Soon Hi (2009) "Nishimatsu Plans Compensation for Chinese Wartime Laborers". *The Asahi Shimbun*, May 2.

アジアの声 (第8集) <七三一部隊> 戦争犠牲者を心に刻む会／編　東方出版 (1994) [Kokoro Kizamu Group (compilation) (1994) *The Voice of Asia: Unit 731*. Tokyo: Tohou Shuppansha, Vol. 8].

Landas, Marc (2004) *The Fallen: A True Story of American POWs and Japanese Wartime Atrocities*. Englewood Cliffs, NJ: John Wiley & Sons, Inc.

Liu, James T.C. (1948) "The Tokyo Trial: Source Materials." *Far Eastern Survey* 17 (14), pp. 168–70.

刘家常，铁汉《日伪蒋战犯改造纪实》春风文艺出版社, 1993 [Liu, Jiachang and Tie Han (1993) *The Record of Transformation of the Japanese and Puppet Jiang War Criminals*. Chunfeng Wen Yi Publishing Co.].

Maga, Timothy P. (2001) *Judgment at Tokyo: The Japanese War Crimes Trials*. Kentucky: University Press of Kentucky.

Masalski, Kathleen Woods (2001) "Examining the Japanese History Textbook Controversies." *Japan Digest*, November.

松村高夫、郭洪茂、李力、江田いづみ、江田憲治 (1997) <戦争と疫病―7 3 1 部隊のもたらしたもの> 本の友社 [Matsumura, Takao, Guo Hongmao, Li Li, Eda Izumi and Eda Kenji (1997) *War and Disease – Those Brought On by Unit 731*. Hon-no-Tomosha Publishing Co.].

Minear, Richard H. (1971) *Victor's Justice: The Tokyo War Crimes Trial*. Princeton, NJ: Princeton University Press.

Mitscherlich, Alexander and Fred Mielke (1949) *Wissenschaft ohne Menschlichkeit: Medizinische und eugenische Irrwege unter Diktatur, Bürokratie und Krieg*. Heidelberg [*Science without Humanity: False Directions of Medicine and Eugenics under Dictatorship, Bureaucracy and War*. Heidelberg].

Museum of Tolerance Online Multimedia Learning Center (1997) *36 Questions About the Holocaust*. The Simon Wiesenthal Center [online]. <http://motlc.wiesenthal.com/site/pp.asp?c=gvKVLcMVIuG&b=394663> (Accessed January 3, 2007).

National Archives Collection of Records of Allied Operational and Occupational Headquarters, World War II. Record Group 331, *Records of Trials and Clemency Petitions for Accused Japanese War Criminals Tried at Yokohama, Japan, by a Military Commission Appointed by the Commanding General, Eighth Army, 1946–1948*. Microfilm Publication M1726, 59 rolls.

Navy Department (1937) *Naval Courts and Boards*. Washington, D.C.: Government Printing Office.

Nie, Jing-Bao (2004) "The West's Dismissal of the Khabarovsk Trial as 'Communist Propaganda': Ideology, Evidence and International Bioethics." *Journal of Bioethical Inquiry*, 1 (1), pp. 32–42.

Nishimura, Takeshi, to CI&E, GHQ, SCAP, SCAP (1946) *Report on War Criminals*, original letter accusing YAMAGUCHI Motoji, WAKAMATSU Yujiro, & HOZAKA fnu of dissection of prisoners of the Allied Forces by Unit 100; Record Group 331, Entry 1331, Box 1772. National Archives Building, Maryland, August 23.

Powell, John W. (1980) "Japan's Germ Warfare: The U.S. Cover-up of a War Crime." *Bulletin of Concerned Asian Scholars*, 12 (4), pp. 2–17.

Powell, John W. (1981) "A Hidden Chapter in History." *Bulletin of Atomic Scientists*, 37 (8), pp. 44–52.

Prévost, Ann Marie (1992) "Race and War Crimes: The 1945 War Crimes Trial of General Tomoyuki Yamashita." *Human Rights Quarterly*, 14 (3), pp. 303–38.

Röling, Bert V.A. and C. F. Rüter (ed.) (1977) *The Tokyo Judgment: The International Military Tribunal for the Far East (IMTFE). 29 April 1946–12 November 1948*. Amsterdam: University Press Amsterdam.

Spurlock, Paul E. (1950) "The Yokohama War Crimes Trials: The Truth about a Misunderstood Subject." *American Bar Association Journal*, 36 (5), pp. 387–89, 436–37.

Stewart, William H. (1986) *Ghost Fleet of the Truck Lagoon*. Montana: Pictorial Histories Publishing Co.

Stratford, Stephen (2007) "Stephen's Study Room: British Military & Criminal History in the period 1900–999" [online]. <http://www.stephen-stratford.co.uk/ukjaptrials.htm> (Accessed February 20, 2007).

Sutton, David Nelson (1946) "Bacteria Warfare" WO 208/4291, War Office, Directorate of Military Operations and Intelligence and Directorate of Military Intelligence, Japanese Biological Warfare in China, Public Record Office, April 23.

Sutton, David Nelson (1950) "The Trial of Tojo: The Most Important Trial in All History?" *American Bar Association Journal*, 36 (2), pp. 93–96.

Taylor, Telford (1949) *Final report to the Secretary of the Army on the Nuremberg War Crimes Trials under Control Council law No. 10*. Washington, D.C.: Government Printing Office, in *The Avalon Project: Control Council Law No. 10* [online]. <http://www.yale.edu/lawweb/avalon/imt/imt10.htm> (Accessed February 15, 2007).

"The Nishimatsu Case" (2009) *The Asahi Shimbun* [Editorial], July 20.

Ueki, Hiroshi, SCAP, to G-2, ATIS, General MacArthur (October 11, 1946) *Motoji YAMAGUCHI et al.* ATIS Translation #23836 of letter [3rd version] by Hiroshi UEKI accusing Shiro ISHII of establishing human experimental station in Harbin and executed Allied POWs; Record Group 331, Entry 1294, Box 1434, DOC ID#23836, Folder # 18. National Archives Building, Maryland.

Underwood, William (2007) "Japan's Top Court Poised to Kill Lawsuits by Chinese War Victims." *The Asia-Pacific Journal* [online]. <http://japanfocus.org/-William-Underwood/2369> (Accessed September 4, 2009, March 2).

United States Holocaust Memorial Museum. *Online Exhibitions: The Doctors Trial* [online]. <http://www.ushmm.org/research/doctors/index.html> (Accessed January 9, 2007).

U.S. House (2007) Committee on Foreign Affairs, Subcommittee on International Organizations, Human Rights, and Oversight. *House Resolution, 121* (July 30) 110th Congress. Washington 2007: Government Printing Office.

U.S. House Committee on Veterans' Affairs, Subcommittee on Compensation, Pension, and Insurance (1986) *Treatment of American Prisoners of War in Manchuria.* 99th Congress, 2nd Session, September 17. Washington, D.C.: Government Printing Office.

United States of America vs. Asano, Shimpei et al. File No. unnumbered dated September 22, 1947 (Vol. I), roll 16 in National Archives Collection of Records of the Office of the Judge Advocate General (Navy), Record Group 125, *Navy JAG Case Files of Pacific Area War Crimes Trials, 1944–1949*, Microfilm Publication C72, 16 rolls.

United States of America vs. Iwanmai, Hiroshi et al. File No. 160413 dated June 10, 1947, roll 8 in National Archives Collection of Records of the Office of the Judge Advocate General (Navy), Record Group 125, *Navy JAG Case Files of Pacific Area War Crimes Trials, 1944–1949*, Microfilm Publication C72, 16 rolls.

United States of America vs. Kajuro, Aihara et al. Case No. 290. "Review of the Staff Judge Advocate" dated May 2, 1949 in National Archives Collection of Records of Reviews of the Yokohama Class B and Class C War Crimes Trials by the U.S. Eighth Army Judge Advocate, 1946–1949, Record Group 331, *Records of Allied Operational and Occupation Headquarters, World War II*, Microfilm Publication M1112, five rolls.

Wallach, Evan J. (1999) "The Procedural and Evidentiary Rules of the Post World War II War Crimes Trials: Did They Provide an Outline For International Legal Procedure?" *Columbia Journal of Transnational Law*, 37 (11), pp. 851–883.

王战平（主编）《正义的审判-最高人民法院特别军事法庭审判日本战犯记实》人民法院出版社, 1991。 [Wang, Zhanping (ed.) (1991) *The Just Trial – Records of the Special Military Tribunal of the People's Supreme Court.* People's Court Publishing Co.].

"人骨問題と何か？" (2003) 軍医学校跡地で発見された人骨問題を究明する会. ["What is the Problem of Human Remains?" (online since 2003) Organization investigating the problem of human remains found at the former site of the Military Medical University] [online]. <http://www.geocities.jp/technopolis_9073/zinkotuhp/document.htm> (Accessed February 9, 2007).

Williams, Peter and David Wallace (1989) *Unit 731: Japan's Secret Biological Warfare in World War II.* New York: The Free Press.

Working, Russell and Bonna Chernyakova (2001) "The Trial of Unit 731." *The Moscow Times.* April 27.

Wu, Tianwei (2005) *The Failure of the Tokyo Trial.* Century of China, copyright 1995 [online]. <http://www.centurychina.com/wiihist/japdeny/tokyo_trial.html> (Accessed March 6, 2005).

Xiong, Tong (ed.) (2009) "Japan's Construction Firm Pays $2.74 Mln to Wartime Chinese Laborers" October 23, 2009. *China View*, October 23 online. <http://news.xinhuanet.com/english/2009–10/23/content_12309262.htm> (Accessed October 23, 2009).

Yang, Daqing (2007) "Documentary Evidence and Studies of Japanese War Crimes: An Interim Assessment." In *Researching Japanese War Crimes: Introductory Essays*. Maryland: Interagency Working Group (IWG), The U.S. National Archives and Records Administration.

张辅麟，田敬宝，夏芒，张岩峰《中国教育改造日本战犯实录》吉林人民主版社 2005。 [Zhang, Fulin, Tian Jingbao, Xia Mang and Zhang Yanfeng (2005) *Factual Record of China's Educational Transformation of Japanese War Criminals*. Jilin People's Publishing Co.].

中国网 (2005) "中国审判日本战犯" 4月22日。[*Zhongguowang* (2005) "China Tries Japanese War Criminals" April 22]. [online]. <http://www.china.com.cn/chinese/MATERIAL/845231.htm> (accessed February 1, 2007).

3 Research on humans at the Khabarovsk War Crimes Trial

A historical and ethical examination

Boris G. Yudin

This chapter deals with the trial of Japanese biowarfare scientists which took place in Khabarovsk, in the Russian Far East, on December 25–30, 1949. One of the points of indictment against the 12 Japanese military defendants referred to "criminal experiments on living humans" performed during the Second World War in Manchuria. This was the first time these experiments, which had been carried out with extreme cruelty over a 15-year period, had been investigated by a court. Aspects of the trial, such as its setting, timing, its rapid execution, and the leniency of the sentences handed down by the court, are discussed.

At the end of 1949, on December 25–30, in Khabarovsk, one of the biggest cities in the Soviet Far East, a trial took place of Japanese biowarfare scientists. Up until now the trial has been rather poorly covered in the literature of the Second World War in the East. This is true notably for Russian sources – despite the fact that the trial was organized by the Soviet authorities and was intended to achieve a number of political and ideological goals.

In this chapter, I present data which provide a window on the Russian perspective to the lead-up to the Khabarovsk Trial, the trial itself, and its outcome. The primary focus of inquiry is the medical experiments performed on human subjects by Japanese scientists that were elucidated at the trial. I also discuss the premises and efficacy of the Japanese wartime program of bacteriological warfare. In addition, I pose the question: How was it possible – from the moral point of view – to carry out such experiments?

The road to Khabarovsk

The final months of 1949 were marked by a number of events, played out in the international arena as well as the Pacific region, which were relevant to the Khabarovsk Trial. On August 23, the Soviet Union successfully carried out its first nuclear weapons test. On October 1, the People's Republic of China was created. The flame of the Cold War, which had been set alight with Winston Churchill's speech of March 1946, burned more and more brightly. On December 21, Josef Stalin, the Soviet dictator, marked his seventieth birthday. His jubilee was commemorated far and wide, and some traces of the celebration can even be found in the published materials of the Khabarovsk Trial. Yet, the most influential event had occurred the previous year. The trial at Khabarovsk was preceded by the International Military Tribunal for the Far East, carried out in Tokyo from May 3, 1946 to November 12, 1948. The Tokyo Tribunal had conducted its affairs in the international arena, with the participation of prosecutors and judges representing 11 powers which had been involved in the war against Japan.

Some signs of the growing conflict between the two superpowers – the U.S.S.R. and the U.S.A. – were revealed at the Tokyo Tribunal. For instance, in his speech at the Khabarovsk Trial, State Counsel for the Prosecution L. Smirnov noted:

> the prosecutor of the Nanking city court presented information to the International Military Tribunal in Tokyo, in which it had been specifically mentioned that Unit "Tama" – one of the most secret divisions of the Japanese Army – had systematically carried out experiments on living humans, inoculating them with poisoned serum.

This information about Japanese atrocities attracted the attention of the International Military Tribunal, which requested that American prosecutors, representing the Kuomintang government of China at the Tokyo trial, submit further evidence on the criminal activities of the "Tama" Unit.

Soon afterward, the Soviet prosecutor at the International Military Tribunal transmitted written testimony by [Major General] Kawashima [Kiyoshi] and [Major] Karasawa [Tomio] regarding the malicious experiments performed on living human subjects to the American Chief Prosecutor, Joseph Keenan.

It seemed, however, that some influential figures were attempting to prevent disclosure of the monstrous crimes committed by Japanese military personnel, and documents describing similar experiments carried out by the "Tama" and Ishii Units were not presented to the Tribunal (The Khabarovsk Trial, 1950: 441–442).

Investigators from a number of countries, including Russia, agree that in the course of the Tokyo Tribunal, the United States, which played a decisive role in the trials, took steps to prevent the airing of war crime charges against those involved in human experimentation. The Japanese historian of science, Tsuneishi Keiichi, notes that the American military began investigating these activities in September 1945. However, this initial investigation was aimed not at amassing evidence for prosecutions but at gathering scientific data acquired in the course of Japanese biological and chemical weapons research. None of the Japanese military personnel who had provided such information were subsequently tried as war criminals. "In other words, they were granted immunity from prosecution in exchange for supplying their research data" (Tsuneishi, 2005).

However, at the end of 1946, the Soviets gave notice of their intention to investigate claims of human experimentation and biological warfare. In response, the Americans began a more comprehensive study of the issues. One result of this new investigation was the Hill and Victor report, dated December 12, 1947. Tsuneishi reproduces the conclusion of the report, where the emphasis fell once more on the scientific value of the Japanese experiments:

Evidence gathered in this investigation . . . represents data which have been obtained by Japanese scientists at the expenditure of many millions of dollars and years of work. Information had accrued with respect to human susceptibility to those diseases as indicated by specific infectious doses of bacteria. *Such information could not be obtained in our own laboratories because of scruples attached to human experimentation.*

(Hill 1947, emphasis added)

According to G. Permyakov, the chief Russian-Japanese interpreter at the Khabarovsk Trial, the Soviet authorities were disappointed with some aspects of the Tokyo International Tribunal. He recalled that in 1946, the Soviet prosecutor at the Tribunal, S. Golunsky, had proposed the submission of a large number of documents describing the bacteriological crimes of the Kwantung Army in Manchuria. Yet, U.S. prosecutors had opposed adding these materials to the file. Consequently, once the Tokyo Trial ended in November 1948, the Soviet authorities decided to institute further proceedings.

The Soviets were also keen to study the Japanese biowarfare program for their own military purposes. After the war with Japan was over, the Soviets and Americans engaged in sharp competition to obtain Japanese research data. This story, however, is much better known from the U.S. than from the U.S.S.R. side. Up until now, publications on Soviet biological weapon programs have been few. Ken Alibek, one of the leading Soviet specialists in bacteriological weapons (now living in the U.S.), states that evidence supplied by former Japanese prisoners and documents seized by the Soviet Army was sent to Moscow for detailed study. These documents included working drawings of factories for the production of biological weapons; these factories were

bigger and more advanced than those in our country at that time. In Sverdlovsk [a major industrial center in the Ural mountains, now Ekaterinburg], a new military research complex was built by order of Stalin. In its construction, Soviet engineers and designers were indebted to drawings and knowledge gained from the Japanese.

(Alibek, 2003: 60)

The Russian historian of science Eduard Kolchinsky writes of the reluctance of the Soviet scientists involved in these developments to make public their activities in the field, and notes that their silence cannot be fully explained by the secrecy required by their research activities:

Like their American colleagues involved in the development of biological weapons . . . Soviet scientists, remembering the fate of Japanese and German experimenters on humans, preferred to keep silent about their contributions to the advancement of the country's defense capability. In this respect they differed sharply from the domestic and Western creators of atomic and hydrogen weapons, missiles etc.

(Kolchinsky, 2007: 397)

During and after the War, the Red Army imprisoned about 600,000 Japanese military personnel. The KGB had the immense task of seeking out those prisoners involved in bacteriological warfare research. Their success was considerable and even some of the gendarmes whose task was to dispatch prisoners for experiments were identified (see Supotnitzky, 2006). Military interpreter Georgy Permyakov recalled:

> In 1946, cipher messages from Moscow were received. We were requested to gather materials on bacteriological warfare. At the same time we were "digging up" Unit 731 and we ascertained that there were three generals in our prisoners-of-war camp who were in charge of these activities [Kajitsuka, Kawashima, and Takahashi]. They began giving evidence, but it did not come all at once.
>
> Altogether we talked with 1000 prisoners. Starting with evidence gleaned from the lower ranks, we proceeded to interrogate the senior ranks. Once this evidence was gathered, we were able to confront these three generals and force them to give further evidence. We went to Harbin and interrogated the Chinese. We gathered a huge amount of data and were proud of this achievement. All this data was prepared for the Tokyo Tribunal – the Eastern "Nuremberg". However, none of it was used.
>
> (Permyakov, 2000)

Then, on October 20, 1949 Permyakov, along with 20 other experienced interpreters, was ordered to a meeting convened by Colonel [first name unknown] Karlin, who had been empowered by the Ministry of the Interior of the U.S.S.R. to bring legal charges against a number of officers of the Japanese Army who had used bacteriological weapons during the war. Permyakov noted that, for reasons of personal safety, the identities of Karlin and himself were kept secret. This explains why Permyakov, unlike other interpreters, was never mentioned by name in the published version of the *Materials*.

The preliminary investigation lasted a little over two months: "The Japanese were initially kept in the Khabarovsk prison . . . High-ranking investigators came from Moscow. . . . The Japanese told everything they knew, without pressure. The interrogations lasted from 9 a.m. till 12 p.m. Investigators, interpreters, prisoners – everybody was worn out" (Permyakov, 2000). As we shall see, the Soviet authorities had important reasons for expediting matters.

Setting the scene for the trial

At the Khabarovsk Trial, 12 Japanese military personnel were accused of the manufacture and use of bacteriological weapons during the Second World War. They were: General Yamada Otozo, former Commander-in-Chief of the Kwantung Army; Lt.-General Kajitsuka Ryuiji, former Chief of Medical Administration of the Kwantung Army; Lt.-General Takahashi Takaatsu, former Chief of the Veterinary Division of the Kwantung Army; Major General Kawashima Kiyoshi, former Chief of the Department of Bacteriological Production, Unit 731; Major Karasawa Tomio, former Chief of a section in the Department of Bacteriological Production of Unit 731; Lt.-Colonel Nishi Toshihide, former Chief of Branch 673 of Unit 731; Major Onoue Masao, former Chief of Branch 643 of Unit 731; Major General Sato Shunji, former Chief of Medical Services, Canton Branch, 5th Army; Lt. Hirazakura Zensaku, a former researcher in Unit 100; Senior Sergeant Mitomo Kazuo, a former member of Unit 100; Corporal Kikuchi Norimitsu, a former medical orderly in Branch 643 of Unit 731; and Private Kurushima Yuji, a former laboratory orderly in Branch 162 of Unit 731.

The charges against them were based on extenstion to Japan of Article 1 of the Decree of the Presidium of the Supreme Soviet of the U.S.S.R., "On measures of punishment for German Fascist criminals guilty of the murder and torture of Soviet civilians and Red Army prisoners of war; also for spies and traitors to the Fatherland among Soviet citizens and their accomplices" (April 19, 1943). It is important to note the extreme severity of the Decree (see, for instance, Ulitzky, 2000: 29). Article 1 states that sentences handed down under previous instruments (which had included the death penalty) were of insufficient severity for "the most infamous evil deeds." In this context, a special means of capital punishment – hanging, which in some cases was to be carried out publicly – was introduced. The Decree also authorized punishments, such as terms of penal servitude lasting 15 to 20 years. It is interesting to note that despite the fact from 1943 until 1952 no fewer than 40,000 persons, including at least 25,209 foreigners, were sentenced under this Decree (Epiphanov, 2001: 73), the Decree itself was classified. Neither the accused nor their counsel were given the opportunity to become acquainted with it. However, on May 26, 1947, following the end of the war and cases entailed by it, the death penalty was canceled by the Decree of the Presidium of the Supreme Soviet of the U.S.S.R.

The timing of the trial deserves special comment. As we have seen, the Khabarovsk Trial began more than a year after the completion of the Tokyo Trials at the end of 1949. In Permyakov's opinion, it was necessary to end the trial before the New Year:

> Moscow forced the investigators to hurry. It was known in high quarters in the Ministry of the Interior that the death penalty would be restored the following year. That is why the people at the top requested the completion of the Khabarovsk bacteriological trial before the end of 1949 – at that time some awkward talks were planned between Moscow and Tokyo on the fate of Japanese POWs. And it is clear that Japan was especially concerned about [the status of senior] officers from the Kwantung and Korean Armies.
>
> (Permyakov, 2000)

The last evening session of the court, held on December 30, finished late at night when the verdicts were announced. We may conclude that, from the very beginning of the preparations for the trial, it had been predetermined that the defendants would not receive harsh punishments. Indeed, on January 12, 1950, the death penalty was restored in the Soviet Union. On that day the Decree of the Presidium of the Supreme Soviet of the U.S.S.R., "On use of the death penalty for traitors to the Fatherland, spies, and subversive saboteurs," was issued. In a departure from the Decree of May 26, 1947, this Decree permitted the use of the death penalty for those who committed especially heinous crimes against the State.

In Khabarovsk, the cases were heard by the Military Tribunal of the Primorsky Military District, presided over by Major General of Justice D. Chertkov. The bill of indictment, dated December 16, 1949, was signed by the Military Prosecutor of the Primorsky Military District, Colonel of Justice A. Berezovsky. As mentioned above, L. Smirnov, State Legal Advisor third class, was State Counsel for the Prosecution at the trial. Although each defendant was provided with a Soviet defender, these defenders played secondary, mainly decorative roles – a situation characteristic of the Soviet juridical system in general.

An expert commission on bacteriological and medical issues, headed by Nickolay N. Zhukov-Verezhnikov, also participated in the trial. The commission comprised six members, experts in epidemiology, immunology, microbiology, parasitology, and veterinary science. Nickolay Zhukov-Verezhnikov, a microbiologist and immunologist, had been an Academician of the Academy of Medical Sciences of the U.S.S.R. since 1948 and, at the time of the Khabarovsk Trial, was Vice-President of the Academy. He was researching methods of prophylaxis against plague and cholera, research which was set against a background of controversy and debate. In August 1948, only about a year before the Khabarovsk Trial, a dramatic Session of the All-Union Academy of Agricultural Science, named after Lenin (VASHNIL), had been held. At the Session, genetics was sharply criticized and rejected by Trofim Lysenko and his followers as a "bourgeois pseudo-science." Some rather exotic "scientific" theories were promulgated in the years of Lysenko's domination over Soviet biology. One of them, on the potential transformation of the plague pathogen into pseudo-tuberculosis, was proposed by Zhukov-Verezhnikov, who was an active supporter of Lysenko's theories (see Domaradsky, 1995).

Officially, the trial was carried out "with open doors." The hearings took place in the District House of Officers of the Red Army. According to G. Permyakov, attending the sittings of the court was relatively easy: it was only necessary to buy an entrance ticket. However, the journalist Evg. Sholokh claimed that special permission was necessary to observe the trial – which seems more plausible, given accepted practice at the time. Many who could not obtain tickets gathered near the House of Officers, where the trial took place, to hear radio broadcasts of the proceedings.

The indictments handed down at the Khabarovsk Trial fell into four areas: the organization of dedicated units for the preparation and implementation of bacteriological warfare; the commission of criminal experiments on living human subjects; the use of bacteriological weapons in the war against China; and activities undertaken in preparation for bacteriological warfare against the U.S.S.R. (The Khabarovsk Trial, 1950: 7–27). Only the second of these areas, human experimentation, will be discussed in this chapter. Charges of "personal participation" in the human experimentation program were brought against four of the defendants (Kawashima, Karasawa, Nishi, and Mitomo). Three others (Yamada, Kajitsuka, and Takahashi) were accused of knowingly permitting the experiments to proceed.

Crime and punishment

Nine of the accused were charged with crimes committed while they were serving with the notorious Unit 731. The Unit was created in 1936 by a secret decree of the Japanese Emperor and organized by Lt.-General Ishii Shiro. For security reasons, its predecessor had been named the "Water Supply and Prophylaxis Board of the Kwantung Army." Unit 731 was located near Pingfan railway station, 20 kilometers from the city of Harbin in northeastern China. According to the bill of indictment, by early 1939 a large-scale military camp with many laboratories and service buildings had been constructed. The staff numbered around 3000 personnel (The Khabarovsk Trial, 1950: 8).

Unit 731 consisted of eight divisions. Human experimentation was carried out within Division 1, the main function of which was the investigation and growing of pathogens for bacteriological warfare. In the course of this research many experiments on animals and humans were carried out. For this purpose – experimentation on human subjects in a "laboratory setting" – a prison compound was constructed inside the camp with the capacity to hold between 300 and 400 people. The object of these experiments was the production of bacteria capable of infecting humans with plague, cholera, gas-gangrene, anthrax, typhoid, paratyphoid, and other diseases.

According to evidence provided by one of the accused, Kawashima Kiyoshi, who headed Division 1 for some time, approximately 3000 people were killed in Unit 731 between 1940 and 1945 through infection with deadly bacteria. Kawashima claimed not to know the number of prisoners killed before 1940 (The Khabarovsk Trial, 1950: 19). For the most part, the experiments were directed toward the development of bacteriological weapons intended to infect humans. However, other experiments were also carried out, including depriving subjects of food and water, inducing frostbite to the hands, and the injection of animal blood into humans. During his preliminary testimony Kawashima stated:

> Constant experiments on living human subjects – Russian and Chinese prisoners – were conducted. They were transported to Unit 731 by Japanese gendarmerie in Manchuria – to test bacteriological warfare samples as well as to investigate ways of treating epidemic diseases in the Unit. Unit 731 had a dedicated prison for these detainees, where "experimental humans" were kept in stringent conditions including isolation; these subjects were habitually known as "logs" [*maruta* in Japanese]. I myself heard such names for test subjects used many times by the commander of Unit 731, General Ishii.
>
> (The Khabarovsk Trial, 1950: 55–56)

When interrogated at the trial, Kawashima once again referred to these subjects as "logs." When asked why Manchuria had been chosen as the site for bacteriological warfare research, he answered that Manchuria was most suitable for experimentation into bacteriological warfare because of the plentiful quantity of "test material" – people who could be used for experiments and were referred to as "logs." Kawashima also explained that these subjects were not held in the Unit's prison under their names, but were listed as numbers (The Khabarovsk Trial, 1950: 259).

In another case, Kawashima was cited as saying that the name "logs" was used "for security reasons" (The Khabarovsk Trial, 1950: 15). We shall return to this point below.

Alongside the experiments conducted in a "laboratory setting," trials were also carried out on testing grounds administered by Unit 731 and under battle conditions. In his testimony, Kawashima stated:

> In June 1941, I . . . took part in the testing of bombs filled with plague fleas at the Unit's testing ground near Anda railway station. In the course of the experiment, bacteriological bombs delivered from the air were tested on 10 to 15 prisoners who were tied to stakes in the ground.
>
> (The Khabarovsk Trial, 1950: 56)

When interrogated at a preliminary hearing, another accused, Nishi Toshihide, stated:

> It was known to me that (planned) experiments involving compulsory infection with deadly bacteria took place on Russian and Chinese subjects (including prisoners of war from the Unit's prison). . . .
>
> These experiments were carried out throughout the year; after the research subjects died, they were burned in a crematorium created for this purpose.
>
> Also, I know that . . . between January and March 1945, experiments exposing Russian and Chinese prisoners to typhus were carried out in the prison. In a separate experiment, five Chinese prisoners were exposed to the plague utilizing infected fleas at a testing ground near Anda in October 1944. In addition, frostbite experiments on human extremities were conducted at Unit 731 in the winter of 1943–44.
>
> Furthermore, in January 1945 ten Chinese prisoners were exposed to gas gangrene with my participation. The goal of this experiment was to ascertain the potential impact of exposure to gas gangrene under conditions of $-20\,^\circ$C frost. Ten Chinese prisoners of war were tied to individual stakes 10 or 20 meters away from a shrapnel bomb contaminated with gas gangrene.
>
> To prevent the immediate deaths of the prisoners their heads and backs were protected with special metal shields and thick quilts, leaving the legs and buttocks exposed. After an electric current was switched on, the bomb was exploded and the area where the prisoners were placed was saturated with shrapnel contaminated by gas gangrene. As a result, all of the test subjects

were wounded in the legs or buttocks and lived an additional seven days before dying in severe pain.

(The Khabarovsk Trial, 1950: 61–62)

During the hearings of arguments at the trial, State Counsel for the Prosecution L. Smirnov stated:

> It has been proved that, in Unit 731, inhuman experiments on living human subjects were carried out not only for research into bacteriological warfare. There were also other, no less inhuman and painful experiments, which . . . were carried out on a larger scale. These experiments were aimed at determining the limits of a human organism's endurance under specific conditions, and at studying . . . the prevention and treatment of non-infectious diseases. . . .
>
> To carry out such experiments . . . Unit 731 was equipped with a pressure chamber in which the limits of the human organism's endurance of high altitudes were ascertained. . . . People placed in this pressure chamber died a slow death involving unimaginable torment.

(The Khabarovsk Trial, 1950: 431)

The indictment prepared for the trial described the fate of those prisoners who happened to survive an experiment:

> If a prisoner recovered following his or her contamination with lethal bacteria, it did not save them from repeat experiments, which were continued until their death as a result of further contamination. Contaminated persons were treated, and different methods of treatment were subsequently studied. They were normally fed and, *following their full recovery*, they were used for a subsequent experiment, utilizing another kind of bacteria. In any case, no one left this death factory alive.

(The Khabarovsk Trial, 1950: 17, emphasis added)

Three of the 12 Japanese military personnel indicted were accused of conducting human experiments while members of Unit 100, which was located in Mogaton, 10 kilometers south of Changchun city, also in northeastern China. Unit 100 was charged, among other duties, with researching new military uses for bacteria and developing acute poisons for the mass extermination of people. Experiments for these purposes were carried out on both animals and living human subjects.

At the Khabarovsk Trial, defendant Mitomo Kazuo, formerly of Unit 100, testified that experiments on living humans were carried out between August and September 1944. These experiments, using Russian and Chinese prisoners, consisted of giving test subjects imperceptible amounts of soporifics and poisons. There were seven or eight Russian and Chinese test subjects. Among the medications used in these experiments were Korean bindweed, heroin, and castor oil seeds. These poisons were mixed in with their food. Each test subject received food poisoned in this way five or six times for a period of two weeks. Within the fortnight, all the test subjects became very weak and it was impossible to use them for further experiments. In order to maintain secrecy, they were all killed.

Mitomo was then subject to detailed questioning by the court:

Question: How was [the killing] done?
Answer: By order of researcher Matsui, one Russian test subject was killed by an injection with one tenth of a gram of potassium cyanide.
Question: Who killed him?
Answer: I injected him with potassium cyanide.
Question: What did you do with the corpse of this Russian?
Answer: I dissected the corpse at the Unit's cattle cemetery.
Question: What did you do with the corpse afterwards?
Answer: I buried it.
Question: Where was the grave dug?
Answer: In the cattle cemetery behind the Unit's buildings.
Question: In the same place where cattle carcasses were buried?
Answer: In the same place, but in another burial site (Stir, buzz of indignation in the hall.)
Question: Tell us, how did you accomplish the murder?
Answer: As a result of previous instructions issued by Matsui, the test subjects already had diarrhea. This diarrhea was the basis for the injection of potassium cyanide.
Question: Does that mean you deceived the test subject? After telling him you were giving him an injection for the sake of treatment, in reality you were injecting him with potassium cyanide?
Answer: Correct.

(The Khabarovsk Trial, 1950: 322–323)

During its session of December 28, 1949, the Court put four questions to the Forensic Medical Expert Commission. The Commission concluded:

all studies [carried out by Units 731, 100, and 1644] were concluded with evaluations of the experimental effectiveness of different kinds of weapons or delivery systems. In these experiments . . . living human subjects were used as "guinea pigs." Bacteriological weapons were regarded as suitable for testing in battlefield conditions . . . if the experiments conducted in the testing grounds led to . . . the forcible contamination and deaths of people. Hence, bombs filled with plague and anthrax bacteria infected many test subjects. The efficacy of bombs filled with plague fleas was studied.

(The Khabarovsk Trial, 1950: 396)

The verdict of the Court was announced on the evening of December 30, 1949. All 12 defendants were found guilty and sentenced to various terms in labor camps. In his closing speech, the State Counsel for the Prosecution requested sentences of 25 years of imprisonment (the maximum sentence at that time) for Yamada, Kajitsuka, Takahashi, Kawashima, and Sato, with sentences ranging from 15 to 20 years for Karasawa, Nishi, Onoue, Hirazakura, and Mitomo. He demanded up to three years' imprisonment for both Kikuchi and Kurushima. The usual practice of the Soviet justice system at that time was that the Court's verdict just rubber-stamped any recommendations made by the prosecution. In this case, however, there was some divergence from these unspoken practices: Sato (20 years), Onoue (12 years), Hirazakura (10 years) and Kikuchi (two years) were all given lighter sentences than those demanded by the prosecution.

Many observers have sought explanations for the unusual leniency of the Khabarovsk Court decision. It became clear to G. Permyakov that, when the death penalty was reinstated in early 1950, those convicted of bacteriological warfare crimes during the trial would be spared capital punishment, even though it was richly deserved. Permyakov remarked that the temporary exemption provided by the earlier Decree had been necessary to keep them alive (Permyakov, 2000), but why was such lenient treatment felt to be necessary? In 2001, journalists R. Working and N. Chernyakova put forward this explanation: "Clearly, Stalin was afraid that Japan would kill Soviet POWs if the Japanese military physicians were executed" (Working and Chernyakova, 2001). However, there are problems with this theory. During the War with Nazi Germany, Stalin had categorized all POWs (including his own son) as traitors. Soviet POWs liberated by the Red Army were, for the most part, dispatched from German prison camps straight to Soviet labor camps. Thus, it would be difficult to imagine Stalin harboring fears about the fate of Soviet prisoners in Japan. Furthermore, it is hard to imagine that there were any Soviet POWs still detained by Japan by the end of 1949.

More recently, E. Sholokh has offered another reason for the lenient treatment: the reason was the same as for the Americans, who had also managed to capture leaders from the Unit. The light sentences were handed down in exchange for the very useful information disclosed by the Japanese prisoners. "Otherwise," writes Sholokh, "it would be difficult to understand such humaneness shown by the Soviet justice and special services systems" (Sholokh, 2004). This seems the most convincing explanation – the unusually light sentences handed down at Khabarovsk were a form of barter. The Japanese convicts would receive only light punishment in exchange for information about bacteriological weapons – information that could prove invaluable to the Soviet Union's own developing biowarfare program.

Another fate was in store for those mid-level operatives of Unit 731 who were not convicted at the trial. M. Supotnitzky retells the story first told by G. Permyakov. On June 2, 1950, Permyakov received an order to come to Khabarovsk-2 railroad station where he was confronted by a huge number of red carriages. He was told that these carriages held Japanese POWs who had worked at Unit 731 and other sites involved in bacteriological research. The Soviet Union had decided to pass these individuals on to China, and Permyakov was to accompany them as he was fluent in both Japanese and Chinese. It turned out that the Japanese did not know that they were en route to China. In all, there were 1002 people on the train. For 16 years, Permyakov knew nothing of their fate. However, following the shooting incident on Damansky Island (March 1969) which took place in the period of severe tensions between the USSR and China, Permyakov read in the English communist newspaper, the *Morning Star*, that these Japanese prisoners had been placed on probation. With their help, the Chinese had opened their own research center for the development of bacteriological weapons. Since the *Morning Star* was supported with Soviet money, Permyakov concluded that this information had been deliberately fed to the newspaper from the U.S.S.R. (Supotnitzky, 2006: Book 2, 569).

The reliability of data and evidence disclosed at the trial

The Khabarovsk Trial has turned out to be one of the most controversial episodes in the history of the Second World War in the East. Some authors are inclined to dismiss it as nothing more than an example of Soviet propaganda, the kind of rhetoric which was so widespread during the Cold War. Thus, in his review of the first edition of one of the best-known books on Japanese biological warfare, *Factories of Death* by Sheldon Harris, J. Vance reproached the author: "The one weakness in his evidence may be the extensive use of the proceedings of the Russian BW show trial at Khabarovsk in 1949" (Vance, 1995: 452). Later, when the second edition of *Factories of Death* was published, L. Fouraker expressed the same view:

> Harris relies . . . on a translated record of a Soviet trial of accused Japanese war criminals. . . . This suspect source is the basis for a great many of the details of Harris's narrative. . . . Without secondary substantiation, I would tend to put all of the Khabarovsk trial information in the questionable category.
>
> (Fouraker, 2004: 2)

An opposing point of view has gained ground recently, the proponents of which maintain that a great deal of irrefutable data was presented at the trial. According to bioethicist Nie Jing-Bao, "the trial established beyond reasonable doubt the basic facts about Japanese BW war crimes including systematic cruel human experimentation, and its conclusions turned out to be remarkably accurate" (Nie, 2006: 25). This second position seems most plausible, and I want here to propose some secondary substantiation for it, using a rather specific methodology.

Unlike the authors cited here, I can rely on my own personal experience of the Soviet system – for more than 40 years I lived in the Soviet Union and was submerged in a political and social reality which was to a great extent produced by Soviet propaganda. At that time, anything more than bare survival depended on a person's ability to develop and cultivate a peculiar skill, which would allow one to extract grains of more-or-less accurate knowledge from a huge body of deliberately distorted information. Even propaganda needs to be based on some real facts and events, which are then interpreted perversely. Aware that such manipulation took place on a constant and predictable basis, Soviet citizens needed to develop corresponding "countermeasures" and to employ them systematically. There was a more-or-less limited set of methods and tricks used by the state to manufacture the disinformation it put out. Thus, if one knew, first, that a particular event had taken place (or even could have taken place), second, that the official information about it was inevitably distorted, and third, that some particular tricks from the state's restricted propaganda repertoire had in all likelihood been used, one would have some chance of extracting those few pieces of knowledge that had been distorted in the process. However, a couple of caveats should be mentioned at this point. While Soviet citizens grew very adept at deploying these deciphering skills they were not infallible. In addition, because such skills were based on subjective personal experience, it was difficult to make them reproducible and objective.

The trial took place in the extraordinary frame of reference which was the Soviet system of justice. Although this system included the roles of accused, judge, prosecutor, defender, and so on, their meaning had little in common with legal practices found elsewhere. For instance, as we have seen, the functions of a defender were negligible – it was never expected that a defender would try to convince the Court of a client's innocence. The task of a defender was mainly to seek out mitigating circumstances. At the same time, the actual status of a prosecutor placed him on a higher level than a judge, whose verdict usually faithfully reproduced the prosecutor's indictment. The verdict in the Khabarovsk Trial diverged somewhat from this norm. Bearing in mind that, for the Soviet authorities, the trial's chief importance lay in its political significance, it is at least possible to understand the function of much of the ideological rhetoric that colored the speeches of many its participants. The published materials of the trial, as well as the rather rare first-hand recollections of it, allow us to conclude that the behavior of its participants was to a considerable extent staged – first of all, in the ease with which accused as well as witnesses admitted almost all the charges. Nevertheless, such divergence from the legal standards accepted in Western countries does not necessarily imply falsifications and distortions at the level of fact.

While Nie Jing-Bao draws attention to the "many problems and shortcomings associated with the operation of the Khabarovsk trial itself" (Nie, 2004: 38) and notes such features as the deliberate exclusion of international observers and the use of propaganda, I support his views on the basic validity of the trial. We need to draw a clear distinction between all these details of the legal process on the one hand, and the great quantity of evidence and factual material presented at Khabarovsk on the other.

My personal experience gained over a long period immersed in the Soviet propaganda system convinces me that it would have been impossible to fabricate, without any real grounds, the vast amount of evidence presented at the trial. Soviet history was rich in *causes célèbres* which received a great deal of publicity. It is instructive to compare the Khabarovsk materials with the famous political trials of the 1930s, which were widely reported in Soviet newspapers, when so-called "enemies of the people" were on the docket. The materials produced at these trials contained many more unfounded invectives and much less factual material than was the case at Khabarovsk. Moreover, many of the alleged crimes of these "enemies of the people" simply defied credibility and common sense.

In fact, I have been able to confirm only one factual error from among the many alleged by those who dismiss the significance of the Khabarovsk Trial – an anecdote that was supposedly "taken from the trial record" concerning "the distribution of bacteria-laden chocolates to Chinese children" (Vance, 1995: 452; the same story is reproduced in Fouraker, 2004: 2). I could find no mention of this story in the Russian version of the "Materials"; it is included, however, in Chapter 1 of the memoirs of Morimura Seiichi, *The Devil's Gluttony* (Morimura, 1983: 6).

Offensive medicine

Having considered some examples of human experimentation presented at the Khabarovsk Trial, we turn now to the rationale behind such practices developed by the medical arm of the Japanese military – pre-eminently by Ishii Shiro, head of Unit 731. The Soviet jurist Mark Raginsky presented a striking piece of evidence at the trial. Describing the activities of the anti-epidemic laboratory in Tokyo, Raginsky produced evidence from "the former worker of the laboratory, a Captain of Medical Services, who spoke at the Khabarovsk Trial under the pseudonym Nakagava Posirii" (Raginsky, 1985: 166). According to Posirii, Ishii Shiro once told the laboratory personnel: "military medicine consists not only of treatment and prevention, but genuine military medicine is designed for offensive warfare" (Raginsky, 1985: 167).

This unorthodox understanding of medicine found its embodiment in a very extensive program of research, which included aggressive experimentation on humans. Yet Japan's efforts to develop effective bacteriological weapons were far from successful.

Russian biologist Mikhail Supotnitzky, the author of a two-volume history of the plague (Supotnitzky, 2006), discusses some of the difficulties in artificially inducing epidemic diseases in human populations. He argues that "the failure of Ishii lay not in the lack of the lethal potential of bacteria and viruses, but in the fact that it is too deeply hidden by nature." He added that the experimenters had chosen unrealistic scenarios for their trials:

> The Japanese succeeded in exploding ceramic bombs at preset altitudes over the geographically flat testing grounds, detonating them on prisoners bound to stakes. These prisoners, in their turn, "waited" until the plagues fleas crawled onto them. However, it would be impossible [to provoke an epidemic] against an actively resisting enemy, especially over large tracts of countryside.
>
> (Supotnitzky, 2006: Vol. 2, 547)

Indeed, according to Supotnitzky, Japanese efforts at inducing epidemics were far from successful:

Official Chinese sources, which were inclined to exaggeration, noted that in total the Japanese subjected 11 major towns in different districts to bacteriological attacks. . . . In 1952, China estimated that 700 people had been the victims of an artificially induced plague between 1940 and 1944. . . . It turns out that this was a smaller number than those Chinese infected as "logs"! As for the Soviet troops, there were no cases of disease at all, despite the fact that they carried out military operations in natural strongholds of infection and entered cities enveloped in plague. Artificially induced bubonic plague "refused" to create pulmonary complications among the Chinese and did not form self-replicating foci within populations.

(Supotnitzky, 2006: 539)

In a Web article reprinted in the journal *Japan Focus*, Tsuneishi Keiichi reaches similar conclusions on the limited effectiveness of Ishii's program. Describing one of its early stages, the large-scale attack on the city of Ningbo on October 27, 1940, Tsuneishi notes:

This attack, killing more than one hundred people, was the most lethal in this series of attacks on Chinese cities. However, when one considers that the attack was carried out by heavy bombers on a risky low-altitude run, these results have to be considered a military failure.

There were two primary reasons for this failure. First, the bacteria used was so infectious that it immediately set off alarms among its victims. Second, the effort suffered from exaggerated expectations of the ability to artificially spark an epidemic. . . . It was expected that pathogens dropped in a densely populated area like Ningbo would quickly spread [from] person to person, but these expectations were betrayed.

(Tsuneishi, 2005)

Tsuneishi then gives a similar assessment of some of the subsequent stages of the program:

In April [1942], Japan launched the Zhejiang campaign. In this campaign, Ishii and company carried out massive biological weapons attacks. Cholera bacteria was the main pathogen employed, and the attacks resulted in more than 10,000 casualties. It has also been reported that some victims contracted dysentery and the plague. More than 1700 soldiers died, mostly from cholera. This would have been considered a great success for the Ishii group, but for the fact that all of the victims were Japanese soldiers.

(Tsuneishi, 2005)

It is worth noting at this point that some commentators have sought to uphold the effectiveness of the Japanese biological warfare tests. According to an estimate included by Sheldon Harris in *Factories of Death*, "By the end of 1942 the casualty count in the open tests surely fell into the six-figure range" (Harris, 2002: 104;

reproduced in Nie, 2004: 36). However, one of the reviewers of *Factories of Death* noted that Harris had borrowed casualty figures from an unreliable source, namely David Bergamini's journalistic and unscholarly book published in 1971 (Fouraker, 2004: 2).

Supotnitzky notes that Ishii regularly exaggerated the significance of his unit's work to the Kwantung Army's command. Indeed, during the Khabarovsk Trial one of the witnesses, Colonel Tamura, former head of the Personnel Department of the Kwantung Army, testified:

> Ishii told me about the effectiveness of bacteria on human test subjects in experiments in laboratory settings as well as in field conditions, and claimed that bacteriological weaponry was the most powerful weapon in the hands of the Kwantung Army. He informed me that Unit 731 was on full alert and if required . . . the Unit would be ready to deluge enemy troops with huge masses of deadly bacteria; and that the Unit could also use the air force to carry out military operations against the enemy's rear and over its cities.
>
> (The Khabarovsk Trial, 1950: 349)

Later, Tamura claimed to have reported on the Unit's preparedness for bacteriological warfare to the Commander-in-Chief of the Kwantung Army, General Yamada.

Supotnitzky's response to these reports is dismissive:

> While Ishii was talking about his 10 old airplanes, the Soviet Army was preparing for war against Japan with 3800 airplanes of the latest design.
>
> Let us now consider whether it really was possible to have harmed Soviet troops using Japanese bacteriological weapons. Let us suppose that a Japanese plane had forced its way through the air defense system and attacked Soviet troop emplacements. Suppose that the air temperature and humidity were at optimal levels for flea activity. Suppose that the fleas were adequately protected and that, when the bombs exploded, they were not blown to pieces. Suppose further that our soldiers failed to notice that these plague-infected fleas were biting them. Even under such optimal conditions, the Japanese military would not achieve the results they anticipated from bacteriological attacks. Even before the war, many Russian and Chinese inhabitants of Harbin were aware of the function of the "hospital" near Pingfan. The General Consulate of the USSR regularly received information about it. In 1945 it was no secret that Japan had carried out bacteriological warfare. . . . Thus, it is not surprising that the Soviet Army was thoroughly prepared for bacteriological attacks in advance. Personnel of the Far Eastern Military District were immunized with highly effective plague vaccine.
>
> (Supotnitzky, 2006: Vol. 2, 549–550)

We may conclude, first, that it was impossible for the Japanese to carry out the development of bacteriological weapons without a sustained increase in the numbers of human test subjects, and second, that the whole project was doomed to failure.

Maruta technology

We turn now from the discussion of empirical data on the human experimentation conducted by Unit 731 to pose the question: What were the ethical values and moral premises that made it possible to perform *without scruples* these experiments on a mass – or even industrial – scale? The question can be reformulated: What understanding of a human being is held by those who regard it as permissible to subject large numbers of people to torture and atrocities? While a single act of atrocity might be ascribed to chance, we must assume that experimenters working on such a large scale had developed rationalizations that allowed them to approve this kind of research. Regrettably, this case is far from unique: human history abounds in examples of mass brutality. Yet it allows us to clarify some aspects of the technology of these practices as they were realized in the field of biomedical research.

First of all, the perpetrators need to find a way of drawing a distinction between "us" and "them." "Us" includes those who performed the experiments as well as those perceived by the experimenters to be in the same category. "They" belong to another category and may be treated as to some extent "non-humans." At the moral level, such a premise provides the pretext for setting aside or weakening the efficacy of the golden rule.

The most common ground for such a distinction is race and/or ethnicity. Indeed, in our case this ground was used. In his book *War Without Mercy*, John W. Dower describes the Japanese theory of a racial hierarchy prevalent at the time of the war. According to the theory, there were three levels of beings in Asia: "First the master race, which was Japan, second was the kindred races such as China and Korea, and third was the guest races that were made up of the island people like the Samoans. All the non-Japanese races were seen as lower life forms and should be subservient to Japan" (Dower, 1986: 8). Such a worldview meant that it was possible to sacrifice people who were members of "inferior" ethnic groups.

As we have seen, the question of race played an essential role in the choice of test subjects. There is no mention in the trial materials of any use of Japanese subjects; most of the experiments carried out by Unit 731 were performed on Chinese, members of one of the "kindred races." Thus the race criterion was not the only one used for categorizing people into "us" and "them." Another ground used by the Japanese military was the choice of test subjects from their national enemies, whether actual or potential. The so-called "laws of wartime" were very often interpreted as an excuse for atrocities of various kinds, including the Unit's hideous experiments. An additional justification was developed by Ishii in his view of military medicine as intended not only for the treatment and prevention of disease in humans, but for offensive attacks on them.

There was nothing unusual in the use of such criteria to distinguish between "us" and "them" (which included categories such as prisoners and criminals) in the context of the Japanese biowarfare program. What is unique and deserves to be seen as an important innovation in the field of socio-psychological "technology" is the development of a new category – the use of the Japanese term *maruta* (wooden log) to designate a test subject.

As we have seen, Kawashima testified that the designation "logs" was used "for security reasons." It seems, however, that security or secrecy was far from being the only reason. In his book, Morimura recalled that a former officer from Unit 731 once told him:

> We did not regard "logs" as people – they were even lower than cattle. There was not one scientist or researcher who had even a minimal regard . . . for these "logs." Everybody in the Unit – military personnel as well as civilians – . . . regarded the destruction of these "logs" as something absolutely natural.
>
> (Morimura, 1983: 13)

In this way, the emphasis was placed on the "non-human" nature of the test subjects – they were perceived as nothing more than inanimate material to be tested. Certainly, we can interpret such a categorization in terms of the psychological protection of the researchers and personnel in the Unit. Akiyama, who was a soldier in Unit 731, recalled that it took him some time and a great deal of emotional turmoil before he could become indifferent to the sufferings of those whom he became accustomed to treating as "logs" (Akiyama, 1958: 67). Along with its psycho-emotional significance this "*maruta* technology" had a social meaning. It would be difficult for an individual to treat a human being as a log in only a single instance. However, if the individual (and those around him) were constantly forced to accept such identification, he (and those around him) could be persuaded that there is no real difference between the test subjects and logs.

As is known, in Unit 731 the Japanese resorted to such practice as using numbers – instead of names – for prisoners/research participants. We can designate such practice as *depersonalization*, in which a human being ceased to be perceived as an individual. *Maruta* technology goes further: in this case we can speak even about *dehumanization*, through which prisoners in some essential sense ceased to be perceived as human beings at all. This terminological innovation is a striking example of social construction; with this invention new entities, new objects came into existence. While those designated by the term did share some properties intrinsic to humans, they were not perceived as human in the true sense; rather they were seen as *not-quite-human*. To be sure, the use of a specific word to designate people belonging to some category of "them" is quite common. We may recall, for example, the use of the word "vermin" by Nazis to characterize Jews. What makes this case unique is that the term *maruta* was applied exclusively in the context of biomedical research and its participants.

Morimura provides some insight into this process of dehumanization: "Before they were sent to the Unit by the gendarmerie, despite the cruel interrogations they endured, they were still human beings with tongues who were forced to speak. But once these people were . . . sent to the Unit, they became nothing more than raw material for research – 'logs' " (Morimura, 1983: 5). Among documents presented at the Khabarovsk Trial were excerpts from a set of guidelines on the interrogation of prisoners of war which describe the use of very severe methods of torture to extract accurate information (The Khabarovsk Trial, 1950: 231–233). Nevertheless, in such cases it was still necessary for the interrogators to perceive the prisoner, despite the fact that he was an enemy, as a person, a human being possessing knowledge, able to understand questions and give answers, and so on.

These specifically human traits were redundant when people were turned into logs as test subjects. It no longer mattered whether they were Japan's enemies or not. From that point on, the main – if not the only – quality which really mattered was the health of these subjects. As has been shown, the Unit's personnel went to considerable efforts to provide those who survived the experiments with the best available treatment and food so as to restore their health in order to prepare them for further trials. This gave rise to a paradoxical situation: actions which in normal, everyday life would be interpreted as expressions of genuine humanity – providing those in need with medical care and food – turned out to be their opposite: the commission of atrocities and preparation for further cruel experimentation. As Morimura wrote: "Healthy 'logs' were required for . . . research. Health became the only quality demanded of these test subjects. Any features more properly defined as human were simply not recognized" (Morimura, 1983: 6). Health and nutrition are among the most basic human needs; yet we can be certain that, if they had been properly informed and asked, the test subjects would not have given their consent to this treatment with its prospects of still further suffering. Thus, the "treatment" offered constituted an additional layer of inhumanity – the satisfaction of basic human needs in order to turn human beings into "logs" once again.

References

Akiyama, H. *Special Army Unit 731*. Moscow, 1958 (in Russian, translated from Japanese).

Alibek, Ken with Handelman Stephen. *Biohazard*. Moscow, 2003 (in Russian).

Bergamini, David. *Japan's Imperial Conspiracy*. New York: William Morrow and Company, 1971.

Domaradsky, I. V. *Inverted*. Moscow, 1995. http://www.domaradsky.ru/life.htm (in Russian).

Dower, John W. *War Without Mercy: Race and Power in the Pacific War*. New York: Pantheon Books, 1986.

Epiphanov, A. E. "Case Studies of Rehabilitation Practices Applied to Foreigners Condemned for War Crimes," *Pravo I Politika* (Law and Politics), 2001, 2 (in Russian).

Fouraker, Lawrence. Review of Sheldon H. Harris, *Factories of Death: Japanese Biological Warfare, 1932–1945, and the American Cover-up*, H-Japan, H-Net Reviews, February 2004. http://www.h-net.msu.edu/reviews/showrev.cgi?path=221861080297858.

Harris, S. H. *Factories of Death: Japanese Biological Warfare 1932–1945 and the American Cover-up*, 2nd edn. New York: Routledge, 2002.

Hill, Edwin V. 1947, *Summary Report on B. W. Investigations*, Camp Detrick, December 12, in Kondo, Shoji, ed., 2003, *CD-ROM Japanese Biological Warfare; Unit 731: Official Declassified Records*, Vol. 6, Tokyo: Kashiwa shobo, 1947.

The Khabarovsk Trial. *Materials of the Trial of Former Servicemen of the Japanese Army Charged with Manufacturing and Employing Bacteriological Weapons*. Moscow: Foreign Language Publishing House, 1950 (in Russian).

Kolchinsky, Eduard I. *Biology in Germany and Russia-USSR During the Social and Political Crises of the First Half of the XX Century*. St. Petersburg, 2007 (in Russian).

Morimura, Seiichi, *The Devil's Gluttony* (Russian translation). Moscow: Progress Publishers, 1983.

Nie, Jing-Bao. "The West's Dismissal of the Khabarovsk Trial as 'Communist Propaganda': Ideology, Evidence and international Bioethics," *Journal of Bioethical Inquiry*, 2004, 1, 1, 32–42.

Nie, Jing-Bao. "The United States Cover-up of Japanese Wartime Medical Atrocities: Complicity Committed in the National Interest and Two Proposals for Contemporary Action," *American Journal of Bioethics*, 2006, 6, 3, 21–33.

Permyakov, Georgy. "Death Zone," *Tikhookeanskaya zvezda* [Pacific Ocean's Star], February 29, 2000 (in Russian).

Raginsky, M. Yu. *Militarists in the Dock. From Materials Presented at the Tokyo and Khabarovsk Trials*. Moscow: Publishing House, "Juridical Literature," 1985 (in Russian).

Sholokh, Eug. "The Infernal Kitchen of 'Daddy' Ishii Shiro," *Konkurent.ru, Weekly*, 50, December 21, 2004 (in Russian).

Supotnitzky, Mikhail V. and Supotnitzkaya, Nadezhda S. *Studies in the History of the Plague*, 2 vols. Moscow: Vuzovskaya Kniga Publishing House, 2006 (in Russian).

Tsuneishi, Keiichi. Unit 731 and the Japanese Imperial Army's Biological Warfare Program. http://www.tokyoprogressive.org/index/weblog/comments/unit731-and-the-japanese-imperial-armys-biological-warfare-program, November 23, 2005.

Ulitzky, S.Ya. *The Struggle against Crime during the Patriotic War*. Vladivostok, Far Eastern University Publishing House, 2000 (in Russian).

Vance, Jonathan F. "Book Review of Sheldon H. Harris, *Factories of Death: Japanese Biological Warfare, 1932–1945, and the American Cover-up*," *Canadian Bulletin of Medical History/Bulletin canadien d'histoire de la médecine*, 1995, 12, 2, 451–452.

Working, R. and Chernyakova, N. *The Japanese Physicians – Crime and Punishment*. Vladivostok, 1058, December 10, 2001 (in Russian).

Part II

Guilt and responsibility

Individuals and nations

4 Data generated in Japan's biowarfare experiments on human victims in China, 1932–1945, and the ethics of using them

Till Bärnighausen

Introduction

In 1932, the Imperial Japanese Military leadership decided to set up an offensive biological warfare (BW) program (cf. Leitenberg 2003; Tsuneishi 1986; chapters 1–3, this volume). Under the leadership of General Dr. Ishii Shiro,[1] Japan's Kwantung Army built research centers to develop biological weapons in several Chinese cities, including Beiyinhe, Harbin (Unit 731), Nanjing (Unit 1644), Beijing (Unit 1855), Mengjiatun (Unit 100), and Guangzhou (Unit 8604). In these centers, Japanese military scientists isolated viruses and bacteria that were thought to have potential as biological weapons, studied the natural course of the diseases caused by these pathogens, and attempted to increase pathogen lethality. They further tried to develop vaccines to protect against infection with the pathogens and investigated methods to produce the viruses and bacteria in large quantities and to disseminate them through weapon systems. In many of these experiments, the Japanese scientists used prisoners of war and other prisoners as experimental subjects. In order to conduct such human experiments, the research centers – in particular Unit 731 in Harbin – had the functional capabilities of both concentration camps and research laboratories. The victims of the human experiments were routinely killed, autopsied, and incinerated in the crematories of the Japanese BW units. Estimates of the number of victims killed by the units range from 3000 to tens of thousands (see Bärnighausen 2002; Han and Xin 1991; Harris 1994).

The history of the BW units of the Japanese Army has been chronicled elsewhere (Bärnighausen 2002; Han and Xin 1991; Williams and Wallace 1989). Here, I will describe and discuss the human experiments of the Japanese military scientists. The discussion of the relevance and scientific rigor of the experiments and the existence of ethical research alternatives is not intended to relativize that bestiality, but to inform the debate over whether or not the data obtained in the experiments may ever be used for purposes other than historical documentation and ethical condemnation. The technical characteristics of the Japanese experiments will be used to discuss three ethical stances toward the use of unethically obtained data: the "position of strict non-use" (unethically obtained data should never be used under any circumstances), the "position of conditional use" (unethically obtained data may be used in exceptional circumstances), and the "position of unrestricted use" (unethically obtained data may always be used independent of the circumstances of its collection). This chapter draws on and expands previous work by the author (Bärnighausen 2002, 2005, 2007).

Different types of sources give accounts of the human experiments of the Japanese BW units (Bärnighausen 2002). A large number of documents written by American Intelligence officers between 1945 and 1947 provide detailed and scientifically exact descriptions of the human experiments (see, for instance, Bacteriological Warfare Experiments by Japanese 1947; Hill and Victor 1947; Thompson 1946). These descriptions were based on interviews with the Japanese scientists who conducted the experiments (see Bärnighausen 2002 for a detailed description of other publicly available sources on the experiments). The American intelligence documents based on interviews with Japanese military scientists provide the most comprehensive overview of the experiments conducted by the Japanese BW units. Since the interviews were conducted to further the BW knowledge of the American military, they contain detailed descriptions of the questions pursued in the experiments, the methods employed, and the results including data on the numbers of human subjects abused in the experiments, dosages of the infectious agents, the modes of infection, symptoms, and mortality rates. While the accounts are detailed and comprehensive, they lack information that one would expect to find in primary sources. The primary trial protocols, however, are not publicly available and it is unclear whether they still exist. It is thus impossible to confirm the validity of the Japanese reports, in many cases made years after the experiments were conducted. The Japanese military scientists may have distorted their accounts of the human experiments, either to downplay the bestiality of the experiments (in order to avoid prosecution) or to exaggerate the importance of the findings (to increase the interest of the American scientists in their research).

Examining the interview process and the content of the final rounds of interviews (led by Dr. Edwin Hill and Dr. Joseph Victor), it seems unlikely that the Japanese military researchers were trying to diminish the number of Chinese prisoners they had abused and killed. On the contrary, the researchers stated repeatedly that the human experimental victims died or "were sacrificed" during and after the trial – when such a confession did not add any information of scientific interest. For instance, Dr. Kitano Masaji and Dr. Kasahara Shiro, who reported on their human experiments investigating the natural course of epidemic hemorrhagic fever, state that the mortality among Japanese soldiers had been reduced from 30 percent to 15 percent through treatment with intravenous electrolytes, glucose, and insulin. The two researchers then state that "mortality in experimental cases was 100% due to the procedure of sacrificing experimental subjects" ("Songo – Epidemic Hemorrhagic Fever, Interview with Shiro Kasahara and Masaji Kitano" 1947: 42).

It seems more likely that some of the scientists exaggerated the success of their experiments. For instance, Dr. Ishii clearly exaggerated the success of one of his tetanus experiments. He stated that he infected 20 victims with *Clostridium tetani* (or *Bacillus tetani* in the nomenclature of the time) and then gave them a tetanus antitoxin that he had produced. Ishii claims that he was able to cure all 20 victims of his experiment. In addition, he states that the serum was successful in curing symptomatic tetanus in all 30 cases that had occurred among Japanese soldiers ("Tetanus, Interview with Shiro Ishii" 1947: 51). Such a cure ratio is implausible. Given today's intensive care technology, including medication that did not exist at the time, such as modern muscle relaxants, diazepam and beta-blockers, the lethality of tetanus when treated with antiserum is about 20 percent to 30 percent once symptoms have occurred (Stille 1992: 889–890). Thus, Dr. Ishii is likely to have overstated the success of his treatment: "Serum therapy has effectively cured 100% of 50 cases" ("Tetanus, Interview with Shiro Ishii" 1947: 51). While we can only speculate why Dr. Ishii exaggerated the success of the treatment, it seems plausible that he intended to increase the value of the results of the experiments in the eyes of his American interrogators.

While the accounts of the experiments clearly contain some exaggerations, it is unlikely that such distortions were common. For one, the interviewers were medical and biological scientists with extensive experience in BW research, and would thus have questioned implausible claims made by the Japanese scientists. The interviewers were Dr. Murray Sander (a microbiologist who had taught at the College of Physicians and Surgeons at Columbia University before joining the Army where he conducted BW research at Fort Detrick, the BW research center of the U.S. Army Medical Command), Lieutenant Dr. Arvo T. Thompson (a veterinary physician and BW researcher at Fort Detrick), Dr. Norbert Fell (a microbiologist and head of Planning and Pilot Engineering at Fort Detrick), Dr. Edwin Hill (head of the Department of Basic Sciences at Fort Detrick), and Dr. Joseph Victor (a pathologist at Fort Detrick). During the interviews, the interviewers frequently probed statements by the Japanese scientists, but failed to detect implausibility. Moreover, in a number of instances the Japanese army scientists admitted freely that experiments had been failures when they could easily have claimed success, which suggests that the accounts were truthful. For instance, Masuda Tomosada, who researched vaccinations against bacterial dysentery, describes a number of vaccination methods, but admits that none of them had conferred any protection against the disease ("Report on Dysentery, Information by Tomosada Masuda" 1947: 33). Thus, while some Japanese scientists are likely to have misrepresented the success of their experiments (see Dr. Ishii's reporting of the results of his tetanus experiments above), others appear to have truthfully reported their results. This inconsistency suggests that there was no concerted effort by the Japanese scientists to exaggerate the success of their experiments in order to increase the perceived value of the information they shared with the American interrogators, even though individual scientists may have tried to do so.

The bestiality of artificially infecting human beings against their will with disease pathogens and killing them in the course of the experiments is self-evident. Of course, from a pacifist position rejecting any development of weapons to harm or kill people, the experiments conducted by the Japanese military scientists could never have been ethically justified, even if human beings had not been brutally victimized in the course of the experiments. While the Japanese researchers did not succeed in developing a biological weapon that could be applied on a large scale, based on a range of sources (Chinese reports, testimonies during the Khabarovsk war crime trials, and U.S. military intelligence reports), it is clear that the Japanese Army did conduct a number of attacks in China (Deng 1965; Han and Yin 1986; "Intelligence Research Project No. 2263" 1945; "Japanese BW Units, Water Purification Units" 1944; Jia 1985; Jiang 1983; Lou 1987; Materials 1950; Shi 1985; Sun and Ni Weixiong 1984; Tang and Cheng 1985; G. Wang 1985; Z. Wang 1984; Williams and Wallace 1989). Table 4.1 summarizes the BW attacks that the Japanese Army is reported to have carried out in China between 1939 and 1944.

Technicalities: relevance, rigor, and research alternatives

Technical analyses play an important role in the debate on the ethics of using data generated in inhumane experiments (Berger 1990). The question whether data from an experiment should be used will arise only if the experiment was relevant (i.e., it investigated a research question that had not already been answered in previous studies and it had at least two outcomes that could plausibly occur) and conducted rigorously (i.e., it was executed such that the data it generated are both reliable and valid).

The question of ethical research alternatives to unethical experiments is important in the debate on the ethics of using unethically generated data because the benefits of using such data will differ substantially depending on whether ethical alternatives exist. If ethical alternatives do exist, the only benefits that can possibly arise from the use of the unethically obtained data are cost savings because ethical research to replace the unethical experiments does not need to be conducted. If, on the other hand, ethical alternatives do not exist, the benefits of using the unethically obtained data will be as high as the value of the information they contain (which could, for instance, be a life-saving treatment). The value of data will not influence the decision whether it should be permissible to use information generated in an unethical experiment, if decision makers adhere either to the "position of strict non-use" or the "position of unrestricted use." Yet, decision makers adhering to the "position of conditional use" are likely to take the value of the unethically obtained data into account in their evaluation of the ethics of data use.

Relevance

Many of the human experiments conducted by Unit 731 were not relevant because they investigated research hypotheses that had either already been proven to be true or were highly implausible. Irrelevant experiments included trials investigating the nature and effects of typhoid, paratyphoid, cholera, bacterial dysentery, smallpox, botulism, gas gangrene, tularemia, plague, anthrax, epidemic typhus, glanders, tuberculosis, brucellosis, and epidemic hemorrhagic fever. This is illustrated in the following paragraphs.

Table 4.1 BW attacks Japanese BW troops are reported to have carried out in China, 1939–1944

Date	Place	Diseases	Dissemination mode
July, August 1939	Western bank of the Hailar River	Typhoid, paratyphoid, bacterial dysentery	Bacterial suspension introduced into the rivers
Summer 1939	Western bank of the Hailar River	Anthrax	Bullets coated with *Bacillus anthracis*
June 1940	Ningbo, Zhejiang Province	Typhoid, cholera	Bacterial suspensions introduced into rivers and lakes
July 1940	Xinwu, Heilongjiang Province	Cholera	Bacterial suspensions introduced into rivers and lakes
October 1940	Zhuxian, Zhejiang Province	Plague	Rice and wheat grains coated with *Yersinia pestis* and infected with *Yersinia pestis* dropped from airplanes
October 1940	Ningbo, Zhejiang Province	Plague	Wheat grains coated with *Yersinia pestis* dropped from airplanes
November 1940	Xinhua, Zhejiang Province	Plague	Wheat grains coated with *Yersinia pestis* dropped from airplanes
December 1940	Shangyu, Zhejiang Province	Plague	*Yersinia pestis* disseminated from airplanes
December 1940	Tangxi, Zhejiang Province	Plague	*Yersinia pestis* disseminated from airplanes
Spring 1941	Changde, Hunan Province	Plague	Cotton balls contaminated with *Yersinia pestis* dropped from airplanes
April 1941	Xindeng, Hunan Province	Plague	Rice grains, wheat grains, and paper shavings contaminated with *Yersinia pestis* dropped from airplanes
November 1941	Changde, Hunan Province	Plague	Cotton balls contaminated with *Yersinia pestis* dropped from airplanes
December 1941	Zhuji, Zhejiang Province	Plague	Cotton and cloth balls contaminated with *Yersinia pestis* dropped from airplanes

(continued)

Table 4.1 (Continued)

Date	Place	Diseases	Dissemination mode
1942	Ningshan, Suiyuan, Shanxi Province	Plague	Rodents infected with *Yersinia pestis* released
1942	Wuji, Shanzi, Hebei Province	Plague	Mice infected with *Yersinia pestis* released
May 1942	Jiangxi Province	Typhoid	Dropped from airplanes
May 1942	Shangxiao, Zhejiang Province	Typhoid, cholera, bacterial dysentery	Dropped from airplanes
August 1942	Nanyang, Hunan Province	Plague	Grains coated with *Yersinia pestis* dropped from airplanes
August 1942	Hangzhou, Zhejiang Province	Anthrax, typhoid, paratyphoid, cholera, bacterial dysentery	N/A
September 1942	N/A	Typhoid, paratyphoid	Bacterial suspensions injected mantou (Chinese dumplings) distributed to Chinese prisoners of war before release from prison
Winter 1942	Yi'an, Heilongjiang Province	Plague	Fleas infected with *Yersinia pestis* released
November 1943	Changde, Hunan Province	Cholera	Dropped from airplanes
August 1944	N/A	Plague	Mice infected with *Yersinia pestis* released

Note
BW = biological warfare, N/A = not available.

*Examples of irrelevant experiments with research hypotheses
that had already been proven to be true*

Dr. Ishii conducted the following smallpox experiment. He opened the skin vesicles of patients with smallpox, dried the vesicle content, and forced 10 human beings to inhale the dried substance. All 10 victims fell ill. They developed "large geographically shaped erythematous, swollen and hemorrhagic areas on the body measuring up to 20–30 cm [centimeters] in greatest dimension." None of the victims of the experiment developed vesicles. According to Dr. Ishii, "[a]bout four died" due to the disease ("Smallpox, Interview with Dr. Shiro Ishii" 1947: 50). No relevant research question could have been answered with the experiment. The mode of transmission of smallpox (via droplet infection) as well as the clinical appearance and incubation period were well known at the time (Zimmermann 1940: 157–158). The fact that the content of smallpox vesicles was infectious had been proven 1500 years before in China. The early Chinese scientists had drawn fluid from the pustules of patients with smallpox and had introduced the fluid into the nose cavities of healthy human beings. The healthy humans fell ill with a mild form of smallpox disease and were subsequently vaccinated against the disease (Zeiss and Rodenwaldt 1943: 242).

An experiment with *Francisella tularensis* was similarly irrelevant: "Experiments in M were conducted with 10 subjects who were injected s.c. [subcutaneously]. All developed fever lasting as long as 6 months" ("Tularemia, Interview with Dr. Shiro Ishii" 1947: 54). The mode of infection of tularemia and the symptoms of the disease were well known at the time.

Dr. Tabei Kanau, a former member of Unit 731, described another human experiment (with *Salmonella paratyphi* A (stem Kurokawa)) that could not have been expected to – and indeed did not – produce any research finding of value, because the symptoms of paratyphoid, the mode of infection, and the fact that during fever salmonella bacteria may be found in blood and stool samples were general medical knowledge at the time (Zeiss and Rosenwaldt 1943):

> Experiments in M:
> 30 mgm [milligram mass] wet weight were fed in 100 cc [cubic centimeter] 8% sucrose. After an incubation period of 3–6 days, fever and diarrhea appeared lasting five days. Blood and stools are positive during fever and stools remain positive for 7 days after fever subsided. The symptoms may recur over many months.
>
> The disease was highly contagious. When a patient was placed in a room with 3 normal people, the others invariably contracted the disease.
>
> ("Paratyphoid, Interview with Dr. Tabei" 1947: 31)

Another reason for irrelevant experiments was the lack of coordination between the different research groups of Unit 731. Three experiments concerning brucellosis are a case in point. Dr. Ishii conducted the following infection experiment with *Brucella melitensis*: "Experiments in M were carried out by the subcutaneous injection of more than 20 subjects. Does not remember the result of such experiments except that undulant fever followed injection and persisted for many months" (Brucellosis, Interview with Dr. Shiro Ishii 1947: 10).

Dr. Hayakawa, on the other hand, undertook the following Brucellosis infection experiment:

> A subject was injected s.c. with 0.01 mgm of B. melitensis. After an incubation period of between 2–3 weeks, undulant fever appeared. With the fever, blood cultures became positive. The subject was followed for 6 months and had fever episodes throughout that period.
>
> ("Brucellosis, Interview with Dr. Kiyoshi Hayakawa" 1947: 11)

Finally, Dr. Yamanouchi injected 10 healthy human beings subcutaneously with different doses of *Brucella melitensis* (ranging from 0.05 to 5.0 milligram bacteria solution). All of the victims exposed to doses above 0.1 milligram contracted Malta fever, while only half of the patients who had been exposed to doses between 0.05 and 0.1 milligram fell ill. In all victims, the *Brucella melitensis* agglutinin titer rose to levels of about 1/10,000 following exposure ("Brucellosis, Interview with Dr. Yujiro Yamanouchi" 1947: 12).

If Dr. Yamaonouchi, who intended to determine the *dosis infectiosa minima* with his experiment, had known of the results of Hayakawa's experiment, he would have used lower doses in his trial. Dr. Hayakawa had succeeded in infecting an experimental victim with a dose that was one-fifth of the lowest dose used in Dr. Yamanouchi's experiment ("Brucellosis, Interview with Dr. Kiyoshi Hayakawa" 1947: 11). On the other hand, Dr. Ishii's experiment (in which 20 human beings were killed) could not have been expected to lead to any result that could not also have been obtained through Dr. Yamanouchi's experiment.

Examples of irrelevant experiments with highly implausible hypotheses

In order to test the infectiousness of different viruses and bacteria when they were suspended in aerosols, a 26-cubic-meter large gas chamber was built on the premises of Unit 731 ("Aerosols, Interview with Dr. Takahashi" 1947: 6). Bacteria and virus aerosols could be generated within the chamber or blown into the chamber through rubber tubes ("Aerosols, Interview with Dr. Takahashi" 1947: 6; Morimura 1985: 144). Researchers of Unit 731 investigated whether and in what doses the following diseases could be transmitted via inhalation of aerosols of the causative agents of the following diseases: plague, anthrax, epidemic typhus, glanders, smallpox, tuberculosis, bacterial dysentery, typhoid, brucellosis, gas gangrene, cholera, and epidemic hemorrhagic fever. For instance, Dr. Tabei exposed five people in the gas chamber for 10 minutes to an aerosol suspension of *Salmonella typhi* (or *Bacillus typhosus* in the nomenclature of the time). None of the victims developed any symptoms of typhoid, but all of them suffered from a heavy cough with sputum as well as malaise and headaches ("Aerosols, Interview with Dr. Takahashi" 1947: 6–7). At the time, it was well known that plague, anthrax, smallpox, glanders, and tuberculosis were commonly transmitted via the airways, while epidemic typhus and brucellosis are rarely transmitted through inhalation of the causative agents. Finally, bacterial dysentery, gas gangrene, and typhoid cannot – as was well established – be transmitted through inhalation (Zinsser and Bayne-Jones 1939). Of the aerosol experiments with the pathogens causing the 12 diseases listed above, only the experiments with cholera bacteria tested an uncertain, plausible mode of infection. From 1914 to 1930, Professor Trillat from the Institute Pasteur in Paris had shown in a series of experiments that – given a certain ambient pressure, temperature, air velocity, and humidity – chickens could be infected with cholera through inhalation of the bacterium, while such infections in human beings had not been described (Hojo 1941: 19).[2]

It is likely that the Japanese military scientists conducted the above infection experiments in order to discover routes of infection which do not occur in nature (for instance, because naturally occurring doses are too low). Such new infection routes may have been used to construct weapon systems to deliver the BW agents. As we shall see, however, the Japanese scientists must have realized that many of their infection experiments could not reasonably be expected to yield any results relevant to their purpose of developing effective biological weapons.

Rigor

The Japanese military scientists conducted many experiments which lacked scientific rigor. For instance, Dr. Ikeda started to investigate the mode of transmission of epidemic hemorrhagic fever in January 1941 in the following experiment. He collected fleas and lice in an area in Manchuria in which epidemic hemorrhagic fever was endemic. He then let the fleas and lice suck blood from patients who had contracted the disease and placed the insects on the skin of healthy human victims. Two weeks after the exposure, a few of the victims showed symptoms of hemorrhagic fever. The experiment was of doubtful rigor because all experimental victims came from the area in Manchuria in which the fleas and lice had been collected, i.e., from an area in which the disease was endemic. Since the incubation period of epidemic hemorrhagic fever is 12 to 24 days it cannot be decided whether those victims of the experiment who showed signs of the disease had been infected by the exposure to the fleas or lice or had been previously infected via another, naturally occurring mode of infection (Tsuneishi 1986: 91).

Another example of an experiment of questionable scientific rigor is a study conducted by Dr. Kasahara and Dr. Kitano. The two scientists attempted to test the hypothesis of whether mites transmit epidemic hemorrhagic fever:

> 203 mites picked from field mice in that area were emulsified in 2 cc saline and injected s.c. in one man with positive results. Another emulsion containing 60 mites produced no effect in another subject. In this way, the subsequent human material was derived from the first case subject who had been injected with 203 mites. In general, the incubation period was between 2 and 3 weeks. Blood from the first experimental case was drawn during fever

20 days after injection of the mites. 10 cc were injected into a 3rd man as well
as into white mice and monkeys. Subsequent cases were produced either by
blood or blood free extracts of liver, spleen or kidney derived from individuals
sacrificed at various times during the course of the disease. Morphine was
employed for this purpose.

("Songo – Epidemic Hemorrhagic Fever, Interview with
Shiro Kasahara and Masaji Kitano" 1947: 42–43)

Drs. Kasahara and Kitano concluded that mice transmit epidemic hemorrhagic
fever. This conclusion, however, does not follow from the results of the experiment.
Since a completely artificial route of infection had been chosen, the result can only
validly indicate that mice carry the virus but not that they transmit it to humans. In
spite of the invalidity of their conclusions, Dr. Kasahara and Dr. Kitano were able
to publish part of the results of their human experiments. In their publication they
hid the fact that they had used humans in the experiments by claiming they had
used monkeys (Kasahara and Kitano 1943). Although the Japanese military
scientists must have expected that the value of their publication would be lessened
if they did not give details about age, gender, weight, and so on of their "laboratory
animals," they stated simply that they had used "Monkeys," "Formosa monkeys,"
and "Longtail monkeys" (Tsuneishi 1986: 88–89; Wang 1987: 27–28). The
description of their experiment in the 1944 publication is strikingly similar to
the description they gave Dr. Hill and Dr. Victor (see above) – however, the word
"man" was replaced by the word "monkey" (Tsuneishi 1986: 90).

Research alternatives

Examples of relevant experiments with ethical research alternatives involving human beings

A number of experiments conducted by Unit 731 had relevant hypotheses but
could have been undertaken without relying on forced human participation. For
instance, tests to demonstrate whether or not a typhoid immunization was effective
could have been conducted by comparing the naturally occurring incidence rates
in a group of immunized people with incidence rates in a non-immunized control
group. Instead, scientists under the leadership of Dr. Tabei of Unit 731 conducted
the following three immunization experiments. First, 15 Chinese prisoners of war
were given one of three immunizations, which had been developed at different
locations in the Japanese empire (in Dalian, in the Kitasato Laboratory in Tokyo,
and at the Medical University of the Army). The 15 prisoners as well as 15
further victims who had been assigned to a control group were each made to
swallow 100 milligrams of typhoid bacteria. Most of the victims contracted
typhoid; two died of the disease; one committed suicide. According to Tabei
the experiment had been a failure, because none of the immunizations had
conferred protection ("Typhoid, Interview with Dr. Tabei" 1947: 56). Second,
a similar experiment in which 13 immunized and 13 non-immunized prisoners

were each given a dose of 150 milligrams of typhoid bacteria had a more suc
cessful outcome. Five of the immunized, but 12 of the non-immunized prisoners
contracted the disease ("Naval Aspects of Biological Warfare" 1947: 56). Third,
during the war criminal trials at Khabarovsk, one of the Japanese witnesses who
had worked for Tabei's group described the following typhoid experiment at which
he had assisted (in 1943). In the experiment, 50 men were given different
"preventive inoculations" and were then forced to drink "water contaminated with
typhoid germs" (The Khabarovsk Trial 1950: 356–357). In total, 217 people are
reported to have been killed in typhoid experiments which could have been
replaced by ethical research.

Examples of relevant experiments with ethical
research alternatives involving animals

Another type of experiment with ethical research alternatives were studies testing
the infectiousness of fluids or viral cultures. Many of these experiments could
have been replaced by animal studies, because it was known at the time that certain
animals could contract the disease under investigation. For instance, Kasahara and
Kitano did not need to use human victims in their studies of the infectiousness of
the agent causing epidemic hemorrhagic fever (carried out between 1939 and
1945), because Japanese scientists had already discovered that monkeys as well as
rabbits and horses could be infected with the agent ("Songo – Epidemic
Hemorrhagic Fever, Interview with Shiro Kasahara and Masaji Kitano" 1947: 42,
44). Bärnighausen (2002) describes six types of human experiments on the
infectivity of epidemic hemorrhagic fever that could have been replaced by animal
studies. Kasahara and Kitano reported that they killed more than 100 human
beings in these experiments.

For instance, the two scientists showed that liver and spleen tissue emulsions of
people whom they had infected with the pathogen causing epidemic hemorrhagic
fever could infect healthy humans only if the organs were obtained during the
fever phase of the disease. For this purpose, they killed seven people whom they
had infected during the fever phase and compared the infectiousness of their tissue
emulsions with the infectiousness of tissue emulsions of artificially infected
victims who had died – as Hill and Victor word it in their report – of a "natural
death" ("Songo – Epidemic Hemorrhagic Fever, Interview with Shiro Kasahara
and Masaji Kitano" 1947: 43).

The ethics of using of unethically obtained data

The question of whether unethically obtained data may ever be used for scientific
purposes has been discussed with regard to the bestial experiments conducted by
Nazi doctors on Jewish and Gypsy victims in the concentration camps at Dachau,
Auschwitz, Buchenwald, and Sachsenhausen. The negative consequences of any
use other than to expose and condemn a "medicine without humaneness"
(Mitscherlich and Mielke 1995) include the following:

- Using the data means forgoing an opportunity to build – in the explicit non-use of the data – a symbolic memorial to the victims of the barbaric experiments. Data use is like "building on top of Auschwitz" (Mostow 1993–1994).
- Using the data violates the rights of the victims many times over again (Post 1991; Sheldon and Whitely 1989). Using the data derived from the victims' sufferings renders the data user – in an act of moral complicity – the torturer of the victims (Cohen 1990).
- Using the data implies that the humans who were abused and killed in the experiments were "physiological entities" and not human beings. Data use thus would keep alive a "philosophy" that the value of human beings differs (Pozos 2003).
- The data belong to the victims; only they can give us permission for its use (Post 1988).
- Data use may relativize crimes against humanity and honor the perpetrators, because some good has been gleaned from horrendous deeds (Gaylin 1989; Weitzman 1990).
- Data use may signal to future scientists that immoral research is, in fact, rewarded with citation and reference (even if the ethics of the research are simultaneously condemned) (Angell 1990; Schafer 1986).
- Data use would corrupt the institution of medicine itself (Beecher 1966). It would undermine medicine's public legitimacy by signaling to society that science cares about knowledge above anything else (Post 1991). In fact, knowledge "may be less important to decent society than the way it was obtained" (Angell 1990).

Three ethical positions have evolved on the use of unethically obtained data. First, a "position of strict non-use" holds that unethically obtained data should never be used because the negative consequences of such use always outweigh any good that could be salvaged from data use under any circumstances (Angell 1990; Beecher 1966; Gaylin 1989; Post 1991). Second, a "position of conditional use" allows that unethically obtained data may be used in exceptional circumstances (e.g., a cure for an otherwise incurable disease is contained in the data) given that certain conditions are met (e.g., the means by which the data were obtained is condemned in any publication of the data) (Moe 1989; Neter 1980; Post 1991; Sheldon and Whitely 1989). Third, a "position of unrestricted use" states that data of scientific value should always be available to be used because there are no absolute ethics and each potential user should decide for him- or herself whether data use can be justified. This position requires that publication of the data is always accompanied by detailed accounts of the research methods used to generate the data, so that the reader can make an informed decision on the ethics of data use (Singer 1980).

Even proponents of the "position of unrestricted use" would never consider using a large proportion of the data obtained in the experiments by the Japanese BW units because the research was irrelevant (e.g., smallpox, botulism, paratyphoid, and brucellosis infection experiments), or the data generated were unreliable or invalid (e.g., infection experiments with the epidemic hemorrhagic fever virus). Proponents of a "position of conditional use" would likely extend the non-use of the Japanese data to results from those experiments for which ethical research alternatives existed (e.g., typhoid vaccination experiments and infection experiments with epidemic hemorrhagic virus). For instance, one type of "position of conditional use" requires that, first, the scientific value of the data is unquestionable; second, publication or citation is accompanied by a strong ethical condemnation of the means by which the data were obtained; and, third, there is no alternative source of information (Moe 1989). In many cases, technical analyses thus obviate the need for an ethical decision on the use of data from some of the inhumane Japanese experiments. However, among the known Japanese experiments, examples exist which require an ethical decision because they generated data that – judging from all publicly available evidence – may be valid and could not be generated through ethical research methods. Such experiments include tuberculosis vaccination trials, studies with mustard gas, and experiments investigating the effects of extreme cold on human beings. These three examples will be analyzed below.

Examples of relevant experiments without ethical alternatives: tuberculosis vaccination experiments

Dr. Futagi Hideo, who conducted tuberculosis vaccination experiments while a member of Unit 731, summarized the results of his research to the American BW experts Hill and Victor as follows:

1 "Comparison of reaction of tuberculin positive and negative individuals to inhalation of 1 mgm *Cl. tuberculosis hominis* revealed significant differences in the clinical course without x-ray changes."
2 "Tuberculin positive individuals were more resistant to infection by inhalation of these bacteria."
3 After inhalation of *Mycobacterium tuberculosis* "Tuberculin negative cases developed positive tuberculin reaction just before bacteria appeared in sputum. Blood cultures were negative in both series."
4 "In tuberculin positive subjects, *Cl. tuberculosis hominis* was much more virulent than BCG (bovine) when injected i.v. [intravenously]."
5 "BCG produced miliary tuberculosis when injected i.v."
6 "Intravenous *Cl. tuberculosis hominis* was less severe clinically, but had greater mortality in tuberculin negative than in tuberculin positive individuals. It produced miliary tuberculosis. The tuberculin reaction became positive in tuberculin negative cases."
7 "*Cl. tuberculosis hominis* produced chronic, progressive inflammation lasting more than 6 months when injected i.c. [intracutaneously] in tuberculin positive individuals. B.C.G. results in similar but less severe infection of shorter duration."

    ("Tuberculosis, Interview with Dr. Hideo Futagi" 1947: 61–64)

During World War II, different scientific teams attempted to determine the degree to which a positive tuberculin test would protect from tuberculosis; whether or not a vaccination with Bacille Calmette-Guérin (BCG) conferred protection and how harmful it could be; and which application mode of BCG should be employed in order to minimize harm to patients (Zeiss and Rodenwaldt 1943: 176–178; Zinsser and Bayne-Jones 1939: 454–455). Dr. Futagi's experiments were thus relevant given the knowledge of the time. The tuberculosis vaccination experiments were likely to have been reliable, as may be judged from Dr. Futagi's descriptions in the Hill and Victor document. Finally, had Dr. Futagi restricted his research to the investigation of naturally occurring cases rather than abusing humans against their will in the experiments, he would not have been able to realistically obtain the above results. A standard textbook of hygiene and infectious diseases of the time summarizes the difficulty of tuberculosis research as follows (after posing the question whether the BCG vaccination confers any protection at all): "As with all questions relating to tuberculosis, only observation over decades and sound statistics may bring clarification" (Zeiss and Rodenwaldt 1943: 178). Dr. Futagi's ethically reprehensible human experiments (as in all experiments of Unit 731, all human subjects were eventually killed) had an advantage over ethical experiments addressing the same questions in that they reduced the length of time needed to obtain meaningful results. From a practical perspective, ethical experiments were virtually impossible to complete, while Futagi's experiments could be easily completed in a comparatively short period of time. In addition, the experiments enabled the researchers to derive results that were far more detailed and powerful than could have been obtained in ethical research, because the mode of infection and the exposure doses were controlled. The benefits to society derived from the results of the inhumane tuberculosis experiments might have been quite large, because the research was relevant to finding effective protection against a common, highly burdensome, and potentially deadly infectious disease.

Examples of relevant experiments without ethical alternatives: mustard gas experiments

A second example of research conducted by members of Unit 731, which was relevant, likely sufficiently rigorous, and not reproducible with ethical research methods are the experiments with mustard gas. In September 1940, members of Unit 731 chained 16 human beings to poles in an open-air experimentation field close to Harbin. The experimentation field was divided into three areas. Experimental victims in the first area wore "no caps, no masks, regular cloths, underwear, and slippers"; the victims in the second and third area wore "army trousers"; and those in the third area also wore gas masks. After the "objects" had been chained to the poles, Japanese soldiers attacked the field with mustard gas bombs using canons and grenade throwers. "The shooting time lasted for 40 minutes: 15 minutes of shooting, 15 minutes break, 10 minutes shooting." Next, the experimental victims were unchained and transported back to the prisons of Unit 731, so that military physicians could examine their health status.

Laboratory examinations added information on the health effects of mustard gas attacks. For instance, the scientists examined the fluid from the blisters that had formed on the skin of the victims 12 hours after the attack and found that on average one milliliter of fluid contained 20–50 cells, 52.9 percent of which were polymorpho-nuclear leucocytes, 41.2 percent were lymphocytes, and 5.9 percent monocytes (Matsumara 1986: 49). The scientists then conducted a number of follow-up experiments. For instance, they injected fluid from the blisters on the skin of the initial victims into the skin on the upper arms or the corneas of additional victims in order to investigate whether the fluid had poisonous properties.

The results of the mustard gas experiments were not only relevant for the design of offensive chemical weapons, but also for the treatment of victims of attacks with such weapons. Judging from the publicly available data, the experiments yielded meticulous descriptions of the clinical symptoms and laboratory parameters at frequent intervals after attacks with chemical weapons that had been carried out under controlled conditions. Obviously, such experiments can never be conducted ethically.

Examples of relevant experiments without ethical alternatives: frost bite experiments

Another type of relevant and rigorous research without ethical alternatives is the freezing experiments conducted by a research group under Dr. Yoshimura Hisato at Unit 731. These experiments were of incredible cruelty. The scientists forced prisoners to stand motionless for 20 to 30 minutes in a –30 to –40 degrees Celsius environment, while exposing a naked finger, hand, foot, arm, leg, nose, or scrotum to the cold (Han 1986: 20–21). The scientists used a ventilator to generate air currents of different velocities in order to accelerate the freezing process (Han 1986: 20–21; Morimura 1985: 103).

Starting in 1943, Dr. Yoshimura conducted cold experiments in a special laboratory building on the premises of Unit 731. The laboratory allowed the scientists to keep experimental conditions (such as temperature) constant and to conduct freezing experiments throughout the year (Cao 1951: 10–11; Han and Xin 1991: 116; Morimura 1985: 103). Despite the immense cruelty of the experiments, Yoshimura and his colleagues were able to publish some of their data in the English-language *Japanese Journal of Physiology* after presenting them at the 21st (in 1942), 22nd (in 1943), and 25th (in 1948) meeting of the Japanese Physiological Society (Yoshimura and Iida 1952a, 1952b, 1952c).

In these publications, the scientists do not explicitly mention some of the most inhumane aspects of their experiments, namely that all of the experimental subjects were forced against their will to participate and were killed following completion of the studies. However, those who read the article should have been highly suspicious of the nature of the experiments. For one, the trial participants were "Chinese coolies" and "Chinese pupils," while the researchers were Japanese, and the experiments had been conducted during the Second Sino-Japanese War and World War II, when Japan had invaded large parts of northeastern China. Moreover, the participants included children under 15 years of age and a baby (Yoshimura and Iida 1952b: 177–178):

> The temperature reaction in ice-water was examined on about 100 Chinese coolies from 15 to 74 years old and on about 20 Chinese pupils of 7 to 14 years. . . . The maximum reactivity was found at the ages of 25 to 29 years, and, as the age became younger and older, the reactivity generally decreased more and more, except that in childhood it was higher than in puberty. Thus the general aspect of change of reactivity with age was similar to that of the other physiological functions. Though detailed studies could not be attained on children below 6 years of age, some observations were carried out on a baby. As is seen in fig. 2, the reaction was detected even on the 3rd day after birth, and it increased rapidly with the lapse of days until at last it was nearly fixed after a month or so.

A number of later studies cite the three articles published by Yoshimura and colleagues in 1952 (Bridgman 1991; Hirai et al. 1968; Konda et al. 1981; Miura et al. 1977; Nelms and Soper 1962; Sawada et al. 2000; Spurr et al. 1955; Tanaka 1971a, 1971b). The authors of these articles and other medically trained readers would have realized that the experiments had caused the participants considerable pain. During the experiments, the middle finger, the whole hand, the toe, or lower leg of a victim was immersed into water of 0 degrees Celsius for either 30 or 60 minutes. The water was regularly stirred in order to maintain 0 degrees around the immersed body part and the skin temperature of the body part was measured every minute. The temperature curves show a fall from normal body temperature to around 5 degrees Celsius in the first 10 minutes and then an oscillation around 5 degrees Celsius for the remainder of the experiment (i.e., up to either 30 or 60 minutes). Exposure to such temperatures for these lengths of time causes enormous pain. Indeed, Sawada Shinichi, Araki Shunichi, and Yokoyama Kazuhito (2000: 85) describe the pain caused by Yoshimura's procedure as follows:

> As mentioned above, Yoshimura et al. proposed a local cold tolerance test, because the CIVD [cold-induced vasodilation] reactivity is closely related to an individual's frostbite resistance. This test method has, however, consisted of 30-min immersion of fingers in ice water (0° C [Celsius]). Under this test condition, most of the participants have tended to feel much pain and distress, and some have either fainted or had to withdraw prematurely from the experiment. We, therefore, previously proposed a simplified and less painful test for evaluating local cold tolerance as a substitute for Yoshimura's method.

Unlike follow-up studies, which used Yoshimura's local cold tolerance test, not one participant withdrew from the original study, suggesting that the participants did not have the choice to withdraw.

Some of the results of the experiments described in the three 1952 articles by Yoshimura and colleagues were relevant for medical practice. The reported effects of environmental factors (such as wind velocity or humidity) and individual factors (such as diet or sleep) on resistance to extreme cold could help to minimize cold-related injury. The experiments may also have been conducted reliably. The Japanese military scientists meticulously recorded the temperatures of each of the victims and controlled a large number of individual and environmental factors that are known to influence resistance to cold. Further, no research alternative existed for the experiments. In addition to the extreme pain experienced by the individuals forced to participate in the experiments, some of the victims suffered vasospasms that can completely block the blood supply to the affected body parts, causing necroses (Ulmer 1997: 721) – an unacceptable consequence in ethically conducted research.

As the examples of the tuberculosis vaccination, mustard gas, and freezing experiments show, at least some of the data generated by Unit 731 may be considered for publication or use by proponents of a "position of conditional use." Certainly, the information contained in the data is not sufficient to fully establish reliability. For instance, no information on the victims' weight, body fat, health status, current medication, or smoking history – all of which may influence cold resistance – is provided in the published articles. However, since the publicly available data on the freezing experiments are only secondary data, it cannot be ruled out that such information does in fact exist in the primary sources. In addition, even if the Japanese scientists had not documented some factors, the relevant information could possibly be inferred or generated from other sources.

The uncertainty about the existence of data that is not yet publicly available renders the case of Unit 731 more complex than other cases of unethically obtained data that have been discussed in the literature. The publicly available data are sufficient to evaluate some of the experiments as certainly irrelevant, unreliable, or reproducible with ethical experiments. For other experiments, it may be established that the research question pursued was relevant and that no ethical research could replicate the barbaric human experiments. While some doubt might remain about the reliability of this subset of experiments, it cannot be ruled out that they were conducted with sufficient scientific rigor to generate valid results. In this context, it is important to know that Hill and Victor as well as the State–War–Navy Coordinating Subcommittee for the Far East (SWNCC) evaluated the data they had obtained from the Japanese military scientists as highly valuable. For instance, Hill and Victor (1947: 5) write:

Evidence gathered in this investigation has greatly supplemented and amplified previous aspects of this field. It represents data that have been obtained by Japanese scientists at the expenditure of many millions of dollars and years of work. . . . These data were secured with a total outlay of ¥ 250,000 to date, a mere pittance by comparison with the actual cost of the studies.

In their evaluation, Hill and Victor stress the fact that the experiments could not be replicated in the United States: "Such information could not be obtained in our own laboratories because of scruples attached to human experimentation" (Hill and Victor 1947: 5).

The SWNCC, in turn, implicitly attributes value to the data in proposing a rationale for why Russian prosecutors, who had demanded access to the Japanese scientists (arguing that they had obtained evidence that these scientists had committed war crimes), should be denied such access:

> This Japanese information is the only known source of data from scientifically controlled experiments showing the direct effect of BW agents on man. In the past it has been necessary to evaluate the effects of BW agents on man from data obtained through animal experimentation. Such evaluation is inconclusive and far less complete than results obtained from certain types of human experimentation.
>
> (SWNCC 1947: 7)

The data that have been made publicly available to date at the Library of Congress and the National Archives in Suitland, Maryland, are certainly of value to the scientist studying the history of biological warfare and human experimentation. It is of only questionable value for medical science and practice. As shown above, a large proportion of the publicly known experiments were either irrelevant or unreliable; other experiments provided evidence of relevant research, but would require additional information to be of direct scientific value. Because the American BW specialists Hill and Victor as well as the SWNCC attached high value to the data, it seems likely that only a proportion of the data secured by Hill and Victor has to date been declassified.

Given the content of the publicly available information on the experiments and the uncertainty about the existence of additional data, the case of the Japanese BW units offers a (currently) unique opportunity for a debate on the ethics of the use of unethically obtained data. The problem posed by the Japanese experiments demands an ethical decision in a situation where there is evidence, but not certain evidence, that the data obtained in some of the most barbaric human experiments known are, in fact, of scientific value.[3] Behind such an imperfect veil of ignorance (Rawls 1971), a decision for one of the three positions on the use of unethically obtained data outlined above carries more ethical weight than if we had either complete certainty about the scientific value of the data or no evidence that such data existed. In the first case, technical arguments about the reliability and validity of the data might lead to the same action recommendations as ethical arguments about data use or non-use, and thus reduce the burden on the ethical argument to prove its conclusion. In the latter case, the ethical arguments have no urgency, and the defenders of any position are free to imagine extreme examples – however implausible – that make it hard for proponents of an opposing view to maintain their position. (For instance, proponents of a "position of conditional use" may ask adherents of a "position of strict non-use" if they would maintain their stance if the unethically obtained data contained a cure for all cancers.)

Two counter-arguments might be brought forward against the claim that the case of the Japanese BW units is distinctive owing to its specific mix of knowledge and uncertainty. First, it may be argued that all data from the inhumane Japanese experiments are worthless to civil society – irrespective of the reliability and validity of the findings – because the purpose of the experiments was to develop offensive biological weapons. This claim can be easily refuted. For one, not all of the experiments conducted by Unit 731 were concerned with a goal of producing offensive BW (e.g., the freezing experiments). Further, results of BW research are commonly useful for both offensive and defensive BW, as well as for non-military purposes (Leitenberg 2003). A case in point is the vaccination research conducted by Unit 731. The fact that an army conducting offensive BW will need effective vaccinations to protect its own soldiers does not preclude the use of the same vaccination in defending a country against a BW attack or in preventing naturally occurring infections.

The second argument might hold that "good science" can never come from unethical experiments. It may not be a coincidence that a large proportion of the research conducted by the Nazi physicians in German concentration camps and by the Japanese military physicians in China has no scientific value. For one, research that brutally abuses human subjects must lack the normal quality controls built into ethical scientific endeavors. Neither the Nazi physicians nor the Japanese military scientists could discuss their research with international colleagues or routinely submit their findings for publication. Neither obtained the funding for their research from scientific institutions but from a wartime bureaucracy and the army. Consequently, these researchers lacked an integral part of good science: criticism and approval from the larger research community. Moreover, researchers, whose conscience did not prevent them from killing other human beings in brutal experiments, may be more likely to distort or falsify scientific results than researchers who refused to partake in such experiments.

However, while many of the experiments conducted by Unit 731 may indeed have lacked scientific rigor, it does not necessarily follow that all of the experiments produced useless data. Evidence that results of some of the experiments may have had scientific value includes articles published by members of Unit 731 and the U.S. Intelligence reports documenting the interest of American BW researchers in the findings. Further (indirect) evidence that some of the Japanese BW research had scientific merit may be seen in the remarkable careers of many of the Japanese scientists upon their return from occupied China (Williams and Wallace 1989: 236–242); former members of Unit 731 rose to some of the highest positions in Japanese academic medicine. For instance, after World War II Dr. Kasahara, who conducted many of the barbaric experiments described above, became Chief Pathologist of the renowned Kitasato Institute in Tokyo and later rose to the position of Vice-President of the Institute. Dr. Yoshimura, who killed hundreds of human beings in the frostbite experiments described above, became President of the Medical Faculty of Kyoto University as well as Scientific Advisor to the Japanese Antarctic expedition and President of the Japanese Society for Meteorology (Han and Xin 1991: 332–352; Tsuneishi 1986: 22; Who's Who in Contemporary Japan 1963: 155; Williams & Wallace 1989: 236–242).

In the (current) case of the Japanese BW experiments – characterized by uncertainty about both the scientific value of many of the findings and the existence of further data – I believe the "position of strict non-use" to be preferable over the other two ethical stances on using unethically obtained data. Certainly, any data which have not yet been made public by either the Japanese or the American government should be made public immediately, so that it can be incorporated into historical accounts of the Japanese BW units. Such a demand, however, would lose its ethical force if it were not accompanied by a declaration that – without exception – the data will not be used for scientific or practical purposes. Leaving open the possibility to use the data would render the victims of the experiments also victims of our decision to demand public disclosure of all the information on the experiments. Unconditional non-use, on the other hand, would have an invaluable symbolic meaning as a memorial to the victims. It would also imply a symbolic punishment of the scientists of Unit 731, who were allowed to pursue renowned careers after World War II, in many cases by exploiting the experience and building on the research results obtained by killing Chinese and Russian prisoners of war (Bärnighausen 2007). Finally, a decision to adhere to a "position of strict non-use" rather than a "position of conditional use" would draw a stark symbolic contrast to the pragmatic stance taken by the U.S. government and military that led to the decision to grant freedom from prosecution to the Japanese military scientists in exchange for unethically obtained data:

> It is recognized that by informing Ishii and his associates that the information to be obtained regarding BW will be retained in intelligence channels and will not be employed as war crimes evidence, this government may at a later date be seriously embarrassed. However, the Army Department and Air Force Members strongly believe that this information, particularly that which will finally be obtained from the Japanese with respect to the effect of BW on humans, is of such importance to the security of this country that the risk of subsequent embarrassment should be taken.
> (Special Staff, United States Army Civilian Affairs Division 1947: 1)

Notes

1   In this chapter, the reader should note that many sources give the name of Japanese with the surname last, such as Shiro Ishii. As in the rest of the book, however, Japanese names are given in the text with the surname first, such as Ishii Shiro.

2   In contrast to his colleagues at the L'Institute Pasteur, Professor Nicolle, Professor Trillat was convinced that biological warfare would be possible if certain conditions were met simultaneously: "Pour qu'elle (la guerre bacteriologique) réussisse, il faut en effet un ensemble de conditions qui ne se trouvent pas réunies en tous temps" (Sudre, cited in Committee Imperial Defence 1938: 35).

3   While the case of the Japanese BW units offers an important example on which to debate the use of unethically obtained data, many other cases of abuse of humans

in medical experiments exist, as described in several chapters in this book. It is important to note that abuses of unwilling or unaware victims in medical experiments were not confined to countries under fascist or para-fascist rule – even though some of the worst crimes against humanity were committed in Nazi Germany and Imperial Japan – but have occurred as well under communism and in democracies. Examples include the poison tests on Gulag prisoners in the Soviet Union (Birstein 2004), and the Tuskegee syphilis study (Tuskegee Syphilis Study Legacy Committee 1996) and human radiation experiments (Advisory Committee on Human Radiation Experiments 1995) in the United States. The discussion of the Japanese case may thus be relevant to other past abuses and likely – even if one dares to hope otherwise – to future abuses.

References

Advisory Committee on Human Radiation Experiments 1995, *Final Report*, October, Washington.

"Aerosols, Interview with Dr. Takahashi" 1947, in *Summary Report on BW Investigation*, ed. E. Hill and J. Victor, December 12, RG 395, Entry 6909-C, National Archives, Suitland Reference Branch, Maryland, pp. 6–7.

Angell, M. 1990, "The Nazi Hypothermia Experiments and Unethical Research Today", *New England Journal of Medicine*, pp. 1462–1464.

"Bacteriological Warfare Experiments by Japanese" 1947, January 17, General Headquarters, Far East Command, Military Intelligence Section, General Staff, Record Group 395, National Archives, College Park, Maryland.

Bärnighausen, T. 2002, *Medizinische Humanexperimente der japanischen Truppen für biologische Kriegsführung in China 1932–1945 [Medical Human Experiments of the Japanese Troops for Biological Warfare in China 1932–1945]*, Peter Lang, Frankfurt a.M.

Bärnighausen, T. 2005, "Barbaric Research: Japanese Human Experiments in Occupied China – Relevance; Alternatives; Ethics", in *Man, Medicine and the State: The Human Body as an Object of Government Sponsored Research, 1920–1970*, ed. W. Eckart, Franz Steiner Publishing Company, Stuttgart, pp. 167–197.

Bärnighausen, T. 2007, "Communicating 'Tainted Science': The Japanese Biological Warfare Experiments on Human Subjects in China", in *History of Medical Ethics and the Ethics of Human Experimentation*, ed. A. Frewer and U. Schmidt, Franz Steiner Publishing Company, Stuttgart, pp. 117–144.

Beecher, H. 1966, "Ethics and Clinical Research", *New England Journal of Medicine*, 274, pp. 1354–1360.

Berger, R. 1990, "Nazi Science – The Dachau Hypothermia Experiments", *New England Journal of Medicine*, 322, pp. 1435–1440.

Birstein, V. 2004, *The Perversion of Knowledge: The True Story of Soviet Science*, Westview Press, Boulder, CO.

"Botulism, Interview with Dr. Shiro Ishii" 1947, in *Summary Report on BW Investigation*, ed. E. Hill and J. Victor, December 12, RG 395, Entry 6909-C, National Archives, Suitland Reference Branch, Maryland, p. 9.

Bridgman, S. 1991, "Peripheral Cold Acclimatization in Antarctic Scuba Divers", *Aviation, Space, and Environmental Medicine*, 62, pp. 733–738.

"Brucellosis, Interview with Dr. Kiyoshi Hayakawa" 1947, in *Summary Report on BW Investigation*, ed. E. Hill and J. Victor, December 12, RG 395, Entry 6909-C, National Archives, Suitland Reference Branch, Maryland, p. 11.

"Brucellosis, Interview with Dr. Shiro Ishii" 1947, in *Summary Report on BW Investigation*, ed. E. Hill and J. Victor, December 12, RG 395, Entry 6909-C, National Archives, Suitland Reference Branch, Maryland, p. 10.

"Brucellosis, Interview with Dr. Yujiro Yamanouchi" 1947, in *Summary Report on BW Investigation*, ed. E. Hill and J. Victor, December 12, RG 395, Entry 6909-C, National Archives, Suitland Reference Branch, Maryland, p. 12.

Cao, Yuan. 1951, *Rikou xijunzhan baoxing* [*The Crime of Japanese Bacteriological Warfare*], Tonglian shudian, Shanghai.

Cohen, B. 1990, "The Ethics of Using Medical Data from Nazi Experiments", *Journal of Halacha Contemporary Society*, spring, pp. 103–126.

Committee Imperial Defence, Subcommittee on Emergency Public Health Laboratory Services 1938, *Memorandum on the Practicability of the Bacteriological Weapon in Future Warfare*, December 12, London.

Deng, Y. 1965, "Rikou zai Changde jinxing shuyi xijunzhan jingguo" ["The Course of the Biological War with Plague Bacteria Conducted by the Japanese Bandits"], *Hunan wenshi ziliao* [*Collection of Historical Materials of Hunan Province*], 18, pp. 62–68.

Gaylin, W. 1989, "Nazi Data: Dissociation from Evil", *Hastings Center Report*, p. 18.

"Germ Tests on POWs Charged to Japanese" 1982, *Washington Post*, April 5, p. A12.

Han, X. 1986, "Rijun 731 budui faxisi baoxing jilu" ["Collection of the Fascistic Atrocities of Unit 731 of the Japanese Army"], *Heilongjiang wenshi ziliao* [*Historical Sources of the Province Heilongjiang*], 1–35.

Han, X and Xin, P. 1991, *Rijun 731 budui zuieshi* [*Historical Documents of Heilongjiang, Volume 31, a History of the Crimes of Unit 731 of the Japanese Army*], Heilongjiang Chubanshe, Harbin.

Han, X. and Yin, Q. 1986, "Qinhua rijun di 731 buduilide laogong" ["The Use of Chinese Labor in Unit 731 of the Japanese Army"], *Anhui wenshi ziliao* [*Historical Sources of the Province Heilongjiang*], 22, pp. 150–164.

Harris, S. 1994, *Factories of Death: Japanese Biological Warfare 1932–1945 and the American Cover-up*, Routledge, London.

Hill, E. and Victor, J. 1947, *Summary Report on BW Investigation*, December 12, RG 395, Entry 6909-C, National Archives, Suitland Reference Branch, Maryland.

Hirai, K., Inoue, T. and Yoshimura, H. 1968, "Studies on Effect of Heat Content on the Vascular Hunting Reaction to Cold, and the Reaction of Women Divers", *Nippon Seirigaku Zasshi [Japanese Physiological Journal]*, 30, pp. 12–21.

Hojo, E. 1941, "Über den Bakterienkrieg" ["About the Bacteria War"], H 10–25/1, National Military Archive, Freiburg im Breisgau, Germany.

"Influenza, Interview with Dr. Shiro Ishii" 1947, in *Summary Report on BW Investigation*, ed. E. Hill and J. Victor, December 12, RG 395, Entry 6909-C, National Archives, Suitland Reference Branch, Maryland, p. 36.

"Intelligence Research Project No. 2263" 1945, Japanese Biological Warfare 1045, July 26, Record Group 226, Entry 146, Box 253, Folder 3502, National Archives, Washington, D.C.

"Interrogation of Dr. Kiyoshi Ota" 1946, General Headquarters United States Armed Forces, Pacific Office of the Chief Chemical Officer, December 2, Entry 295, Box 9, Record Group 112, National Archives, College Park, Maryland.

"Interview with Dr. Kozo Okamoto" 1947, in *Summary Report on BW Investigation*, ed. E. Hill and J. Victor, December 12, RG 395, Entry 6909-C, National Archives, Suitland Reference Branch, Maryland, p. 32.

Jia, F. 1985, "Wo qinyan kandao rikou feiji hongzha Baojide canzhuang" ["I Have Seen with My Own Eyes how the Planes of the Japanese Bandits Bombarded Baoji"], *Baojishi wenshi ziliao* [*Historial Materials of Baoji City*], 3, pp. 42–45.

Jiang, Y. 1983, "Can wurendaode xijunzhan: Ningbo shuyi can'an diaocha" ["The Cruel, Inhumane Bacterial War: Investigation of the Plague in Ningbo"], *Congheng*, 2, pp.127–133.

Kasahara, S. and Kitano, M. 1943, "Studies on Pathogen of Epidemic Hemorrhagic Fever", *Japanese Journal of Pathology*, 33, pp. 476–483.

The Khabarovsk Trial. 1950, *Materials on the Trial of Former Servicemen of the Japanese Army Charged with Manufacturing and Employing Biological Weapons*, Foreign Language Publishing House, Moscow.

Konda, N., Shiraki, K., Sagawa, S. and Ohta, Y. 1981, "Cold-induced Vasodilation Reaction of Skin Vessels at 2 ATA", *Journal of UOEH*, 3, pp. 207–213.

Leitenberg, M. 2003, "Distinguishing Offensive from Defensive Biological Weapons Research", *Critical Reviews in Microbiology*, 29, pp. 223–257.

Lou, F. 1987, "Li rikou shuyi huanzhede canzhuang" ["The Miserable Appearance of the Patients Suffering from the Plague Brought by the Japanese Bandits"], *Dongyangshi wenshi ziliao* [*Historical Sources of Dongyang City*], 5, p. 186.

Matsumara, T. 1986, " '731 budui' de shiyan baogaoshu" ["The Laboratory Book of 'Unit 731' "], *Heilongjiang wenshi ziliao* [*Historical Sources of Heilongjiang Province*], pp. 36–86.

Mitscherlich, A. and Mielke, F. (eds) 1995, *Medizin ohne Menschlichkeit. Dokument des Nürnberger Ärzteprozesses* [*Medicine Without Humaneness. Documents of the Nuremburg War Criminal Trials*], Fischer Verlag, Frankfurt a.M.

Miura, T., Kimotsuki, K., Tominaga, Y. and Suzuki, Y. 1977, "Effect of Environmental Conditions on the Cold-induced Vasodilation of Office Workers and Forestry Workers", *Journal of Science of Labor*, 53, pp. 75–81.

Moe, K. 1989, "Should the Nazi Data be Cited?", *Hastings Center Report*, pp. 5–7.

Morimura, S. 1983, *Emode baoshi* [*The Devil's Gluttony*], Part 2, Jilin Renmin Chubanshe, Changchun.

Morimura, S. 1985, *Shiren moku* [*The Devil's Gluttony*], Part 3, Qunzhong Chubanshe, Beijing.

Mostow, P. 1993–1994, " 'Like Building on Top of Auschwitz': On the Symbolic Meaning of Using Data from the Nazi Experiments, and on Nonuse as a Form of Memorial", *Journal of Law and Religion*, 2, pp. 403–431.

"Naval Aspects of Biological Warfare" 1947, August 5, General Records of the Department of the Navy 1798–1747, Formerly Top Secret General Correspondence of the CNO/ Secretary of the Navy 1944–1947, CNO Top Secret, Record Group 330, Box 55, National Archives, Washington, D.C.

Nelms, J. and Soper, D. 1962, "Cold Vasodilatation and Cold Acclimatization in the Hands of British Fish Filleters", *Journal of Applied Physiology*, 17, pp. 444–448.

Neter, E. 1980, "Ethics and Editors: Commentary", *Hastings Center Report*, p. 23.

Ogata, K., Harada, K. and Kamota, M. 1952, "Influence of a Large Amount of Sodium Chloride Ingestion on the Basal Metabolism and on Resistance to Cold and Frost-bite", *Japanese Journal of Physiology*, 2, pp. 303–309.

"Paratyphoid, Interview with Dr. Tabei" 1947, in *Summary Report on BW Investigation*, ed. E. Hill and J. Victor, December 12, RG 395, Entry 6909-C, National Archives, Suitland Reference Branch, Maryland, p. 31.

Post, S. 1988, "Nazi Data and the Rights of Jews", *Journal of Law and Religion*, 6, pp. 429–433.

Post, S. 1991, "The Echo of Nuremberg: Nazi Data and Ethics", *Journal of Medical Ethics*, 17, pp. 42–44.

Pozos, R. 2003, "Nazi Hypothermia Research: Should the Data be Used?", in *Military Medical Ethics*, Vol. 2, ed. T. Beam and L. Sparacino, Borden Institute, Walter Reed Army Medical Center, Washington, D.C., pp. 437–462.

Rawls, J. 1971, *A Theory of Justice*, Belknap Press of Harvard University Press, Boston, IL.

"Report on Dysentery, Information by Tomosada Masuda" 1947, in *Summary Report on BW Investigation*, ed. E. Hill and J. Victor, December 12, RG 395, Entry 6909-C, National Archives, Suitland Reference Branch, Maryland, p. 33.

Sawada, S., Araki, S. and Yokoyama, K. 2000, "Changes in Cold-induced Vasodilatation, Pain and Cold Sensation in Fingers Caused by Repeated Finger Cooling in a Cool Environment", *Industrial Health*, 38, pp.79–86.

Schafer, A. 1986, "On Using Nazi Data: The Case Against", *Dialogue Canadian Philosophical Association*, 25, pp. 413–419.

Sheldon, M. and Whitely, W. 1989, "Nazi Data: Dissociation from Evil", *Hastings Center Report*, pp. 16–17.

Shi, A. 1985, "Lishuixian renjian shuyi liuxing jianli" ["A Short History of the Spread of the Plague Among the Residents of Lishui County"], *Lishui wenshi ziliao* [*Historical Sources Lishui County*], 2, pp. 186–188.

Singer, E. 1980, "Ethics and Editors: Commentary", *Hastings Center Report*, p. 24.

"Smallpox, Interview with Dr. Shiro Ishii" 1947, in *Summary Report on BW Investigation*, ed. E. Hill and J. Victor, December 12, RG 395, Entry 6909-C, National Archives, Suitland Reference Branch, Maryland, p. 50.

"Songo – Epidemic Hemorrhagic Fever, Interview with Shiro Kasahara and Masaji Kitano" 1947, in *Summary Report on BW Investigation*, ed. E. Hill and J. Victor, December 12, RG 395, Entry 6909-C, National Archives, Suitland Reference Branch, Maryland, pp. 42–44.

Special Staff, United States Army Civilian Affairs Division 1947, "Interrogation of Certain Japanese by Russian Prosecutor", September 26, 17/18/B, Box 628, Entry 468, National Archives, Washington, D.C.

Spurr, G., Hutt, B. and Horvath, S. 1955, "The Effects of Age on Finger Temperature Responses to Local Cooling", *American Heart Journal*, 50, pp. 551–555.

State–War–Navy Coordinating Subcommittee for the Far East (SWNCC Subcommittee) 1947, "Interrogation of Certain Japanese by Russian Prosecutor", August 1, Appendix A, 17/18/B, Box 628, Entry 468, National Archives, Washington, D.C.

Stille, W. 1992, "Bakterielle Krankheiten des ZNS", in *Lehrbuch der Inneren Medizin* [*Textbook of Internal Medicine*], ed. W. Siegenthaler, W. Kaufmann, H. Hornbostel and H. Waller, Georg Thieme, Stuttgart, pp. 889–890.

Sun, J. and Ni, W. 1984, "Ningbode shuyi canhuo: riben qinhua zhanzhengzhongde zuixing – Ningbo shuyide fasheng he jingguo" ["The Horrible Plague Catastrophe in Ningbo: The War Crimes of the Japanese Invaders – The Outbreak and Course of the Plague in Ningbo"], *Ningbo wenshi ziliao* [*Historical Materials of Ningbo City*], 2, pp. 174–180.

Tanaka, M. 1971a, "Experimental Studies on Human Reaction to Cold – Different Vascular Hunting Reaction of Workers to Cold", *Bulletin of Tokyo Medical and Dental University*, 18, pp. 169–177.

Tanaka, M. 1971b, "Experimental Studies on Human Reaction to Cold – Differences in the Vascular Hunting Reaction to Cold According to Sex, Season, and Environmental Temperature", *Bulletin of Tokyo Medical and Dental University*, 18, pp. 269–280.

Tang, G. and Cheng, S. 1985, "Lishuicheng shuyibing liuxingde huiyi" ["Memories of the Spread of the Plague in Lishui County"], *Lishui wenshi ziliao* [*Historical Sources of Lishui County*], 2, pp. 189–190.

"Tetanus, Interview with Shiro Ishii" 1947, in *Summary Report on BW Investigation*, ed. E. Hill and J. Victor, December 12, RG 395, Entry 6909-C, National Archives, Suitland Reference Branch, Maryland, p. 51.

Thompson, A. 1946, "Report on Japanese Biological Warfare", May 31, 57 4926 Cy 1, Library of Congress, Science and Technical Reports Section, Washington, D.C.

Tsuneishi, K. 1986, "The Research Guarded by Military Secrecy – The Isolation of the E. H. F. Virus in Japanese Biological Warfare Unit", *Historia Scientiarum*, 30, pp. 79–92.

"Tuberculosis, Interview with Dr. Hideo Futagi" 1947, in *Summary Report on BW Investigation*, ed. E. Hill and J. Victor, December 12, RG 395, Entry 6909-C, National Archives, Suitland Reference Branch, Maryland, pp. 61–64.

"Tularemia, Interview with Dr. Shiro Ishii" 1947, in *Summary Report on BW Investigation*, ed. E. Hill and J. Victor, December 12, RG 395, Entry 6909-C, National Archives, Suitland Reference Branch, Maryland, p. 54.

Tuskegee Syphilis Study Legacy Committee 1996, *Final Report of the Tuskegee Syphilis Study Legacy Committee*, May 20.

"Typhoid, Interview with Dr. Tabei" 1947, in *Summary Report on BW Investigation*, ed. E. Hill and J. Victor, December 12, RG 395, Entry 6909-C, National Archives, Suitland Reference Branch, Maryland, p. 56.

Ulmer, H. 1997, "Umweltphysiologie" ["Environmental physiology"], in *Physiologie des Menschen* [*Human Physiology*], ed. R. Schmidt and G. Thews, Springer Verlag, Berlin, pp. 697–716.

Wang, G. 1985, "Riben diguozhuyi jinxing xijunzhande zui'e" ["The Crimes of the Implementation of the Bacterial War of the Japanese Imperialists"], *Baojishi wenshi ziliao* [*Historical Materials of Baoji City*], 3, pp. 39–41.

Wang, S. 1987, " 'Sunwure' de jinxi: Riben qinlüezhe zui'ede renti shiyan" ["Past and Present of "Sunwu Fever": The Criminal Human Experiments of the Japanese Invaders"], *Sunwu wenshi ziliao* [*Historical Sources of Sunwu County*], 2, pp. 22–29.

Wang, Z. 1984, "Kangri zhanzheng shiqi Ningbo shuyi jishi" ["Report on the Plague during the Resistance War against the Japanese"], *Ningbo wenshi ziliao* [*Historical Materials of Ningbo City*], 2, pp. 181–195.

Watts, J. 2002, "Victims of Japan's Notorious Unit 731 Sue", *The Lancet*, 360, p. 628.

Weitzman, M. 1990, "The Ethics of Using Nazi Medical Data: A Jewish Perspective", *Second Opinion*, pp. 27–38.

Who's Who in Contemporary Japan 1963, Japanese Politics Economy Research Institute, Tokyo.

Williams, P. and Wallace, D. 1989, *Unit 731: The Japanese Army's Secret of Secrets*, The Free Press, New York.

Yoshimura, H. and Iida, T. 1952a, "Studies on the Reactivity of Skin Vessels to Extreme Cold I. A Point Test on the Resistance against Frost Bite", *Japanese Journal of Physiology*, 2, pp. 147–159.

Yoshimura, H. and Iida, T. 1952b, "Studies on the Reactivity of Skin Vessels to Extreme Cold II. Factors Governing the Individual Difference of the Reactivity, or the Resistance against Frostbite", *Japanese Journal of Physiology*, 2, pp. 177–185.

Yoshimura, H. and Iida, T. 1952c, "Studies on the Reactivity of Skin Vessels to Extreme Cold. III. Effects of Diets on the Reactivity of Skin Vessels to Cold", *Japanese Journal of Physiology*, 2, pp. 310–315.

Zeiss, H. and Rodenwaldt, E. 1943, *Einführung in die Hygiene und Seuchenlehre* [*Introduction to Hygiene and Epidemics*], Ferdinand Enke Verlag, Stuttgart.

Zimmermann, E. 1940, *Mikrobiologie, Erkennung und Bekämpfung der Infektionskrankheiten* [*Microbiology, Detection and Combating Infectious Diseases*], Ferdinand Enke Verlag, Stuttgart.

Zinsser, H. and Bayne-Jones, S. 1939, *A Textbook of Bacteriology*, D. Appleton-Century Company, London and New York.

5   Discovering traces of humanity

Taking individual responsibility for medical atrocities

Nanyan Guo

Introduction

The medical atrocities committed by the Ishii network and the Medical School of Kyushu Imperial University during the Second World War reflect a severe erosion of morality and humanity. The death sentences meted out to thousands of experimental victims for the sake of "medical research" violated the basic principles of medicine, whose goals historically have been the relief of pain, the saving of life, and the restoration of humanity.

The discourse of these medical atrocities incorporates a voluminous literature of reminiscences and confessions detailing the ways in which the atrocities were carried out. However, among them there are only a few examples of ethical reflection by participants and consideration for the suffering and dignity of victims, and even fewer cases where the perpetrators felt unwilling or unable to continue their participation in the atrocities. This phenomenon leads us to consider both their rare manifestations of humanity and the ready discarding of empathy as a result of the careerism or nationalism that pervaded both the Japanese Army and the medical establishment.

In order to understand how and why a tiny minority of people managed to keep their humanity intact in such circumstances, this chapter will focus on examples of individuals who rejected the atrocities they were involved in and who showed remorse toward the victims. First, we will examine the ways in which the atrocities in question were commonly justified and denied. Second, we will assess the significance of what remained of morality in the minds of particular individuals. Finally, we analyze the mechanisms by which an individual's moral choices make a decisive difference in such extreme situations. The major materials on which my research is based include participants' confessions, witness testimonies, documentary writings, scholarly studies, and non-fiction novels and fictional treatments have been published in Japan.

It is important to state at the outset that the materials discussed here all draw on postwar accounts. Testimonials gathered after the war may fail to accurately reflect what the participants actually thought in the process of committing their atrocities. It is nevertheless important to analyze these reminiscences as they indicate what some perpetrators may have thought at the time, or at least what they wished they had thought. Such a "wish" is itself a sign of an awakened morality either because of being forced to confess in Chinese prisons, or through the pressures of postwar Japanese society, or self reflection. Nevertheless, this "wish" is the major focus of this chapter.

An outline of the atrocities and the postwar trials

The "medical atrocities" carried out by Japan during the Second World War include the development of biological and chemical weapons, the utilization of biological warfare, and the use of human vivisection for medical and educational purposes. Most of these atrocities were committed by the Ishii network which consisted of Unit 731 (Harbin), Unit 100 (Changchun), Unit 516 (Qiqihar), Unit 1855 (Beijing), Unit 1644 (Nanjing), Unit 8604 (Guangzhou), the Preventive Research Laboratory (Tokyo), and Unit 9420 (Singapore). There was vivisection which was carried out at Kyushu Imperial University Medical School before the end of the Second World War.

Only a few of those who committed these atrocities were tried after the War. In December 1949, following the Khabarovsk Trial 12 persons were sentenced to terms of imprisonment ranging from 25 to two years. However, all were returned to Japan by 1956, except for one man, Karasawa Tomio, who committed suicide before their departure for Japan (Kondo 2002: 186–187). In August 1948, the allied occupation force in Japan, GHQ, conducted the Yokohama Trials over atrocities carried out at the Kyushu Imperial University Medical School in which eight American airmen, survivors from a downed B-29 bomber, were vivisected for "medical practice" between May and June 1945 (Sugamo homu iinkai 1981: 237–239). Five defendants were sentenced to death and three to life imprisonment. However, all the sentences were commuted in 1950. In China, in 1956, military tribunals in Shenyang tried a surgeon officer, Sakakibara Hideo, for his leadership role in the Linkou Branch of Unit 731 in addition to other Japanese war criminals (Guo 1995: 336, 346), but all were returned to Japan by 1964.

The U.S. Army Chemical Corps located in Camp Detrick in Frederick, Maryland, was given permission by the U.S. government to grant Ishii Shiro and his colleagues immunity from war crimes in exchange for their research data. The U.S. did not know that human experiments had been conducted by the Japanese until late 1946, when the Soviets revealed information gained from Japanese prisoners held in the Soviet Union. The Soviets sought extradition of Ishii and his colleagues in order to gain access to the research data already obtained by the U.S. They also threatened that if the U.S. did not agree to this arrangement, they would disclose the Japanese atrocities at the International Military Tribunal for the Far East in Tokyo (1946–1948).

Although the U.S. authorities well understood that the immunity granted to Ishii was at odds with the Nuremberg Trials where Nazi doctors had been prosecuted for inhuman experiments, the U.S. nevertheless granted him and his colleagues immunity. According to the report by Edwin V. Hill, "Such information could not be obtained in our own laboratories because of scruples attached to human experimentation. These data were secured with a total outlay of ¥250,000 ($695) to date, a mere pittance by comparison with the actual cost of the studies" (Hill 1947). Hill's line of reasoning indicates that the U.S. shared the same logic as the Japanese medical researchers who justified human experiments for "medical research" purposes that overrode humane values. This rhetoric of "the end justifying the means" suggests that both sides in the war had lost their moral compass. Similar phonomena may be seen from comfort women issues, mass slaughter of Chinese civilians, U.S. firebombing of Japanese cities and the use of nuclear bombs on Hiroshima and Nagasaki.

With the protection of the U.S., and without coming under any further scrutiny, most Japanese military doctors and researchers involved in human experimentation survived – and, indeed, thrived – well into the postwar period. Some became university presidents, faculty deans, prominent professors, heads of private research institutes and medical associations, and so on. Others, however, adopted low profiles to work in local clinics or public health institutes, perhaps in an attempt to atone for what they had done during the War.

Denials and justifications

Denials and justifications of wartime medical atrocities are commonplace in Japan. The most often repeated pretexts are "the national interest," "the Emperor's command", and the need for "scientific research." These justifications all figure in the statements made by five members of the Ishii network after the war:

1　"There is nothing shameful in what I did at Unit 731. . . . The Soviet Union was also conducting research into germ weapons . . . I was doing this for Japan, and I am not ashamed at all of what I did" (Hiyama 1980: 105).
2　"We fought for our country. What was wrong with using *maruta* [literally, 'logs'] as experimental material for the benefit of Japan? What do you people know about this, if you didn't go to the war?" (Morimura 1985, 2004: 50).
3　"We believed that the war was conducted in order to bring wealth to Japan, which was a poor country in those days, and to bring peace to Asia . . . therefore we believed that *maruta* were not human beings. They were even lower than animals. . . . No one in Unit 731 ever had any sympathy for them. To all of us, they deserved to die" (Morimura 1983, 1995a: 58).
4　"Because my older brother was killed by the Chinese, I did not have any sympathy for *maruta*" (731 Research Society 1996: 79).
5　"Although I wielded the surgical knife for almost four years, I did not have even the slightest sense of guilt. Everyone believed we were doing this for the Emperor" (Nihon jido 1983, 2000: 26).

It is clear from these statements that these five individuals did not perceive any humanity in their victims. The national interest was paramount, and their morality was narrowed to a single focus: what would benefit Japan. In the first statement, the speaker chooses to believe that it was perfectly right to carry out these experiments because another country was doing the same. Choosing his words carefully, he mentions only the Soviet Union and not the United States. He emphasizes his pride in his work at Unit 731. It seems the "moral support" he gained from national policy, feelings of racial superiority, and army orders was so strong that he could comfortably set aside any individual morality. The following four statements echo his value premises. Any possible doubt, hesitation, or sympathy was completely eliminated. Their consciences remained numb. If a few perpetrators ever felt at all sorry for their victims, it is only because the victims at least resembled animals; as one female member of Unit 731 recalled, "Whenever I saw the smoke coming from the chimney I always joined my hands to pray for their souls, even though we called them 'black-headed rats' " (Gunji 1982a: 154). These statements all reveal the troubling fact that their wartime mentality remained intact after the War, with the term *maruta* being repeatedly used. It seems that these perpetrators lacked any self-reflection on the state of their consciences as individuals and continued to ignore the human value and dignity of their victims. In so doing, they set aside the opportunity to restore their own humanity which had been grossly eroded during the War. Of course, some people's public denials might have been defensive reactions which do not necessarily reflect their deeper feelings.

Another common rationale was the "development of medical science" for the benefit of postwar society. The author of the documentary novel *Nomi to Saikin* (*Lice and Bombs*), Yoshimura Akira, writes that most Japanese surgeons dreamed of conducting human experiments, and three surgeons from Japanese national universities made a special visit to a Kwantung Army Unit in Manchuria in order to have the opportunity of examining human necks in cross-section immediately after decapitation. Their academic "curiosity" and "enthusiasm" even impressed the army chief (Yoshimura 1975: 30–31). One former military doctor stated: "I must emphasize that the research results gained by military surgeons during the war greatly contributed to medical developments in the post-war period" (Ishida 1982: 47). When the logic of "the end justifies the means" is applied, the atrocities were easily excused for the tangible gains they seemingly accrued.

Generally speaking, both during and after the War, only a few perpetrators publicly claimed an awakening of conscience as a result of reflection over war atrocities they had committed. Among 2000 patients at the Konodai Army Hospital, a research center for mental illness that operated from 1937 until 1945, only two persons were reportedly affected by their memories of slaughtering Chinese; both repeatedly saw the faces of their Chinese victims in their dreams (Noda 1998: 342–343). According to new research, in the same hospital around 31 out of 374 patients had symptoms related to an abiding sense of guilt of killing Chinese (Shimizu 2006, 2007: 229, 233). It seems that only a small minority developed mental illness because of their consciousness of crimes. A few people from Unit 731 disclosed the trauma they suffered. One member confessed that he was traumatized by his experience of vivisecting a Chinese woman who suddenly woke up owing to inadequate anesthesia. Another member said that two kinds of sound had stuck in his ears all his life: one is the sound of the beating of a victim's heart which was just taken out and was measured by a table balance, and the other is the sound of prisoners' fetters (Nishino 2002: 221–222).

A residual belief in human values

Although it was very uncommon for military medical personnel to show any respect for their victims' humanity, some individuals did so. One Unit 731 member, Chida Hideo, could not cope with the atrocities involved in human experimentation and suffered a mental breakdown. He could not understand why so many Chinese had to be sacrificed in such a gruesome way in order to "save Japanese soldiers' lives." He told his superior about his misgivings, and was fortunate enough to be allowed to transfer to another department to avoid further distress where he was not directly involved in human experiments (731 Research Society 1996: 104–108).

There were also individuals who remained unconvinced by what they were ordered to do in Unit 731. A junior member of the unit, Tsuruta Kanetoshi, who served in Nomonhan on the Russian–Manchurian border between May and September 1939, the site of a Japanese–Russian clash, was ordered to pour typhoid bacilli into a river in order to poison local residents. When later asked by Ishii Shiro in person how he felt about the War, he replied unhesitatingly, "It's better not to go to war." Because of telling the truth of his mind, Tsuruta was punished by being made to feed lice on his own body for three days (731 Research Society 1996: 67–68).

A few brave individuals placed humanity above all other considerations in such circumstances. One Unit 516 member recalled that his unit had a rare atmosphere of freedom, and that when "technician lieutenant S.Y.," a graduate of Osaka University, was ordered to participate in a gas experiment on prisoners, S.Y. "rejected the order by telling his boss, Captain N, that he was a Catholic, and therefore could not participate in such inhuman experiments." His disobedience was overlooked by the captain (Morimura 1983, 1995b: 62–64). This example suggests that the humane religious beliefs held by an individual, combined with a relatively relaxed environment, could give someone the strength of will to reject participation in atrocities. At the same time, we should not forget that, according to its members' testimonies, Unit 516 ruthlessly sacrificed many lives through gas experiments (Morimura 1983, 1995b: 56–70).

This case resembles that of Doi Takeo, the author of *Amae no Kozo* (*The Anatomy of Dependence*), who told his superior when he was conscripted, "I am a Christian, therefore I will not kill anyone" (Endo 2000: 390). Neither S.Y. nor Doi was persecuted for their religious beliefs and their rejection of acts involving doing harm to others. These examples suggest that an individual with a firmly established moral code has the potential to resist inhumanity and become a catalyst for change. Sometimes, disobedience does win out.

Sometimes, such moral resistance was expressed in more private terms. Hayashi Atsumi, a military surgeon and a Christian, wrote in his diary for December 28, 1942: "The essence of medicine must be a religious state of selflessness . . .

otherwise it can only degrade the medical practitioner." After the war, Hayashi criticized a colleague who conducted vivisection solely out of curiosity (Mizutani 1997: 67–69). These individuals managed to keep their morality intact by either publicly stating or privately recording their opposition to medical atrocities. Their resistance is a ray of light in the darkness.

Others protested internally, in their own minds, against the atrocities, if not to their superiors. A member of Unit 1644 stated: "When I saw the blackened face of the *maruta* after his blood had been completely drained, I wondered how someone could do such a thing to him . . . What had the *maruta* done to deserve these atrocities . . . I wanted to treat them like human beings" (Matsumoto 1996: 188–190). A member of Unit 731 often gave prisoners cigarettes before they were killed:

> What did these Chinese people feel? I trembled when I imagined myself in the same situation . . . I wanted to apologize to each one of them when I was assisting with the injections that were forced upon them . . . I couldn't understand how Japanese could perform these experiments without a sense of guilt. I couldn't believe that our soldiers would be made safer by those deadly experiments . . . I still can't forget those Chinese faces after 40 years.
>
> (Senda 1996: 104–109)

Their innate sense of morality helped these operatives refuse to "understand" the atrocities they were involved in. What is the purpose of draining a person's blood? How can lethal experiments save lives? If we would reject such a cruel death for ourselves, why do we inflict it on others? Why can't the Chinese be treated like human beings? These simple questions removed all justification for the medical atrocities in the minds of these individuals.

Some participants might have felt uncomfortable at the beginning, but gradually accustomed themselves to participation in the gruesome experiments. For instance, one Unit 731 member recalled:

> When I pulled the knife out of his body, blood dropped on my hand. I can never forget that moment. I could not eat my dinner that day, and I had nightmares for the whole week. Although I didn't regard the Chinese as human beings, I hated cutting them up like this. However I could not disobey the order.
>
> (Hoshi 2002: 187–188)

This individual's perception of the low value to be placed on the lives of Chinese made it possible for him to continue to obey orders, even if he was clearly aware of the inhumanity of the experiments.

Although not brave enough to either criticize or disobey orders, some perpetrators showed their sympathy for the victims. A number of reminiscences reveal their inner voices. A former prison guard recalls his feelings toward two female prisoners who were experimental subjects, along with a small child. "With tears in their eyes, the grandmother and the mother both begged me to free the little child, and said they were ready to die at any time through any experiment (if only the child could be saved)." Their words resounded in his heart, as he had recently lost his 2-year-old daughter to measles. The only comfort he could offer was this reply: "OK, I'll consult my boss" (Kamiya 1998: 82). Even though the guard could offer no practical assistance, his expression of sympathy and willingness to help must have given some hope to the women. To be given hope is to be treated like a human being. Respecting people's humanity requires the ability to imagine their suffering. In this case, the guard's pain at losing his daughter enabled him to imagine the agony experienced by the women.

Some perpetrators even managed to experience empathy, feeling their victims' suffering as if it were happening to themselves. One Unit 516 member witnessed the death of a mother and her daughter being poisoned by gas. "The cruel thing is that I was even holding a stopwatch to measure the time that it took them to die. . . . After 37 years, I can still clearly see the mother's soft hands covering the child's head to protect her from the prussic acid gas in the chamber" (Morimura 1983, 1995b: 70–71). His detailed description of the victims' facial expressions reveals his understanding of their fear and despair during the killing process, an experience which had kept his conscience awake for four decades.

Similarly, a truck driver for Unit 731 recalled his feelings one day after he had driven a group of prisoners to an open field for gas experiments; the victims "happily and deeply breathed in the fresh air and bathed in the sunlight with glittering eyes, not knowing they would die in just a few hours." At that moment, he could not help feeling that "they *were* human beings" too, and he could no longer treat them as *maruta* (Koshi 1983: 51–52). His glimpse of their short-lived enjoyment gave him an opportunity to understand their feelings and therefore to "re-humanize" them. This reminds us of a famous war novel by Ooka Shohei (1909–1988), *Furyoki* (*Taken Captive*), set in the Philippines and published in 1948. The main character cannot bring himself to shoot a young American soldier who is approaching him unaware that he is hiding close by in the jungle. The author analyzes the protagonist's reasons for not pulling the trigger, stating that he was touched by the soldier's ruddy complexion and fresh, youthful looks, rather than being motivated by love for human beings (Ooka 1994: 19–27). A glance at the soldier's face – part of his unique individuality – made a critical difference to the protagonist's fateful decision.

However, this compassionate inner voice is rarely heard in the postwar reminiscence literature of the medical atrocities. The majority of the perpetrators chose to turn a blind eye to the suffering faces of their victims. In pushing aside their victims' humanity, these "well-educated" professionals (professors, doctors, researchers, technicians, medical assistants, and so on) were also forsaking their own humanity and occupational ethics. This "double immorality" is a leading characteristic of the wartime medical atrocities.

Nevertheless, after the war, the ability to regret one's actions and to be critical of the past was restored to some individuals. According to one Unit 731 operative:

Those military surgeons had a hunger for vivisection. . . . After most of the internal organs had been removed, the body looked like a dark and empty sack. Of course the heart was still beating. . . . The surgeon then looked just like a demon. . . . Although I was someone who read a lot of literature and had relatively liberal ideas at that time, I had no desire to stop the vivisection, even though I felt a bit sorry for the *maruta*.

(Koshi 1983: 117–122)

One military surgeon, who worked in Shanxin, China, during the War and practiced vivisection on at least 14 victims, was captured by the Chinese Army. In prison camp, he was asked to read a letter from a woman whose son was killed by him for medical purposes.

For the first time I felt an unspeakable sense of guilt . . . I had deprived her of her son . . . I used to think that everything I did was for the war effort, but now I believe that even the death penalty is not sufficient enough for me. . . . How much pain the Chinese must have suffered. How sad their families must have felt!

(Nishizato 2002: 160; Yoshikai and Yuasa 1981, 1996: 92, 253)

Such a sense of guilt meant that some perpetrators were unable to continue their "medical research" after the War. Although Akimoto Sueo, the author of *Yi no rinri o tou* [*Questioning Medical Ethics*], who joined the Ishii network in 1944, did not participate directly in human experimentation, he later regretted being part of the network and decided not to resume his post at the University of Tokyo as a medical researcher after the War. Rather, he sought to atone for his actions by working as a doctor in a local health center to help improve public health (Tsuneishi 1994: 19–20). Akimoto stated that he would regret his part in the atrocities until his death (Williams and Wallace 1989, 2003: 271).

Others were so burdened by their guilt that the prospect of living a normal life after the War was unbearable. One medical scientist, Okamoto Kei, from the Epidemic Research Institute of Tokyo Imperial University, left a brief but revealing suicide note: "I know my crime" (*Ware wagatsumi o shiru*) (Nishizato 2002: 175; Shibata 1998: 212; Tsuneishi and Asano 1982). Another perpetrator, Karasawa Tomio, who was sentenced to 20 years' imprisonment at the Khabarovsk Trial, hung himself in a laundry room shortly before he was due to be repatriated to Japan in 1956 (Aoki 2005: 372).

This kind of regret and guilt, experienced at the individual level, may be seen as genuinely redemptive because it does not originate from an order of the state or the government, but rather in the individual's soul. The people discussed above eventually managed to escape from the collective mentality which surrounded them, and began to think, feel, and act as individuals.

According to Ishii Harumi, the daughter of Ishii Shiro, shortly before his death from cancer of the pharynx in 1959 Ishii was baptized by a Roman Catholic priest, Hermann Heuvers, who was teaching at Sophia University in Tokyo, and received a Christian name, "Joseph." Although when she was interviewed Harumi failed to explain why her father had decided to become a Christian, she continued to state that her father seemed to be "relieved" following his baptism (Williams and Wallace 1989, 2003: 279). Although Ishii's baptism has never been confirmed by any documentary evidence (Aoki 2005: 374), his desire for baptism suggests that he felt guilty for his wartime medical atrocities and was searching for forgiveness. It would be interesting to know how his sense of guilt came to be formed, if such was indeed the case.

The necessity for human experimentation?

The "advancement of medical science" was repeatedly used as a justification for experiments on living human subjects. As we have seen, one military surgeon emphasized the medical gains to be made from human experimentation (Ishida 1982: 47). However, this justification has been questioned by other participants and scholars.

One Unit 731 member did not believe that the experiments could be scientifically justified. He said,

> When I thought about what was being done in Unit 731, I realized there was no research that had to be conducted through human experiments. All those experiments could have been done on animal subjects. In fact, the sole purpose served by the "experiments" carried out by Unit 731 was human slaughter.
>
> (Gunji 1982b: 233)

Another Unit 731 operative stated:

> Military doctors were using their prerogative to perform vivisection. They lacked self-reflection. They were only motivated by curiosity. . . . In reality, the structure of the body can be easily determined from medical textbooks rather than by cutting open a living body. And the organs that were supposed to be observed could be destroyed when making incisions.
>
> (Akimoto 1983: 129–139, 146)

The futility of human vivisection and the real motivation behind it are reinforced by further examples. In the northern part of Shanxi province, one military doctor specializing in internal medicine ordered his subordinates to vivisect a Chinese farmer "in order to determine the position and shape of his appendix." When he failed to locate it, he shot the farmer with his pistol (Hoshi 2002: 32). One medical researcher criticized the Kyushu atrocities in similar terms: "The vivisection at Kyushu Imperial University was done so poorly and carelessly that there was nothing to be documented at all. No record remained. The vivisection was nothing more than wholesale slaughter" (Kawakami 1965: 488).

Tsuneishi Keiichi, a distinguished scholar of the history of science and a contributor to this volume, sees no merit in human experiments.

Superficially, there appeared to have been some progress made in research because so much had been invested in military medicine. But in wartime, so much was sacrificed and wasted. A comparable level of progress could have been easily achieved in peacetime through reasonable resource allocation and animal experiments.

(Tsuneishi 1998: 214)

Tsuneishi also points out that the Japanese program was marred by flaws in the scientific methods adopted:

Scientifically, the experimental results only show the differences between individual victims and lack statistical validity because the number of subjects was limited. Their findings from various experiments produced only a rough outline of the physical conditions experienced by individuals. The data produced by the Ishii network lack scientific value. . . . Besides, their experiments involving dry blood plasma for transfusion, water purifying machines, penicillin, BCG vaccine, plague vaccine, typhus vaccine, cholera vaccine and tetanus serum were redundant, as these products were already being utilized overseas.

(Tsuneishi 1995: 179–180, 198)

Tsuneishi also states that the treatment for frostbite devised by Yoshimura Hisato through human experimentation was already practiced by Russian doctors in the nineteenth century (Tsuneishi 1994: 290). He further indicates that the pursuit of "scientific" results in the absence of any human feeling produces only a sense of "self-satisfaction" in scientific researchers which, if taken to an extreme, will end up destroying the world (Tsuneishi 2002: 82).

Tsuneishi's comments make it clear that these experiments served only to enhance the reputations of some medical researchers by increasing their research output and promoting them to the top echelons of the medical establishment. However, we must be cautious about arguing whether the experiments were "useful" or "necessary," because if some results can be categorized in this way, the door leading to the justification of inhuman experiments is open once again. The vital point is that an unconditional value should be placed on human life, leaving no room to condone any inhuman experimentation undertaken for any reason whatsoever.

Individual responsibility

The medical atrocities conducted by the Ishii network certainly raise questions as to who should bear responsibility and who should be punished. A Unit 731 member, who was sentenced to ten years' imprisonment at the Khabarovsk Trial, told the court: "I hope that those who are guilty of preparing to conduct bacteriological warfare and bear most responsibility for these preparations, namely, the Japanese Emperor Hirohito, Lieutenant General Ishii and Major

General Wakamatsu, will be severely punished" (Foreign Languages Publishing House 1950: 519). However, those on the lower rungs of the military ladder, who actually carried out the atrocities, must bear responsibility too, as they are the people who perfected the "art" of slaughtering human beings with their medical knowledge, abilities, curiosity, ambition, cruelty, eagerness, and creativity, often going far beyond their leaders' expectations. Without their efforts, no order could have been executed. Thus, the sins of the Emperor and the failure of national policy cannot be used to exonerate individual perpetrators from responsibility. Noda Masaaki records that, after the war, one soldier realized while in a Chinese prison that each individual must question his own responsibility for his actions before blaming his superiors (Noda 1998: 164).

As the Japanese novelist Morimura Seiichi, author of *Akuma no hoshoku* (*Devils' Gluttony*) on Unit 731, poignantly asks:

> Were those countless experiments really conducted as a result of a "collective madness"? Didn't we see the careful calculation of individuals and the spirit of exploration exhibited by medical researchers at work in those experiments? Were not those experiments actually performed for their own sake rather than for the "nation"? These questions were answered by the fact that, after the war, these experimental results were all used for the benefit of the researchers involved. The atrocities were conducted by individuals under the cloak of the "nation". That explains why they did not want to confess anything that might be disadvantageous to themselves, why they tried to hide or mitigate their crimes, and showed absolutely no regret.
>
> (Morimura 1985, 2004: 251–252)

Morimura rightly points out the culpability of each individual involved. The sad reality is that so few of the perpetrators came to regret their crimes, continually protecting themselves by recourse to one excuse after another – from the "Emperor's command," "national policy," and "orders from above" to "scientific research".

Although it was not easy for those involved to disobey orders, it was not impossible to do so, as we have already seen. One participant in the Kyushu Imperial University atrocities stated:

> No matter what kind of situation we were faced with, as long as we insisted, we could have prevented the atrocities from happening. . . . Compared with those who were arrested by the police for their anti-war activities, it would have been much easier for us to refuse to participate in the vivisection experiments. We cannot say that we did not have a choice.
>
> (Kamisaka 1979: 255)

Although such a voice is rare, it is witness to the real possibility of choice possessed by each individual. It was not because the participants did not *have* a choice, but rather because they did not try to *make* a choice. In the situation they faced, it must have been much safer to obey orders – and much easier to cast aside humanity and morality rather than reject unethical behavior.

It is an alarming fact that only a handful of perpetrators have ever expressed their guilt. Of course, some regrets may have been very private and will never be made public for fear of the embarrassment associated with disclosing a shameful past. It is ironic that, in order to hear a perpetrator's real voice, we have to turn to fiction, and to two works in particular, *The Sea and Poison* and *Song of Sadness*, by Japanese novelist Endo Shusaku (1923–1996), both of which are based on the Kyushu Imperial University atrocities.

The protagonist of *Umi to dokuyaku* [*The Sea and Poison*] (Endo 1971), Suguro, is given the option of declining his boss's invitation to participate in the vivisection. However, because he is tired of the war chaos, has no hope for peace, and has become indifferent to most events around him, he passively accepts the offer (pp. 122–124). Still, as the procedure is about to begin, he is desperate to get away, but the loud laughter of the military officers present "sounded like a thick wall and blocked his escape" (p. 130). He remains in the operating room, leaning motionlessly against the wall for most of the time (pp. 137, 143). Although not an active participant, he becomes the sole observer of the whole process of the vivisection of two American soldiers. Hearing one of them groan, he suddenly feels a sense of "powerlessness" and "humiliation." Although telling himself, "I did not do anything . . .", Suguro still hears a rhythmic voice in his ears, repeating the refrain "killed, killed, killed" (p. 147). Leaving the operating room, he descends the stairs listening to the sound of his own steps. "Two hours ago, the American soldiers also walked up these stairs without knowing what would befall them," he muses. "The good-natured face of the prisoner with chestnut hair will probably soon vanish from the surgeons' minds. But it can't disappear from my mind. I can't forget" (pp. 147–148).

Suguro's colleague Toda, who had actively participated in the vivisection, tells him: "As a result of the deaths of these prisoners, we know how to treat thousands of patients with tuberculosis. We did not kill him. We revived him. Conscience can change depending on which perspective you take." Toda continues: "I don't think those who are going to punish us would be any different if they were put in the same situation." Toda represents the attitudes of real perpetrators who try to justify whatever atrocities they have committed, but Suguro is not convinced by Toda's arguments. By telling himself "I can't forget," he has already chosen a lasting moral punishment for himself.

The Sea and Poison was adapted for the cinema in 1986 in a black-and-white feature film with the same title by director Kumai Kei. It was awarded the top prize for a Japanese film by film magazine *Kinema Junpo* and won the Silver Bear award at the 37th Berlin International Film Festival in 1987. The director interprets the "sea" in the novel as a "symbol" of the spirit and way of life of the Japanese people who "are not looking for anything supremely meaningful, but are happy to live in the world of the gods by following a conformist path" (Kumai 1987: 294). Endo later states that he wrote the novel because he wanted to show the weakness of human beings, since he himself probably would not have had the strength to maintain his belief in justice either under such circumstances (Endo 1998: 138). Nevertheless, he does not get bogged down in lamenting human weakness but rather seeks to create a character who possesses the ability for self-reflection.

The same character appeared in a further novel, *Kanashimi no uta* (*Song of Sadness*), twenty years later, in 1978. Following an abortion operation, Suguro recalls what had happened 30 years early in another operating theatre. "That time, the long corridor was deadly quiet, too, and the windows of the hospital corridor were veiled in darkness when he left the operating room, just like today. Since that evening, everything in his life has changed. Meanwhile, something that would never change was being born inside him" (Endo 1981, 2003: 58). This immutable "something" may be interpreted as his newly shaped sense of morality. In this novel, Suguro is constantly criticized by the people surrounding him. The journalist who relentlessly questions him, however, is described as a character who himself is lacking in self-reflection. This narrative technique makes it hard for readers to believe that the journalist would act any differently if placed in the same situation. Tortured by his growing sense of guilt and social pressures, Suguro eventually chooses to commit suicide. His death symbolizes the ultimate punishment – one which he imposes on himself. These two novels reveal the depth of the protagonist's soul, which is full of regret, guilt, and self-loathing because of his attendence at the vivisection.

Through the character of Suguro, Endo depicts a double movement of the psyche – on the one hand describing an individual's difficulty in maintaining a consistent moral standard, and, on the other, depicting his newly regained sense of morality through a constant recalling of the past and undergoing self-reflection. Through these two novels, Endo sheds some light on Japan's medical establish-ment, which has still not recovered from a catastrophic loss of humanity. Meanwhile, Endo also attempts to fill a gap in modern Japanese literature which, he believes, has never made the effort to probe deeply into the human soul (Endo 2000: 54). This lack of personal introspection is unlikely to be a purely literary phenomenon, but is a psychological reality in Japan and other countries. Although Suguro is a fictional character, the process of his psychological development reveals a possibility of redemption for individuals through self-reflection and restoration of morality. This is a significant means by which an individual can take responsibility for his or her actions.

Conclusion

According to Tsuneishi, "Ishii's network was not something that happened in the past, but rather it still exists in the present medical establishment in Japan. If we fail to reveal the atrocities of the past, similar atrocities can be easily repeated" (Tsuneishi 1994: 292). Moreover, I would add that the kind of "atrocity" Tsuneishi has in mind is universal, not unique to a particular nation, a particular race, or a particular time. When we study medical atrocities, we cannot be satisfied with blaming the culprits and external causes. All people, including those from victimized countries, need to examine the state of their own morality. "What would

I do if I were put in a similar situation?" "Would I refuse to participate in such atrocities?" "Would I be brave enough to refuse to obey orders?" If our answers are equivocal, then we know that the seeds of similar crimes lie in our minds too.

It is important to realize that the cycle of collective violence can be broken by the moral courage and humanity of individuals. If an individual can imagine and identify with other people's suffering, and sustain his or her moral beliefs in the face of it, then it is possible that unethical instructions can be rejected or ignored, or at least evaded. Numerous examples of individuals saving Jews from Nazi orders for their destruction have already shown that the fundamental humanity within each person can help prevent atrocities (Glover 2001: 381–393). That is why we need to learn from the attitudes of those who regard a human life as the most precious thing.

References

Akimoto, Sueo 秋元寿恵夫 1983, *Questioning Medical Ethics: My Experiences with Unit 731* 医の倫理を問う―第731部隊での体験から, Tokyo: Keiso shobo.

Aoki, Fukiko 青木富貴子 2005, *731*, Tokyo: Shinchosha.

Endo, Shusaku 遠藤周作 1971, *The Sea and Poison* 海と毒薬, Tokyo: Kodansha. English version: *The Sea and Poison*, trans. Michael Gallagher, London: Peter Owen, 1972. Quotations are my translation.

Endo, Shusaku 遠藤周作 1981, *Song of Sadness* 悲しみの歌, Tokyo: Shinchosha, 2003 new edition. English version: *Song of Sadness*, trans. Teruyu Shimizu, Ann Arbor, MI: Center for Japanese Studies, University of Michigan, 2003. Quotations are my translation.

Endo, Shusaku 遠藤周作 1998, *Futile Essays* 読んでもタメにならないエッセイ, Tokyo: Kodansha.

Endo, Shusaku 遠藤周作 2000a, "My Dissatisfaction with Modern Japanese Literature" 現代日本文学に対する私の不満, in *Complete Literary Works of Endo Shusaku* 遠藤周作文学全集 Vol. 13, Tokyo: Shinchosha.

Endo, Shusaku 遠藤周作 2000b, "A Recollection of the Showa Period" 昭和―思い出のひとつ, in *Complete Literary Works of Endo Shusaku* 遠藤周作文学全集 Vol. 13, Tokyo: Shinchosha.

Glover, Jonathan 2001, *Humanity: A Moral History of the Twentieth Century*, London: Pimlico.

Gunji, Yoko 郡司陽子 1982a, *My Testimony on Unit 731: Revelations of a Female Member* 証言　七三一石井部隊―今、初めて明かす女子隊員の記録, Tokyo: Tokuma shoten.

Gunji, Yoko 郡司陽子 (ed.) 1982b, "I was a Prisoner of the Chinese Army" わたしは中国軍の捕虜だった―総務部調査課翻訳(情報)班H・M」 *The Truth about Ishii's Germ Troops: Testimony from Participants in Top-secret Tasks* 真相　石井細菌戦部隊―極秘任務を遂行した隊員たちの証言, Tokyo: Tokuma shoten.

Guo, Xiaoye 郭晓晔 1995, *The Great Trials in the East: Documents of Trials of Japanese War Criminals* 东方大审判 审判侵华日军战犯纪实, Beijing: Jiefangjun wenyi chubanshe.

Hill, Edwin V. 1947, *Summary Report on B. W. Investigations*, Camp Detrick, December 12, in Kondo, Shoji, ed., 2003, *CD-ROM Japanese Biological Warfare; Unit 731: Official Declassified Records*, Vol. 6, Tokyo: Kashiwa shobo.

Hiyama, Yoshiaki 檜山良昭 1980, *Chasing the Doctors of the Germ Troops* 細菌部隊の医師を追え, Tokyo: Kodansha.

Hoshi, Touru 星徹 (ed.) 2002, "The Japanese War Criminals who Returned to China" 中国へ『帰郷』した日本人戦犯たち, "Military Police, Military Surgeons and Unit 731" 憲兵、軍医、そして七三一部隊, in *What We Did in China: Testimonies from the Association of Returned Prisoners of War from China*, 私たちが中国でしたこと―中国帰還者連絡会の人びと―, Tokyo: Ryokufu shuppan.

Ishida, Shinsaku 石田新作 1982, *Dedicated to Evil – The Japanese Military Doctors* 悪魔の日本軍医, Tokyo: Yamate shobo.

Kamisaka, Fuyuko 上坂冬子 1979, *Vivisection: The Incident at Kyushu University's Medical School* 生体解剖, Tokyo: Mainichi shimbunsha.

Kamiya, Noriaki 神谷則明 1998, "The Unit 731 from My Father's Story" 父が語った「731」, in *Research on War Responsibility* 季刊戦争責任研究, 19.

Kawakami, Takeshi 川上武 1965, *A History of Modern Japanese Medical Care* 現代日本医療史―開業医制の変遷―, Tokyo: Keiso shobo.

The Khabarovsk Trial 1950, *Materials on the Trial of Former Servicemen of the Japanese Army Charged with Manufacturing and Employing Bacteriological Weapons*, Moscow: Foreign Language Publishing House, in Kondo, Shoji, ed., 2003 *CD-ROM Japanese Biological Warfare; Unit 731: Official Declassified Records*, Tokyo: Kashiwa shobo.

Kondo, Shoji 近藤昭二 2002, "The Covery of Germ War Connected with Post-war Crimes" 戦後の犯罪につながる細菌戦の隠蔽, in Unit 731 and Germ War Trial Campaign Committee 731・細菌戦裁判キャンペーン委員会, ed., *Germ War to be Tried, No. 7* 裁かれる細菌戦　資料集シリーズ No. 7, Tokyo: the Editor.

Koshi, Sadao 越定男 1983, *The Japanese Flag is Soaked in Red Tears: A Confession by a Member of a Unit 731* 日の丸は紅い泪に＜第731部隊員告白記＞, Tokyo: Kyoiku shiryo shuppannkai.

Kumai, Kei 熊井啓 1987, *Film and Poison* 映画と毒薬, Tokyo: Kinema Junppo.

Matsumoto, Hiroshi 松本博 1996, "Human Experiments Conducted in Nanjing Too" 南京でもやっていた人体実験, in 731 Research Society, ed., *The Germ Troops* 細菌戦部隊, Tokyo: Banseisha.

Mizutani, Naoko 水谷尚子 1997, "The Organization and Activities of Unit 1644, with Regard to the Breakout of Pestilence in1942" 一六四四部隊の組織と活動(月)―一九四二年の崇山村ペスト流行をめぐって―, *Senso sekinin kenkyu* 戦争責任研究,, 16.

Morimura, Seiichi 森村誠一 1983, 1995a, new edition, *Devils' Gluttony* 新版　悪魔の飽食, Tokyo: Kadokawa shoten, first edition 1983, revised edition 1995.

Morimura, Seiichi 森村誠一 1983, 1995b, new edition Part II, *Devils' Gluttony* 新版続　悪魔の飽食, Tokyo: Kadokawa shoten, first edition 1983, revised edition 1995.

Morimura, Seiichi 森村誠一 1985, 2004, Part III, *Devils' Gluttony* 悪魔の飽食　第三部, Tokyo: Kadokawa shoten, first edtion 1985, revised edition 2004.

Nihon jido bungakusha kyokai 日本児童文学者協会・日本こどもを守る会 1983, 2000, ed. *Wartime Experiences, Part IV, Unit 731 in Manchuria* 続・語りつぐ戦争体験4　満州第731部隊, Tokyo: Sodo bunka.

Nishino, Rumiko 西野瑠美子 2002, "Memory of and Responsibility for Germ War" 細菌戦における記憶と責任, in Unit 731 and Germ War Trial Campaign Committee 731・細菌戦裁判キャンペーン委員会, ed., *Germ War to be Tried, No. 7* 裁かれる細菌戦資料集シリーズ No. 7, Tokyo: the Editor.

Nishizato, Fuyuko 西里扶甬子 2002, *Biological Army Unit 731: The Japanese Army's War Crimes Exempted from Prosecution by the United States* 生物戦部隊七三一 ― アメリカが免罪した日本軍の戦争犯罪, Tokyo: Kusanone shuppan.

Noda, Masaaki 野田正彰 1998, *War, Crime and Responsibility* 戦争と罪責, Tokyo: Iwanami shoten.

Ooka, Shohei 1994, *Furyoki (Taken Captive)* 俘虜記, *Selected Works of Ooka Shohei*, Tokyo: Chikuma shobo (first published 1948).

Senda, Hideo 千田英男 1996, "The Burden of My Whole Life" 終生の重荷—脳裏にこびりついて離れない断末魔の形相, 731 Research Society, ed., *The Germ War Troops* 細菌戦部隊, Tokyo: Banseisha.

731 Research Society 七三一研究会 (ed.) 1996, *The Germ Warfare Troops* 細菌戦部隊, Tokyo: Banseisha.

Shibata, Shingo 芝田進午 1998, "Ethics and Responsibilities of Medical Personnel" 医学者の倫理と責任 —「医学者」の戦争犯罪の未決済と戦後被害, in Yamaguchi Kenichiro, 山口研一郎, ed., *The Manipulation of Life and Death* 操られる生と死 — 生命の誕生から終焉まで, Tokyo: Shogakukan.

Shimizu, Hiroshi 清水寛 (ed.) 2006, 2007, *The Japanese Imperial Army and Its Soldiers with Mental Illness* 日本帝国陸軍と精神障害兵士, Tokyo: Fuji shuppan, first edition 2006, second edition 2007.

Sugamo homu iinkai 巣鴨法務委員会 1981, *The Truth of Trials of War Criminals* 戦犯裁判の実相, Vol. 1, Tokyo: Fuji shuppan.

Tsuneishi, Keiichi 常石敬一 1994, *Organized Crimes by Medical Researchers: Unit 731 of the Kwantung Army* 医学者たちの組織犯罪— 関東軍第七三一部隊, Tokyo: Asahi shimbunsha.

Tsuneishi, Keiichi 常石敬一 1995, *Unit 731: The Truth about Biological Weapons and Crimes* 七三一部隊　生物兵器犯罪の真実, Tokyo: Kodansha.

Tsuneishi, Keiichi 常石敬一 1998, "Medical Research and War: Questions to Medical Establishment" 医学と戦争—いま、医学会に問われていること, in Saito Takao and Koyama Arifumi, eds, *Lectures on Bioethics* 生命倫理学講義, Tokyo: Nihon hyoronsha.

Tsuneishi, Keiichi 常石敬一 2002, *Crossroads of Conspiracy: An Investigation into the Imperial Bank Incident and Unit 731* 謀略のクロスロード —— 帝銀事件捜査と731部隊, Tokyo: Nihon hyoronsha.

Tsuneishi, Keiichi 常石敬一 and Asano, Tomizo 朝野富三 1982, *Germ Warfare Troops and Two Medical Researchers who Committed Suicide* 細菌戦部隊と自決した二人,の医学者, Tokyo: Shinchosha.

Williams, Peter and David Wallace, 1989/2003, *Unit 731: The Japanese Army's Secret of Secrets*, London: Hodder & Stoughton/Japanese version, Nishizato Fuyuko, trans 七三一部隊の生物兵器とアメリカ — バイオテロの系譜, Kyoto: Kamogawa shuppan, 2003.

Yoshikai, Natsuko and Yuasa Ken 吉開那津子、湯浅謙 1981, 1996, *The Memories That Cannot be Erased: Records of Vivisections Performed by the Japanese Army* 増補新版　消せない記憶—日本軍の生体解剖の記録, first edition 1981, revised edition 1996.

Yoshimura, Akira 吉村昭 1975, *Fleas and Bombs* 蚤と爆弾, Tokyo: Kodansha. Originally published as *Bacteria* 細菌 in 1970.

6 On the altar of nationalism and the nation-state

Japan's wartime medical atrocities, the American cover-up, and postwar Chinese responses

Jing-Bao Nie

One of the most intrinsic and pervasive moral conflicts – universalism vs. parochialism – is intimately bound up with the ascent of science and the rise of the nation-state, two historical phenomena that have shaped the modern and contemporary world as potently as the expansion of capitalism. Advances in science and medicine are often propounded on the basis of a universalist presupposition that they will serve the well-being of humankind. Too often it has been said that science and medicine have no national boundaries – because scientific truth advances beyond artificial geographical divisions and because diseases, bacteria and viruses do not respect the borders of nation-states. At the same time, the emergence of the nation-state and the development of nationalism may be seen as modern forms of an age-old tribalism. While nationalist sentiment has often stimulated the advance and positive social application of scientific and medical knowledge, nationalism can also turn science and medicine, whether voluntarily or involuntarily, into the handmaiden of the nation-state, including its expansionist (internationally) and suppressive (domestically) aims.

Nationalist ideology can significantly increase human capacity to commit extraordinary evils and decrease human capacity to resist and address inhumanity when and after atrocities have occurred. Japan's wartime medical atrocities constitute a paradigmatic case of how human lives and fundamental values such as morality, justice, medical ethics, and scientific integrity can be sacrificed on the altar of nationalism and the nation-state. Although Japan's ambitious military schemes were defeated by joint international efforts and the Japanese biological warfare empire collapsed as a result, justice has never been served with regard to Japan's medical war crimes. While this failure is an outcome of complex historical and political factors in the postwar period, including the United States' cover-up of the physicians' activities, Japanese denial, and the relative silence of successive Chinese governments, are all among the unfortunate events involving different nation-states that have all prioritized national interests over justice and morality. In other words, a key issue has been and remains the spell of nationalism that holds Japan, China, and the United States and other nations in its thrall.

This chapter constitutes both a historical and ethical inquiry. In the first part, it presents the role of nationalist ideology in shaping Japan's wartime medical atrocities as well as in the postwar international failure to address those atrocities, what I called elsewhere the "continuing triumph of inhumanity" (Nie 2004). In the last two sections, it offers a normative account by calling up the Confucian moral imperative, "medicine as the art of humanity," and by stressing the necessity to remain alert to the powerful danger of nationalism for science and medicine.

Nationalism: an ideological foundation for the Japanese atrocities

I begin by examining the rationale for Japanese physicians and scientists to vivisect, experiment upon, and torture thousands of people. In 1936 at the first meeting of Unit 731, a motivational speech given by one of the group's leaders (probably Ishii Shiro, a specialist in bacteria-related fields and the driving engine of the Japanese bacteriological warfare machine) defined the nature of their work as "a double medical thrill." The speaker knew well that "our God-given mission as doctors is to challenge all varieties of disease-causing micro-organisms; to block all roads of intrusion into the human body; to annihilate all foreign matter resident in our bodies; and to devise the most expeditious treatment possible." Nevertheless, he bluntly admitted that the task they were about to take up involved "the complete opposite of these principles." The speaker warned his colleagues that this might cause them "some anguish as doctors." However, he assured them that their research would provide "a double medical thrill" – "one, as a scientist to exert effort to probing for the truth in natural science and research into, and discovery of, the unknown world, and two, as a military person, to successfully build a powerful military weapon against the enemy" (Williams and Wallace 1989: 37–38).

As the speaker himself realized, these two "thrills" or stimuli – the exhilaration of advancing medical science to help humankind fight diseases and the excitement felt in creating an effective biological weapon to help Japan win the war – clash. The speaker's point, however, is that whatever was necessary for Japan's victory was permissible. In the actual pursuit of this "double medical thrill," the creation of a powerful weapon took precedence over all else.

Mass atrocities are always the consequence of individual choices made in the context of a complex mix of ideology and socio-political forces. The ideological foundation which enabled Japanese doctors and scientists to create "factories of death" and conduct numerous barbaric human experiments emerged as the result of a complex process. Here I would like to highlight an all-too-familiar socio-political factor making possible systematic medically sanctioned killing: nationalism. Nationalism was the main ideological pathway to medical war crimes, just as it provided the overarching ideological framework for Japan's war of aggression in the Asia-Pacific in general.

Ishii Shiro (1892–1959) was a fierce nationalist. From his youth, Ishii "openly supported the ultranationalists, espousing their anticapitalist, antibourgeois, antiliberal, and pronational socialist views" (Harris 2002, 18–19). Trained in medicine, he made good use of his connections in the Ministry of Army to launch and develop his career in BW. The Kwantung Army, the real controller of the Japanese puppet state, provided Ishii with generous institutional support for his

BW empire centered in Manchuria (Manchukuo) and extending throughout China and beyond.

Nationalism has been closely entwined with Japan's remarkable pursuit of modernization and modernity including the development of science and technology – what was once called "civilization and enlightenment" – since the Meiji period (Gluck 1985; Shimazu 2006; Mizuno 2008). National consciousness, patriotism, and cultural nationalism, combined with the state Shinto religion, became the core of Japan's newly developed compulsory public education system. As part of this system, "ethics," or moral discipline to be accurate, was a required course, emphasizing loyalty and filial piety to the nation, the state, and the Emperor as the individual's highest civic duty. Militarism was an essential part of this mix. A high nationalist wave arrived around the first Sino-Japanese war of 1894 to 1895 and the 1904 to 1905 war with Russia. Japan's twin victories in these wars further augmented a growing nationalism. As embodied in the notion of *kokutai* (national polity), nationalism reached its peak in the 1930s and 1940s. At home, nationalist extremists carried out a series of terrorist acts, including assassinating prominent politicians, businessmen, and court officials. Nationalism fueled the military expansion that culminated in the invasion of China and other Asian countries and the attack on the American naval base at Pearl Harbor.

In the case of Japanese wartime medical atrocities, nationalism went hand in hand with imperialism and racism. Manchukuo was itself a salient example of how imperialism works together with nationalism in the creation of a modern "nation-state" (Duara 2004). In the Khabarovsk Trial conducted by the Soviet Union in late 1949, one of the accused was Major General of Medical Services Dr. Kawashima Kiyoshi, formerly Head of both the First Division (bacteriological research) and the Fourth Division (mass production and storage of bacteria) of Unit 731. When questioned by the state prosecutor about why preparations for bacteriological warfare were conducted in Japanese-occupied Manchuria rather than in mainland Japan, Kawashima replied that, in addition to the geographical advantages that would make it "easier and more convenient to deploy the bacteriological material from there," there was another major reason, namely convenience of experimentation (The Khabarovsk Trial 1950: 263). That is, "Manchuria was very convenient because there was adequate experimental material there"; in other words, human subjects were available for experimentation – *maruta* (logs of wood or lumber) to use the perpetrators' terminology for their victims.

The widespread image of Japan, often in contrast with Germany, as a country without repentance for its war atrocities, is a stereotype because many Japanese do take the past seriously. The large number of Japanese works on the wartime medical crimes cited in various chapters and listed in the bibliography of this volume clearly reflect the contributions of Japanese who have come to terms with the past. However, Japan remains deeply divided on how to remember war, colonialism, and atrocities. A critical point is that the Japanese government has been largely unrepentant, has failed to engage in self-examination, and prefers to celebrate its military heritage. This official denial is founded basically on a nationalist ideology. The financial and political protection of successive postwar governments allowed most of the individuals who were active in the biological warfare program to lead comfortable lives after the war with many becoming prominent leaders in the medical profession, research, and education. Eventually, some former members of Unit 731 such as Shinozuka [Tamura] Yoshio publicly expressed feelings of deep remorse. But others such as Mizobuchi Toshimi, who participated in destroying all evidence of the Unit's work at the end of the War, and who witnessed the killing of all remaining prisoners with methane gas, have no such regrets. Mizobuchi, who continues to convene the Unit's annual reunion, told ABC's foreign correspondent in 2003: "I am proud of what we did. If I was younger, I'd consider doing it again because it was an interesting unit." Shimizu Keihachiro, a professor at a respected Japanese university, told the same reporter that all of Japan's alleged wartime atrocities, including the Nanjing Massacre and the biological warfare program, are "lies" perpetrated by the Chinese. For Shimizu, "China is the one who did bad things. If Japan did not exist in Asia, China would have been divided up by Western people like Africa was. China has survived because of Japan." He went further: "The Japanese race has never done bad things. That is why we have become such a strong country now" (ABC Foreign Correspondent 2003).

"In the national interest:" the American justification for the cover-up

In the 1980s it became known that, immediately after the War, the U.S. authorities secretly granted the Unit 731 perpetrators, including the prime culprit Ishii, immunity from war crimes prosecution in exchange for scientific data gained from vivisections and human experimentation (Powell 1981; Williams and Wallace 1989; Harris 2002). Even direct payoff was made to perpetrators (Reed 2006). U.S. bioethicist Jonathan Moreno, a former member of President Clinton's advisory committee for handling U.S. government-sponsored human radiation experiments conducted during the Cold War, has characterized the bargain struck by the U.S. authorities with Ishii and his associates as a "deal with devils" (Moreno 2001, 87).

The postwar acts of the U.S. government, both those of commission and omission, have made it an accomplice or accessory after the fact with respect to Japanese wartime medical crimes (Nie 2005). Although American scientists and officials had detailed knowledge about Japan's biological warfare program, including the "secret of secrets" (i.e. human experimentation), and although the U.S. government was at the same time publicly and aggressively bringing many Nazi physicians to justice in the German trials, the U.S. authorities withheld vital information from the International Military Tribunal for the Far East so that Japanese medical war crimes were never prosecuted in the U.S.-controlled Tokyo trial. The American military even made cash payments to obtain the Japanese documents (Tsuneishi 2005; Reed 2006). Moreover, the U.S. authorities publicly poured scorn on irrefutable evidence of Japanese medical atrocities from other sources, notably the Soviet Union's Khabarovsk Trial.

Those U.S. officials who were involved recognized the inconsistencies and double standards in their different treatment of the Nazi and Japanese doctors. For instance, the 1947 report of the subcommittee of the State–War–Navy Coordinating Committee charged with directing information acquired into the appropriate intelligence channels noted that:

> Experiments on human beings similar to those conducted by the Ishii BW group have been condemned as war crimes by the International Military Tribunal for the trial of major Nazi war criminals in its decision handed down at Nuremburg on 30 September 1946. . . . This government is at present prosecuting leading German scientists and medical doctors at Nuremberg for offences which included experiments on human beings which resulted in the suffering and death of those experimented on.
>
> (Harris 2002, 301)

However, far from prosecuting the Unit 731 scientists, the U.S. granted them immunity from prosecution in exchange for valuable scientific data. In his summary report dated December 12, 1947, Dr. Edwin V. Hill, Chief, Basic Sciences, Camp Detrick (headquarters of the U.S. BW program), explained:

> Evidence gathered in this investigation . . . has been obtained by Japanese scientists at the expenditure of many millions of dollars and years of work. Information has accrued with respect of human susceptibility to those diseases as indicated by specific infectious doses of bacteria. Such information could not be obtained in our own laboratories because of scruples attached to human experimentation. These data were secured with a total outlay of ¥ 250,000 to date, a mere pittance by comparison with the actual cost of the studies.
>
> (Harris 2002, 264)

The decision to grant immunity was not made without hesitation. U.S. officials were aware of the possible risks, as Colonel R. M. Cheseldine, a member of the State–War–Navy Coordinating Committee, remarked at a meeting held on September 26, 1947: "This government may at a later date be seriously embarrassed." Still, Cheseldine concluded, "this information, particularly that which will finally be obtained from the Japanese with respect to the effect of BW on humans, is of such importance to the security of this country that the risk of subsequent embarrassment should be taken" (ibid., 303).

The decision-making process by U.S. scientific, military, and government authorities regarding Japanese BW war crimes was marked by a striking absence of ethical or moral considerations. American historian Sheldon Harris (2002, 305) poignantly summarized the issues at stake:

> No one in 1948 was prepared to raise the issue of ethics, or morality, or traditional Western or Judeo-Christian human values in confronting those responsible for the Japanese BW negotiation. The questions of ethics and

morality as they affected scientists in Japan and in the United States never once entered into a single discussion that is recorded in any of the minutes, notes, records of meetings, and so on, from the initial Murray Sanders reports of November 1945 to the Joint Chiefs of Staff cable to General MacArthur on March 13, 1948. In all the considerable documentation that has survived over the more than five decades since the events described, not one individual is chronicled as having said BW human experiments were an abomination and that their perpetrators should be prosecuted.

It was therefore for the sake of the national interest and national security that the U.S. authorities released indictable war criminals. One of the many ironies to emerge from the Japanese BW war crimes and their aftermath is that the intentions of U.S. scientists and officials to extract useful information from the Japanese data were probably never fulfilled.

The American postwar cover-up of Japan's wartime medical atrocities for the sake of the national interest – complicity after the fact, as clearly defined by the common law tradition – not only trampled on morality and justice in general, but has become a historical burden for the U.S. on the international stage. Such fall-out will continue to haunt the U.S. government until it faces up to its actions and takes meaningful steps to rectify them. These should include an official apology by the U.S. government and/or Congress for its cover-up of Japan's medical atrocities and the provision of appropriate financial compensation to the families of victims (Nie 2005).

An excursus: nationalist rhetoric in the Soviet Union's Khabarovsk Trial

From December 23–30, 1949, in Khabarovsk, the Soviet Union conducted an open trial of 12 former Japanese servicemen (eight were physicians and scientists) ranking from Commander-in-Chief of the Kwantung Army, under which Unit 731 operated, to the heads of the Unit's various divisions and as far down the scale of responsibility as laboratory orderlies (see Chapter 3, this volume; also Nie 2004). Despite many shortcomings such as the lack of international participation, the trial proved beyond reasonable doubt that the Japanese Imperial Army had established an extensive biological warfare program, that bacteriological weapons were manufactured and employed, and that Japanese physicians and scientists conducted barbaric experiments on living human beings. Moreover, the Soviet Union made efforts to disseminate the facts verified at the Khabarovsk Trial through diplomatic channels and the media, including the publication of the trial materials in English and other languages. Unfortunately, until the early 1980s the West almost totally dismissed the facts uncovered by this remarkable trial as mere "communist propaganda" (Nie 2004).

The Khabarovsk Trial was the one bright spot in a series of disappointing international responses to Japan's wartime medical atrocities. However, a stridently nationalist tone was evident throughout the trial. For instance, in his final speech,

State Prosecutor Smirnov asserted that, prior to the 1930s, "Peace in the Soviet Far East was maintained only as a result of the genius of Stalin's policy, as a result of the victorious consummation of the Stalin five-year plans, as a result of the vigilant concern displayed by the Bolshevik Party and the Soviet Government for the strengthening of the Soviet Armed Forces" (The Khabarovsk Trial 1950, 407). Moreover, "It was only the crushing blow of the Soviet Armed Forces" that initially "saved mankind from the horrors of bacteriological warfare into which the Hitlerite miscreants were preparing to plunge the world" and that "again saved mankind from the horror of bacteriological warfare" and "with a swift blow shattered the major striking force of criminal Japanese imperialism – the Kwantung Army" (ibid., 411).

To a great extent, considerations of the national interest drove the Soviet investigation. Perhaps for this reason, it never sought active international participation in bringing Japanese war criminals to trial. Its conduct nevertheless contrasts with the U.S. protection of the perpetrators of the biowar program and buying their data.

China's postwar responses

China's postwar response – or lack of adequate response – to Japan's wartime medical atrocities is an intriguing story. The attitudes of successive Chinese governments – both Nationalist and Communist – have perplexed analysts (Harris 2002, 314–317). No Chinese administration has ever rigorously pursued justice on behalf of the Chinese victims. It seems that nationalism or a particular concept of the national interest yet again provides a key to explaining China's relative lack of action over the Japanese BW crimes.

In the Tokyo Trial, only the Soviet representatives consistently pursue the subject of redress for victims. The judge and representative from the Republic of China and the Nationalist Party were basically silent on the subject from start to finish. While the Nanjing Trial held by the Republic of China in 1946 and later trials conducted by the People's Republic of China, especially that in Fushun in 1956, investigated Japanese BW crimes, both the Nationalist and Communist military tribunals failed to rigorously investigate these crimes. The sentences handed down in these trials were even more lenient than those awarded in the Khabarovsk Trial. In contrast to the Doctors' Trial during the Nuremberg Tribunal in which seven of the 23 Nazi physicians and medical administrators charged were sentenced to death by hanging, no Japanese doctors were sentenced to death in any of the Russian and Chinese trials (see Chapter 2, this volume).

How do we account for these discrepancies? This may be impossible to answer in the absence of court and archival records. Some remarks by Mao Zedong provide clues, though they fail to fully clarify the Communist government's standpoint on the subject. In interviews with delegations and individual visitors from Japan between 1955 and 1961, Mao reflected on how China should deal with the legacy of the war with Japan. In the context of the Cold War, he stressed repeatedly that the majority of the Japanese people were China's friends and that American imperialism was the common enemy of the Chinese and Japanese people. Thus Chinese and Japanese should unite to overcome American political and military interference in Asia. In order to move forward, Mao promoted an approach predicated on forgetting, rather than remembering. In his own words to Japanese visitors: "Our ancestors once quarreled, fought with each other. All this can be forgotten now! All this should be forgotten because it is unpleasant stuff. What use is it to keep it in our minds?" Noting that many Japanese visitors referred to the evils of Japan's invasion of China and apologized for it, Mao insisted that it was "not reasonable to demand a payment for past debt. You have apologized. You cannot apologize every day, can you?" (Mao 1994: 226). "Japan is no longer in debt to anyone. Rather, other countries owe Japan" (438). Mao went further, stating that although Japan's invasion into China was of course wrong, it also had some beneficial effects so that in some sense the Chinese owed "thanks" to the Japanese Imperial Army (226). In a meeting with a parliamentary representative from the Japan Socialist Party, Mao explained:

> It is the Japanese warlords who occupied more than half of China, a reality which educated the Chinese people. Otherwise, the Chinese people would still be not awakened, nor united; we would still be living in the mountains [as guerrillas], and would never have come here to Beijing to see the Beijing Opera. It is because of the Japanese Imperial Army, which occupied half of China, that the Chinese people found themselves in a tight corner, woke up, armed themselves to fight, and established many [Communist-led] bases against the Japanese, thus creating the conditions necessary to win the "War of Liberation" [the Communist war against the Nationalist Party]. So the Japanese warlords and monopoly capitalists did us a good turn. If "thanks" are due at all, I would rather thank the Japanese warlords.
>
> (Mao 1994, 460–461; all translations of Mao's words cited here are by Nie)

Mao's remarks, appealing to the Japanese people through his progressive visitors to help break China's isolation and establish China–Japan diplomatic relations, acknowledged Japan's inadvertent contribution to the eventual Communist Party victory, first in the anti-Japanese resistance and subsequently in the civil war with the Guomindang. They reveal Mao's pragmatic strategy of combining realpolitik with an appeal to the nation-state and nationalist sentiment.

Mao's remarks in fact resonate with the thought-provoking thesis on the key role of "peasant nationalism" in revolutionary China (Johnson 1962). This thesis argues that Japanese invasion evoked a nationalist response which resulted not only in Japan's ultimate defeat but contributed to the rise of the Chinese Communist Party. The success of Communist power lay not in the machinations of the international Communist movement, nor its economic (land reform) policies, but in effectively channeling mass nationalism to win support and legitimacy in the face of a ruthless invader.

Indeed, the Communist Chinese state has been continuing to shape and utilize nationalism to mobilize a vast nation and strengthen its claim to legitimacy. In the context of responding or not responding to Japan's wartime medical atrocities, the issue has long become a political tool either to increase nationalist ferment when it is politically useful or to quash calls for justice when the state no longer wishes to make use of mass nationalism to achieve its goals. Zhou Enlai, China's Premier, once disclosed the official reason for the lenient sentences given to the Japanese war criminals and for returning them to Japan after re-education and trials – these war criminals were themselves the victims of war. Moreover, they had the potential to strengthen relations between Japan and China in the long run (again, see Chapter 2, this volume). In other words, leniency, in stark contrast with the ruthlessness of Japan's treatment of the Chinese people, was justified by the overall interests of the Chinese and Japanese people, and even world peace. Zhou played the central role in dealing with Japanese POWs who were re-educated and, in 1956, sent back to Japan. Indeed, many of them subsequently spent a lifetime speaking about their atrocities in China and participating in peace activism, often through the Association of Returnees from China (*Chugoku Kikansha Renrakukai*, abbreviated as *Chukiren*). The approach for which Zhou was primarily responsible may be viewed, as claimed officially, to be a brilliant diplomatic and humanitarian success. Not only has China's clemency helped to open the way toward China–Japan reopening relations, but the return of the soldiers proves highly advantageous in raising issues of war atrocities in ways far more effective than, for example, Chinese criticism of Japan. In addition, the Chinese authorities are right that the captured soldiers were not those who bore the highest responsibilities; indeed, they too were victims, seeing the issue of justice from another angle.

Nevertheless, what I would like to focus on here is the role of nationalist sentiment and ideology. Nationalism, in the forms of state, intellectual or scholarly, and mass nationalism, has overshadowed China's official and popular postwar responses to Japanese wartime medical atrocities. As manifested in standard historical textbooks, academic studies and mass media (e.g., Nan 2005), the anti-Japanese war in general, and Japan's wartime medical atrocities in particular occupy a salient part in the contemporary collective memory of China. This collective memory is fundamentally nationalistic, defining Japanese perpetrators of war crimes as "devils" and "enemies of Chinese people." As a result, the universal dimension of Japanese war crimes is rarely expressed in the nationalist memory. The well-known Unit 731 Criminal Evidence Museum (*Qinhua Rijun Diqisanyi Budui Zhizhen Chenlieguan*) in Harbin, like the Memorial of Nanjing Massacre in Nanjing, is an important site of "patriotic education" (*aiguo zhuyi jiaoyu*). The major reason for remembering Japan's wartime medical atrocities is to sustain and enhance patriotism in the service of realizing the collective Chinese dream, to make the nation wealthy and strong (*fuqiang*).

While both the Nationalist and Communist governments, in part owing to the rivalry between them, never actively pursued war reparations from Japan, in the past decade some Chinese victims of Japanese biological warfare have begun seeking justice and compensation in lower level Japanese courts, supported by non-governmental organizations in China and Japanese lawyers and NGOs (see Nan 2005). This is part of a wider effort to redress war crimes including forced labor, sexual slavery ("comfort women"), and the Nanjing Massacre. However, although tolerating them, the Chinese government has not encouraged these efforts, perhaps because officials believe that activism of this kind might undermine the relationship between the two countries and might also undermine social stability within China.

Interestingly, the recent phenomenon of seeking justice and compensation on behalf of the victims of Japanese war crimes reflects the expansion of Chinese nationalism since the 1980s, and especially since the 1990s. In China, as in Japan and the United States, nationalism pervades modern and contemporary life (Gries 2004; Sleeboom 2004; Zhao 2004; Hughes 2006; Shirk 2007). While Chinese may disagree radically on concrete foreign policy issues, like in many other countries, nationalist sentiment often constitutes a shared common ground. For instance, as we have seen, state nationalism on the one hand and elite and mass nationalisms on the other result in very different approaches to Japan's wartime medical atrocities – the former tending to let the issue rest and the latter seeking justice and compensation. Yet, each of these responses appeals to nationalist sentiment.

Sociologically and ethically, Japanese wartime medical atrocities provide a textbook case of collective and state violence. We may note that despite their very different historical and political contexts, Japanese war crimes and the state and popular violence associated with the Chinese Cultural Revolution of the 1960s and 1970s display certain uncanny similarities. Both campaigns were carried out in the name of good and even holy causes; both sharply constrained freedom of discussion and press; both involved the active participation of ordinary people in extraordinary acts of collective violence, treating fellow human beings as non-humans; and both were facilitated by the state (Nie 2005). It should also be pointed out that, at the same time when they were mercifully treating Japanese war criminals, the party and government of the People's Republic were mercilessly executing thousands of Chinese classified as "class enemies," including landlords, rich peasants, capitalists, and anti-revolutionaries in order to secure the newly established Communist power. And earlier, during China's civil war in which millions of Chinese died, a series of war crimes were committed by Nationalists as well as Communists. For instance, from June to October 1948, the People's Liberation Army besieged Changchun, a northeastern city where Japan's other infamous biological warfare unit (Unit 100) was located. At lease 160,000 civilians died from famine directly resulting from the siege. A Chinese historian whose book on the subject was banned immediately after its publication in 1989 has compared Changchun with Hiroshima: the similar civilian casualties taking nine seconds in one place and five months in another (Zhang 2002, ch. 31; for a journalist report see Jacobs 2009).

It is beyond question that foreign aggression and exploitation, like Japan's brutal invasion, were among the major causes of China's massive social suffering throughout the long twentieth century. It is nevertheless seriously misleading to single out imperialism, colonialism, and the depredations of foreign states and nations as *the* most important cause, as the official Chinese ideology and nationalist discourse often have. On the way to win power and during the course of governing, Chinese states – Nationalist and Communist – have imposed upon Chinese people massive violence and social sufferings, more than those by foreign states. Unfortunately, due partly to the spell of nationalism, the Chinese medical professions and scientific communities are both victims and victimizers in the power exercise of nation-states.

"Medicine as the art of humanity": an old Confucian moral imperative

It is strange that, as noted in the Introduction (see also Nie et al. 2009), international as well as East Asian medical ethics has paid little attention to these atrocities in more than half a century. Even in Japan and China, the subject has been treated as having little relevance to contemporary science, medicine, and medical ethics. Here I do not intend to explore this phenomenon. Rather, I will consider Japan's wartime atrocities in the light of Confucian and East Asian culture in general, and its perspective on health care and morality in particular.

It has been suggested and often believed among contemporary Chinese and Japanese that Japan's wartime medical atrocities were intimately linked with East Asian culture in which such values as collectivism and obedience to secular authorities (such as parents and emperors) are strongly emphasized and even institutionalized (e.g., Tsuchiya 2000). However, this wrongly implies that Japanese war crimes are justifiable according to the dictates of East Asian culture and morality, and that these acts are only wrong in the eyes of Western culture and morality. However, "Japanese doctors' human experimentation is not only an offence against Western morality, against the common sense of humanity, but also *against Asian and Japanese moral principles and ethical ideals*" (Nie 2001: 5, emphasis in original). East Asian cultural and moral traditions should in no sense be regarded as ethically responsible for the human experimentation carried out by the Japanese doctors and the international failure of justice that followed it.

Japan's wartime medical atrocities are an affront to fundamental East Asian moral norms such as compassion (*ci*) in Buddhism, and humanity (*ren*) and righteousness (*yi*) in Confucianism. They even transgress the basic moral concepts of Japanese samurai traditions such as *gi* (justice, rectitude, or morality) and *jin* (humanity, sympathy, virtue). Specifically, they violate a deep-rooted moral principle in East Asian medical ethics traditions drawing on Confucianism, especially Neo-Confucianism – that is, medicine as the art of humanity or humaneness (*yi nai renshu*). One way to resist the increasing power of the contemporary state and nationalism, and their threats to medical professionalism and medical ethics, is to recall this Confucian vision of medical morality.

Partly to enhance the moral and social status of medicine in Confucian society, ancient Chinese medical practitioners promoted the idea of "medicine as the art of humanity." As a core concept in Confucianism, *ren* has different shades of meaning when applied to ethics and politics. It has been translated variously as "humaneness," "benevolence," "perfect virtue," "goodness," "human-heartedness," "love," "altruism," and "humanity." A widely quoted Chinese saying, which can be traced to the eleventh century, avers that "He who lacks the opportunity to work as a good prime minister may work as a good physician." Koizumi Chikahiko, a strong supporter of Ishii and at one time Japan's minister of health, liked to quote a Chinese proverb derived from this saying: "Great doctors tend the country, good doctors tend the people, and lesser doctors heal illness" (Harris 2002: 21). As this latter saying suggests, both medicine and the civil service serve the same Confucian moral goals. Medicine as the art of humanity requires the physician not only to master Confucian teachings but, more importantly, to follow Confucian morals in medical practice. Ming Dynasty physician Gong Tingxian, in his famous "Ten Maxims for Physicians," explains that "physicians must adopt a disposition of humaneness [*renxin*, a heart of humanity]. This is essential. They should make special efforts to assist people of every walk of life so that their good deeds have far-reaching influence" (Unschuld 1979; Nie 2009).

The notion of "medicine as the art of humanity" has been essential for medical ethics in Japan as well. It has been practiced by Japanese doctors over many centuries and is highly valued in Japan today. This is the ethical ideal of "complete dedication to the patient and the art of medicine" articulated by Wada Tokaku, the eighteenth-century Japanese physician and medical philosopher, whose ideals were informed by Buddhism, Daoism-inspired Zen Buddhism in particular, and the samurai code (Matsumoto et al. 2001). In stark contrast, in the eyes of the perpetrators of wartime medical atrocities, the human subjects of their experiments were not patients, not human beings, not even animals – but merely "logs of wood" (*maruta*) or "experimental materials."

The moral imperative of medicine as the art of humanity offers a counter-thesis to the exaltation of nationalism in science. In general, the Confucian universalist ideal of "all people under heaven" as brothers, an ancient Eastern version of internationalism, runs counter to the sweeping tide of nationalism in the modern world. In particular, the old Confucian designation of medicine as a great Dao (Way), medicine as the art of humanity, defines the primary goal of medicine not as glorifying any particular nation-state or group but as serving the general welfare of humanity. In light of this, scientific research and the social application of scientific knowledge must strive to adhere to moral norms. Science and medicine should ultimately be life-affirming. Indeed, the influential but too often violated Confucian political principle of ethical governance (*renzheng*) requires all social policies, including those related to science and medicine, to put people as the highest priority, the ruler as secondary, and the kingdom or nation as the least weighty entity of the three.

Concluding remarks

Nationalism as an ideology has a very dark side with respect to medicine and science. As Japan's wartime medical atrocities and the international postwar responses to them have demonstrated, not only did nationalism provide Japan with an ideological path to medical butchery and thus turn the art of healing into a vehicle for inhumanity, it also served the United States as a justification for exploiting the fruits of evil. Moreover, the failure of the primary victim, China, to deal effectively with the "inhuman medicine" to which it was subjected and to pursue justice for victims is itself directly linked with nationalism. On the altar of the nation-state, all that is good and valuable may be sacrificed: not only human lives, but also morality and justice, humanity and righteousness, to use some potent Confucian terms.

Although the great majority of social thinkers in the nineteenth and the early twentieth centuries anticipated the significance of scientific advances for human life, few foresaw the massive expansion of nationalism and chauvinism or their deadly consequences during this period (Berlin 1998). In fact, most major modern social thinkers including Karl Marx anticipated the opposite: the decline and gradual death of nation-states and the shrinking power of nationalist ideology. Today, the study of nationalism has become a field with voluminous and continuing contributions from scholars from across the humanities and social sciences. On the one hand, it has been widely acknowledged that nations are socially and historically constructed, that they are "imagined communities" (Anderson 1991 [1983]), and that the ideology of nationalism has led to the foundation of nations and nation-states (Hobsbawm 1990) – rather than the other way around as is commonly assumed. At the same time, the sweeping power of nationalism is a contemporary reality that continues to develop and is increasingly felt in every aspect of life, from sport and politics to science and medicine. The comparative histories of England, France, Russia, Germany, the United States, and Japan suggest that nationalism has been crucial to the rise of modernity and national economic growth and represents the real spirit of capitalism (Greenfield 1992, 2001).

Surprisingly, while such disciplines as the history and sociology of science have been institutionalized from the mid-twentieth century, the literature on the interaction of nationalism and science remains fragmentary (Crawford 1992). Surely, studies of such notorious subjects as Nazi medicine and Lysenkoism in the Soviet Union should at least touch on the role of the nation-state and nationalism. But the major focus of these investigations often lies elsewhere – e.g., on the impact of racism, particularly anti-Semitism, and totalitarian attitudes to science and medicine.

At the beginning of the twentieth century (1902), three decades before the development of Japan's bacteriological warfare program, William Osler, one of the greatest physicians of modern times, delivered an address on "Chauvinism in Medicine" to the Canadian Medical Association. Osler defined medicine in terms of four essential features: its noble ancestry, its remarkable solidarity, its progressive character, and its singular beneficence. Doctors' aims are universal – to treat and prevent disease. Chauvinism and nationalism are dangerous for medicine, constituting "the great curse of humanity": "In no other shape has the Demon of Ignorance assumed more hideous proportions; to no other obsession do we yield ourselves more readily" (Osler 2001: 234). Too often, human beings, physicians included, have subordinated the human race to the nation, "forgetting the higher claims of human brotherhood." Osler believed in the beneficent power of medicine, a power that could transcend national boundaries: "There seems to be no limit to the possibilities of scientific medicine; philosophers see, as in some far-off vision, a science from which may come in the prophetic words of the Son of Sirach, 'Peace over all the earth' " (232). For him, "While medicine is everywhere tinctured with national characteristics, the wider aspects of the profession . . . – our common lineage and the community of interests – should always save us from the more vicious aspects of this sin, if it cannot prevent it altogether" (235–236). We "may congratulate ourselves that the worst aspects of nationalism in medicine are disappearing before the broader culture and the more intimate knowledge brought by ever-increasing intercourse" (237). Osler (2001: 249) summed up optimistically:

> The open mind, the free spirit of science . . . the liberal and friendly relationship between different nations and different sections of the same nation, the brotherly feeling which should characterize members of the oldest, most beneficent and universal guild that the race has evolved in its upward progress – these should neutralize the [Chauvinist and nationalist] tendencies upon which I have so lightly touched.

In the aftermath of Nazi medicine and Japan's wartime medical atrocities, as well as numerous unethical examples of medical research and practice elsewhere, one can no longer share the optimism of Osler and his contemporaries a century ago regarding the universal and singular beneficence of medicine, and scientific biomedicine in particular. There are many ethical lessons still to learn from Japan's wartime medical atrocities and the postwar responses to them. The Confucian ideal of medicine as the art of humanity – rather than being merely a means of serving nationalist interests and the political tool of the state – has renewed relevance for our so-called "postmodern" world. Resisting the abuse of science and medicine by the nation-state should be a priority, if not *the* priority, for contemporary medical ethics and medical professionalism. In the modern world, science and medicine can no longer develop – or even survive – without support from the state. However, if they are totally subordinated to the interests and power of the nation-state, science and medicine erode their own moral grounds for existence as autonomous professions.

Acknowledgments

I am grateful for the characteristically insightful comments and helpful suggestions from Professors Arthur Kleinman and Mark Selden in writing and revising this chapter.

References

ABC Foreign Correspondent. 2003. Unit 731. ABC TV, April 22.
Anderson, Benedict. 1991 (revised edition; first edition 1983). *Imagined Communities: Reflections on the Origin and Spread of Nationalism*. London: Verso.

Berlin, Isaiah. 1998. Nationalism: Past Neglect and Present Power. In his *The Proper Study of Mankind: An Anthology of Essays*. New York: Farrar, Straus & Giroux.

Crawford, Elisabeth. 1992. *Nationalism and Internationalism in Science 1880–1939: Four Studies of the Nobel Population*. Cambridge: Cambridge University Press.

Duara, Prasenjit. 2004. *Sovereignty and Authenticity: Manchukuo and the East Asian Modern*. Lanham: Rowman & Littlefield.

Gluck, Carol. 1985. *Japan's Modern Myths: Ideology in the Late Meiji Period*. Princeton, NJ: Princeton University Press.

Greenfield, Liah. 1992. *Nationalism: Five Roads to Modernity*. Cambridge, MA: Harvard University Press.

Greenfield. Liah. 2001. *The Spirit of Capitalism: Nationalism and Economic Growth*. Cambridge, MA: Harvard University Press.

Gries, Peter Hays. 2004. *China's New Nationalism: Pride, Politics, and Diplomacy*. Berkeley: University of California Press.

Harris, S. 2002 (revised edition; first edition 1994). *Factories of Death: Japanese Biological Warfare 1932–1945 and the American Cover-up*. New York: Routledge.

Hobsbawm, E. J. 1990. *Nations and Nationalism since 1780: Programme, Myth, Reality*. Cambridge: Cambridge University Press.

Hughes, Christopher R. 2006. *Chinese Nationalism in the Global Era*. London: Routledge.

Hutchinson, John and Anthony D. Smith. 1994. *Nationalism* (Oxford Reader). Oxford: Oxford University Press.

Jacobs, Andrew. 2009. China is Wordless on Traumas of Communists' Rise. *New York Times*, October 2.

Johnson, Chalmers A. 1962. *Peasant Nationalism and Communist Power: The Emergence of Revolutionary China 1937–1945*. Stanford, CA: Stanford University Press.

The Khabarovsk Trial. 1950. *Materials on the Trial of Former Servicemen of the Japanese Army Charged with Manufacturing and Employing Bacteriological Weapons*. Moscow: Foreign Language Publishing House.

Mao, Zedong. Edited by the Ministry of Foreign Affairs of the PRC and the Research Office of Historical Literature of the Central Committee of the Chinese Communist Party. 1994. *Selected Essays of Mao Zedong on Foreign Affairs*. Beijing: The CCCCP Literature Press and World Knowledge Press.

Matsumoto, Masatoshi, Kazuo Inoue and Eiji Kajii. 2001. "Words of Tohkaku Wada: Medical Heritage in Japan." *Journal of Medical Ethics* 27: 55–58.

Mizuno, Hiromi. 2008. *Science for the Empire: Scientific Nationalism in Modern Japan*. Stanford, CA: Stanford University Press.

Moreno, J.D. 2001. *Undue Risk: Secret State Experiments on Humans*. New York: Routledge.

Nan, Xianghong. 2005. Ultimate Crime: Bacteriological Warfare Not Yet Ended. *Nanfang Zhoumo* (Southern Weekend), July 7.

Nie, J.B. 2001. Challenges of Japanese Doctors' Human Experimentation in China for East-Asian and Chinese Bioethics. *Eubios Journal of Asian and International Bioethics* 11: 3–7. Available online at http://www2.unescobkk.org/eubios/EJ111/ej111d.htm.

Nie, J.B. 2004. The West's Dismissal of the Khabarovsk Trial as "Communist Propaganda": Ideology, Evidence and International Bioethics. *Journal of Bioethics Inquiry* 1(1): 32–42.

Nie, J.B. 2005. State Violence in Twentieth-century China: Some Shared Features of the Japanese Army's Atrocities and the Cultural Revolution's Terror. In Ludger Kühnhardt and Mamoru Takayama, eds, *Menchenrechte, Kulturen und Gewalt: Ansaetze einer Interkulturellen Ethik* [*Human Rights, Cultures, and Violence: Perspectives of Intercultural Ethics*]. Baden-Baden: Nomos.

Nie, J.B. 2006. The United States Cover-up of Japanese Wartime Medical Atrocities: Complicity Committed in the National Interest and Two Proposals for Contemporary Action. *American Journal of Bioethics* 6(3): W21–W33.

Nie, J.B. 2009. The Discourses of Practitioners in China. In R. Baker and L. McCullough, eds, *The Cambridge World History of Medical Ethics*. New York and London: Cambridge University Press.

Nie, J.B., Tsuchiya, T. and Li, L. 2009. Japanese Doctors' Experimentation in China, 1932–1945, and Medical Ethics. In R. Baker and L. McCullough, eds, *The Cambridge World History of Medical Ethics*. New York and London: Cambridge University Press.

Osler, William. 2001. *Osler's "A Way of Life" and Other Addresses*, edited and annotated by Shigeaki Hinohara and Hisae Niki. Durham, NC: Duke University Press.

Powell, J.W. 1981. Japan's Biological Weapons: 1930–1945, A Hidden Chapter in History. *Bulletin of the Atomic Scientists* October: 44–52.

Reed, Christopher. 2006. The United States and the Japanese Mengele: Payoffs and Amnesty for Unit 731 Scientists. *Japan Focus*, August 1, 2006. Available online at http://japanfocus.org/products/topdf/2177.

Shimazu, Naoko (ed). 2006. *Nationalism in Japan*. London: Routledge.

Shirk, Susan. 2007. *China: Fragile Superpower*. Oxford: Oxford University Press.

Sleeboom, Margaret. 2004. *Academic Nations in China and Japan*. London: RoutledgeCurzon.

Tsuchiya, T. 2000. Why Japanese Doctors Performed Human Experiments in China 1933–1945. *Eubios Journal of Asian and International Bioethics* 10: 179–280. Available online at http://www2.unescobkk.org/eubios/EJ106/ej106c.htm.

Tsuneishi, K. 2005. New Facts about US Payoff to Japan's Biological Warfare Unit 731. *Japan Focus*, August 15. Available online at http://japanfocus.org/products/topdf/2209.

Unschuld, Paul. 1979. *Medical Ethics in Imperial China*. Berkeley: University of California Press.

Williams, Peter and David Wallace. 1989. *Unit 731: The Japanese Army's Secret of Secrets*. London: Hodder & Stoughton.

Zhang Zhengrong. 2002 [1989]. *Xuebai Xuehong: Guogong Dongbei Dajuezhan Lishizhengxiang* [*White as Snow, Red as Blood: The Historical Truth of the Decisive Battles of Nationalists and Communist in Northeastern China*]. Hong Kong: Tiandi Tushu.

Zhao, Suisheng. 2004. *A Nation-state by Construction: Dynamics of Modern Chinese Nationalism*. Stanford, CA: Stanford University Press.

Part III

Ethics and historical memory

Parallel lessons from Germany and the U.S.A.

7 Bioethics and exceptionalism

A German example of learning from "medical" atrocities

Ole Döring

Introduction: the current wave of exceptionalism in bioethics

This chapter offers an approach to ethical exceptionalism, which poses a challenge to contemporary bioethics. It re-emphasizes a non-relativistic ethics by setting out a concept of ethics that systematically combines theoretical philosophical reflection with narrative material. The memorial at the former concentration camp of Ravensbrück, with its atrocities in the name of medicine, exemplifies the purpose and constructive meaning of moral learning from experiences of inhumanity. Thus it connects the individual moral account with global community ethics.

The language of medical genomics is loaded with dramatic terminology and metaphors of warfare. The hype surrounding the "Gene Wars," associated with the Human Genome Project, is well documented. It is well understood that premature expectations and the race to secure advantages and opportunities can readily culminate in strategic coalitions between researchers, policy makers, and industry. Recently, this rhetoric seems to have gained new momentum. On the other hand, the World Medical Association has made it very clear that medical ethics under exceptional conditions, as in time of war, are subject to the same basic rules that apply during peacetime, as set out in the Helsinki Declaration and other documents.

Recently, a flurry of activism in the aftermath of the terror attacks of September 11, 2001 has reinvigorated the debate over questions of emergency and triage in biomedical ethics. For example, Michael Gross has introduced a critical framework for analyzing the application of medical ethics under conditions of conflict. On balance, he seems to be leaving the question of whether conflict situations require distinct types of ethics controversially open. Gross explains the stakes clearly enough: "Wartime triage pushes further when casualties overwhelm medical facilities. The question is not when a patient is treated, but who is treated" (Gross 2006: 329).

Others have argued more pointedly for an ethical relativism based on a moral framework that accepts the idea of exceptionalism. "The use of war or warlike powers has to come from the right intentions, i.e. the argument that one wants to protect the people must be serious. . . . War and warlike situations need to be the means of last resort." And, "Extreme situations require extreme, sometimes very unpleasant and very extraordinary means" (Sass 2005: 164).

For the sake of conceptual clarity, we need to remind ourselves that, notwithstanding the merits of such an axiomatic ethics, there is still no proven way of measuring or otherwise positively accounting for "good" or "right" intentions and of distinguishing mere rhetoric or the formal parroting of a moral platform from action that proceeds from genuine moral determination. Thus, research that aims at developing desperately needed social goods (such as medicines) cannot substantially base the ethical justification of morally problematic methodologies on promises or expectations of the resulting benefits – as is evident from the rejection of the maxim that the means justify the ends. The recent direction of bioethical debate calls us to reacquaint ourselves with the fundamentals of moral rationality.

No pragmatic, utilitarian, or otherwise consequential argument can override basic ethical principles. The only rationale for admitting an exception is that particular circumstances allow it exclusively to serve these same principles, albeit in a different manner than under normal circumstances. Obviously, the burden of proof, and the responsibility for any adverse consequences of such an ethical judgment, lies on those who claim the exception. And whether the claim of exceptional circumstances can or cannot be justified in a particular case, it can never be argued that the end justifies the means – and neither should the means contradict the spirit of the end. Thus, from a philosophical perspective, the only justifiable instance of positive exceptionalism turns out to be, on closer inspection, in no way a departure from fundamental ethical imperatives, but rather the opposite – an endorsement of the need to pay close attention to the real and actual requirements of a given principle. It expresses an alert appreciation of the contingency of practice, which occasionally happens to transgress the bounds of moral convention. Hence, in biomedical ethics there can be no exception, for instance, from the inviolability of human dignity, even when circumstances seem to indicate that conventional codes of practice, as morally or legally prescribed, cannot apply. Only in this way can one acknowledge exceptional situations while rejecting relativism.

Given the case in point, the question is clearly, as Gross puts it, whether, "[I]f medicine serves the aims of war its duty to safeguard human life at all cost will suffer?" (Gross 2006: 329). That is to say, whether we can accept the conditional "if" and still affirm the consequences in medical ethics terms. Is it possible, or can it be ethically justified in the first place, for medicine to bind itself to any external cause, such as the goals and necessities of war, or a particular scientific-cum-political agenda?

Again: what medicine?

The narratives crafted for purposes of persuasion in the political arena have created a myth that the biomedical sciences are locked into a permanent struggle at the very frontiers of life and death – albeit figuratively in terms of the survival of a national economy. The latest example of such hype is the fraud committed by Hwang Yoo-Suk and his supporters in South Korea. Following his claims to have achieved human cloning, researchers in the life sciences all over the world did not hesitate to muster every sophisticated political tool at their disposal in order to remove perceived obstacles to research in this area (Gottweis and Triendl 2006).

This case shows how the perception of biomedicine as an exceptional shortcut to health and prosperity can increase the pressure on bioethics to deliver rationales for supporting such streamlined progress. The rhetoric of disaster management claims high stakes (major medical breakthroughs, national pride, or economic prudence) in order to shun moral qualms or conventional scientific virtues such as patience. At the same time, it lowers the *moral* stakes of medicine by shifting the conceptual emphasis from serving human dignity to engineering the physiological aspects of human life. As a consequence, with moral meaning challenged and fear and greed the driving forces behind the ethics "market," bioethics could easily find itself lending support to a vicious spiral of fear and despair rather than reason.

This socio-political backdrop reveals the murky lines of demarcation and slippery slopes encouraging the bending of ethical values and standards in the name of "exceptional opportunity," or even an alleged duty to sacrifice some for the benefit of the many. In other words, again borrowing from Gross, the principal question raised by triage is: "When, exactly, is the patient to be treated?" – not "Who is to be treated?" Clearly, such considerations relate to the implications of the principle of justice in medical ethics.

This chapter is grounded in the assumption that bioethics should focus on humanity and justice, and on the societal conditions that promote confidence in medicine and medical research. It should be acknowledged that, by virtue of its practical character, medicine has always included a focus on emergency and disaster, elements that must be addressed in any consideration of an adequate medical ethics – and in fact have always been understood as vital aspects of medical ethics.

By acknowledging that medicine is destined to be practiced under conditions that regularly require pragmatism, prudence and utilitarian calculations, and a notable degree of uncertainty, we do not thereby admit that such contingencies should define the duty of medicine. I believe that they rather define the challenging situation in which medicine seeks ways to function with dignity. Thus it would be inappropriate and unnecessary – almost disrespectful to the art of medicine – to open up new lines of discussion about exceptional scenarios. It seems more relevant to look for ways of meeting the related institutional, conceptual, and procedural challenges from an ethical perspective. For example, it is more and more obvious that medical need is overwhelming medical facilities in areas such as organ procurement and the allocation of patients for transplantation surgery. Instead of corrupting the ethical impulse by admitting the principle of exceptionalism, medicine should rather inspire efforts to analyze and improve the situation that creates injustice and double standards in the first place.

In a large-scale comparative international study, two historians of medicine have recently made it dramatically evident that honest codes of science and medical ethics are required to combat a "latent amorality that dictatorships [have] found easy to nurture" (Sachse and Walker 2005: 5) among scientists and medical professionals who, isolated within their institutional and administrative cultures, are easily exploited by powerful political agendas. This observation obviously pertains to non-dictatorial political systems as well.

At this structural level, the major contemporary threats to ethical integrity are well described in the words of Sachse and Walker: "Modern science has 'demystified' the world, a process that has led to . . . less inhibition when interacting with nature" (2005: 9) – and less inhibition in viewing other human beings as biological resources for medical purposes. Today, this process does not usually take place under express wartime conditions. However, the rhetoric of warfare is not uncommonly used to justify certain activities – activities which Sachse and Walker have shown bear some resemblance to the successful collaboration between unethical (indeed, criminal) German scientists and medical professionals and the Kaiser Wilhelm Gesellschaft, the forerunner of today's Max Planck Society, during the 1930s and the Second World War.

Such reflections have relevance for the self-understanding of the medical profession and the meaning of medicine. These issues should be addressed within a larger debate about a "healthy society," pondering the different ways in which abuses can become embedded within "normal" life and what they have to tell us about the structures of inhumane practices that begin with "exceptions" and slippery slopes that start off ever so gently. Such a discourse could provide us with a keen historical sense of what matters in medical ethics. The related question of how a "memory culture" might approach the challenge of "learning from the past" so as to make it most meaningful for present-day discussions is also a timely one. It serves to illustrate and reconfirm the struggle for humanity as a universal principle and general virtue.

Making a case

The task of "making sense" of the unspeakable is just the first step in the even larger challenge of making the incomprehensible meaningful for us in a practical way. In this chapter, I would like to use a dual approach, combining theoretical and methodological reflection to explore a concrete example of organized learning.

Theodor Adorno has struck the keynote of the theme of fundamental moral reassertion. "Education after Auschwitz means making our innate inhumanity aware of itself" (der Kälte zum Bewußtsein ihrer selbst zu verhelfen). It holds up the mirror that reflects the way we do *not* want to be. To merely re-educate people to "love thy neighbour" (Umerziehung zur Nächstenliebe) would be to found a moral good on a moral falsehood (das Wahre im Falschen fundieren) (Adorno 1966, 2003). To be satisfied with merely blaming the perpetrators would create an arbitrary distance between "us" and "them." It would give us a temporary reprieve from facing ourselves in the mirror that is the other. But we need more than juridical and ethical judgment. Above all, we need to overcome the crude rationale of "us and them," an opposition that has become a key element of our strategies of inhumanity. If we hope to learn anything from the worst offenders, we must go through the route of their humanity so as to find our common patterns of *in*humanity.

In order to supplement Adorno's primary focus on those who actively committed or passively tolerated the atrocities of the Nazi era, it may be appropriate to contextualize these events and to explore their meaning by highlighting the perspective of the victims. Here I am not referring to those outstanding victims who have become heroes or martyrs for their role in the resistance or by virtue of their impressive deeds, beliefs, or character. My hypothesis is this: understanding "how these things could happen" and attempting to "prevent something like this from happening again" is intimately linked with sympathy for the "ordinary faces" of people who were denied an "ordinary fate."

In order to illustrate what I mean, I want now to refer to the Nazi concentration camp at Ravensbrück. It was one of the sites where "medical" experiments were carried out on prisoners, mainly women, children, and "unwanted" people. The camp was located near the old spa of Fürstenberg, in a beautiful scenic landscape 70 km north of Berlin. Ravensbrück was Germany's largest women's concentration camp. Between 1939 and 1945, approximately 132,000 women from 47 countries were imprisoned there for reasons associated with their race, religion, ideology, or social behavior. More than half were executed or died from malnutrition, sickness, or exhaustion resulting from heavy labor, or from the effects of medical experiments. The camp has been converted into a museum, a memorial site, and an institution for education, research and debate with an international focus and agenda.

Making the unspeakable speak

I would like to begin with a statement written in the form of a poem by one inmate who survived the camp, thus paying my respects to someone with the authority and resolve to speak to us across the years. Any further introduction would be redundant since, for the purposes of this chapter, the text speaks for itself.

To Those Who Hesitate to Ask
Batsheva Dagan

Ask now
Since today
Is tomorrow's yesterday.

Ask now
Since tomorrow,
You suddenly see,
It is already too late!

Ask now
For today
There are witnesses!

Ask now
For tomorrow

All will be expressed in words
Or opinions.

What we shall miss when tomorrow arrives
Is the meeting of eyes and response,
A reply to all questions
In tongues or in faces.

Ask again!
And continue to ask!
Now is the time!
Yesterday shall not return.

Reconstructing a historical context

Historical reconstruction is an attempt to reconstitute the subject matter of our enquiries so that we can appropriate it for practical purposes in a contemporary context. It sets out to re-create the physical circumstances of a given case as a kind of simulacrum and thereby create a comparative base for reflecting on the meaning of humanity in action.

In 1946, 23 doctors, SS (Schutzstaffel, or elite guard) officials, and bureaucrats were tried before the American military court in Nuremberg for their participation in medical experiments on human subjects in concentration camps and research institutions, as well as in "euthanasia" killings. These trials represented merely the tip of the iceberg. Alexander Mitscherlich, who studied the trials on behalf of the West German Chambers of Medicine, was struck by the fact that, during the proceedings, the names of high-ranking scientists and university professors were constantly mentioned. They had taken advantage of their positions to select victims who would serve their own research purposes and other uses. One example of this indirect involvement in Nazi genocide was the case of the renowned neuropathologist Professor Julius Hallervorden, who examined the brains of 697 victims of so-called euthanasia, also euphemistically referred to as "mercy killing," at the Kaiser Wilhelm Institute for Brain Research in Berlin's Buch district. Facing serious charges at Nuremberg, he attempted to reason his way out of responsibility for his actions: "After all, where those brains came from was none of my business" (Lifton 1986: 67–68; cf. Mitscherlich and Mielke 1978).

Toxicologist Wolfgang Wirth helped the German Army develop chemical weapons during his work at the Institute for Pharmacology and Military Toxicology of the Military Medicine Academy in Berlin by evaluating lethal poisonous gas experiments carried out on concentration camp prisoners. Mitscherlich pointed out that, in the Third Reich, a doctor

was able to become a licensed killer and henchman in the public service simply by combining two processes: the aggressiveness of his scientific vocation and the ideology of the dictatorship. There is virtually no difference between seeing a person as a "case" or as a number tattooed on the arm – the double facelessness of a merciless epoch.

(Mitscherlich and Mielke 1978: Preface)

Mitscherlich's book is an early account of the rationale behind such activities – depriving victims of their humanity and addressing them as mere objects, instruments, or impersonal numbers.

Approaching Ravensbrück

Basically, the Ravensbrück camp served as a rationally structured and efficiently organized industrial complex and was designed for multiple purposes. Some elements served the various branches of Germany's conventional wartime industries (involving companies such as IG Farben and Siemens), especially in the areas of armaments and military clothing, while others were dedicated to research (such as developing a scientific basis for improving postwar agriculture, for example, through innovative fertilizers). Another related industry was the systematic killing of unwanted people. Within this context, different "businesses" were developed, including experimentation on human subjects, for the benefit of German medical science – or for other reasons, such as mere curiosity.

Today, Ravensbrück has become a memorial site where a very different kind of research is undertaken, namely educational and historical studies, in order to inform a variety of public education activities. (Similar sites are discussed in Wegner 2000 and 2002.) Among the priorities is the organization of visits by international students and a voluntary support network for the maintenance and reconstruction of the site. The vast collection of evidence on display that the contemporary visitor to the site will encounter can be broken down into numerous macro- and micro-level elements which are nonetheless interrelated and mutually supporting. Examples are:

- Facts about the structure of the camp; details of daily life (trivia) – how industry worked here.
- Systemic rationales – what purposes they served.
- Economic patterns functioning in the camp.
- Political purposes served by the camp.
- The doctors: names, faces, biographies and activities – Who did what?
- Fragments from people's lives – fragments of humanity, including pictures of faces, clothing, intimate items, objects from daily life, poems, songs, literature, music, arts and handicraft (culture) created by inmates under the most unimaginable conditions. These remains tell intimate stories of humanity under adverse circumstances.
- Documents: How did the system respond to internal deviant behavior? For example, some staff members were prosecuted for the rape of German inmates (condemned as "immoral and unmanly behavior") as well as for intercourse with "non-Arians" (seen as transgressing "racial" boundaries).

- Personal stories: What does it feel like to be deprived of humanity?
- Examples of "normal moral behavior" – what German citizens did, and what they could and should have known and done as ordinary citizens to take a stand against evil.
- Not least, every visitor will find her or his own personal story to take away.

Ravensbrück as a site for "medical" experiments

In addition to its role as a concentration camp and a site for the organized mass murder of political and other expendable (mainly female) prisoners, physicians performed biological and chemical research experiments on prisoners. These experiments fell into two main categories: (1) developing the technology for clandestine mass sterilization programs, and (2) experimental chemotherapy. In what follows, I will discuss only one of these areas, as both betray a very similar sense of inhumanity and random futility.

The chemotherapy experiments conducted at Ravensbrück should be seen in a particular historical context. In June 1942, SS Chief Reinhard Heydrich (the "Protector of the Eastern Empire") died following a successful assassination attempt from a wound infection. Prof. Dr. Karl Gebhardt, who was Director of an SS medical clinic and attempted to treat Heydrich, initiated a series of "medical" experiments on prisoners. As a surgeon, Gebhardt had been criticized for applying "scientifically outdated medical methods" (traditional septic therapy or the amputation of infected body parts). When Gebhardt requested the opportunity to prove that these accusations were groundless, his old school-fellow and Head of the SS, Heinrich Himmler, granted him permission to perform the requested experiments and assigned personnel, resources, and prisoners for the task.

The purpose of this research was described as twofold. First, Gebhardt set out to prove that the new chemotherapy (using sulphonamides) would not have been able to save Heydrich and would thus absolve himself from the accusations and possible sanctions he faced. Second, Gebhardt also hoped to prove that sulphonamide-based or indeed other varieties of chemotherapy would not constitute a promising avenue for research on new medical responses to the increasingly serious problem of infectious wounds that were killing soldiers in growing numbers during 1942 and 1943, especially those on the Eastern Front.

The "scientific" component of the research involved analyzing the development of artificially induced wound infection; describing basic traumatic wound infection (such as occurred under battlefield conditions), and the effects of traditional and new medical therapies when combined; and comparing different methods and degrees of wound infection in terms of the composition of the infection. The following methods and procedures were applied in particular to inmates at Ravensbrück:

- Prisoners' lower legs were cut open (without their knowledge or consent).
- Implanting of bacteria, followed by wrapping of the affected limb, took place.

- Experimental aseptic operations were performed, involving the cutting of bone, muscle, and nervous tissue.
- Artificial bacterial infection was applied, using "realistic" fragments of wood, metal, and dirt.
- Subjects were monitored.

> (Sources: Strebel 2003: 256ff., and my own on-site research on several occasions during the spring and summer of 2005)

To anyone exposed to the physical remains of this place and the atmosphere it exudes, this particular case illustrates the banality of evil in terms of the chilling character and utter pointlessness of the experiments carried out. The detailed and routinized organization of inconceivable suffering without the slightest trace of sympathy reduces the human being to an entirely instrumental role within a pointless system of mechanical production, depriving individuals of their humanity and converting them into disposable items on an industrial production line. Tragically, it appears that where there is no expectation of humaneness there is no room for sympathy. This case shows that banality as a form of evil (accompanying more sophisticated and bizarre manifestations) has an intimate relation to the double face of humanity (Bradshaw 1989). We seem to be able to live as caring members of society while, at the same time, organizing ourselves into professional structures capable of overseeing the systematic degradation of human beings.

The purpose and spirit of educational remembering ("Gedenken")

To remember is not simply to follow our duty not to forget. The act of remembrance inspires us to keep a vivid record of the history of humanity. It unravels a thread which has been disturbingly present throughout recorded human activity and which expresses itself most acutely in those areas that include a large component of power and responsibility – such as medicine and medical ethics.

The starting point for creative remembering is to focus on our manifold patterns of activity. Inasmuch as it aims to encourage practical learning, remembering will include some fundamental and serious elements of moral commitment ("Bekenntnis") undertaken by individuals. Clearly, the kind of horror that we have envisaged at Ravensbrück will continue to happen if we fail to muster our moral resolve and take active precautions in light of our daily practice. We need to stay constantly alert in our social and political lives. Since we cannot expect to find easy solutions corresponding to some predetermined (e.g., "historical" or "cultural") understanding of evil, we are required to resort to the myriad patterns of understanding that exist as parts of an explanatory moral patchwork. Such horrors will continue to happen if we fail to take active precautions at the micro, individual level, continually reviewing our daily practice. As a result, the notorious exclamation "J'accuse!" no longer represents a mature attitude when dealing with the past. The starting point for meaningful and morally valuable remembering is found in individual moral commitment ("Bekenntnis").

With a site such as Ravensbrück, the chief purpose of remembering (or memorializing) is to make the experience real for us – that is, for those who were not immediately involved. It should become more real for us than it was for those who found ways of detaching Ravensbrück from the sphere of practical commitment and thus could ignore it or pretend to "live with it." Notably, in Ravensbrück as in other places, we encounter a complementary feature of humanity, revealed in moving examples of individual courage and moral engagement – often in the small but conscious acts of humanity that we owe each other as human beings. For example, the small acts of daily courage of Mrs. Paula Schultz, a pharmacist in the town of Fürstenberg, who smuggled small items and pieces of news in and out of the camp for the benefit of inmates, appear as morally instructive as the better-known cases of Oskar Schindler (Pember 2005) or John Rabe (Wickert 2008), when their respective resources are taken into account.

This moral remembering should be distinguished from attempts to make its objects more realistic, as in the overhyped sounds and visuals we are exposed to in many topical movies. The claim to objectivity and the rendering of history in a four-dimensional framework associated with these productions is fundamentally misleading, because it suggests that we can in fact understand something substantial about what we are watching and that our sympathy with the actors will translate into something meaningful for us. What we can gain in terms of practical learning and understanding from such assumed simulations is of comparatively little value. We cannot feel the agony, think the thoughts, sense the smell and the cold or the taste of despair in any way that formed the subjective and thus real meaning of the original events. We leave such movies with no more than an intellectual or emotional impression of the events they depict, an impression which fails to form a connection within the established and privileged spheres of our own ordinary experience. Certainly, such movies can have an influence on us. However, this does not depend on any sense of "realism," but on our capacity to empathize. We enjoy such entertainment precisely because we feel fundamentally safe – able to keep an intrinsic distance that will not allow what we see to touch our hearts. As a result, we forgo an opportunity to get the task of remembering right.

Remembering involves the attempt to overcome this distance by making the situation as meaningful as possible for us, without pretending that it is meaningful for us in any way that expresses or reflects the real suffering endured by the original victims. It is the process involved, not what we make of it. This is a humble claim that acknowledges the limits of even the most sincere effort to understand what cannot be understood, since it is a priori impossible to reappropriate the full, real, or true meaning of events. Remembering is an absurd endeavor, in the manner of Camus' Sisyphus (Camus 1955). It works through the creation of opportunities for spontaneous moral responses by appealing to our basic moral sense and moral intuition.

The search for such opportunities can be guided by the classical Chinese (Confucian and Daoist) principle of "Wuwei," which dissuades those in power from dictating, propagating, or instilling moral practices, but rather encourages them to create space in which such acts can unfold naturally. Hence, our political and intellectual guardians should avoid interfering with the self-generation of basic moral experience. This is an important principle because the historical fate of Ravensbrück as a memorial is also an example of the political and ideological abuse of remembering, whether as an instrument of "class struggle" during the "Cold War" or to serve any other agenda. Theoretical support for this approach may be found in the Book of Mengzi (Mencius), with its account of the reconstruction of the sources of moral capability and its emphasis on the uninhibited, autonomous character of moral learning from the grass roots (Roetz 1993). This approach to remembering suggests keeping the incidents encountered as minor, simple, surprising, and perhaps as trivial as possible, so as to allow us to feel and build connections between our own reality and the reality of the past.

"We study and teach about it primarily for ethical reasons that are rooted in deep longing for a safer and more humane world. . . . My thesis is that *handle with care* is the most basic ethical implication of interdisciplinary Holocaust education" (Roth 2007). Accordingly, remembering can be a method of fostering ethics that goes well beyond the challenges of a merely prudent and pragmatic ethics debate, reasserting the humane purposes of humanity and defending normative areas that will not bow to relativism. The counter-strategy – creating the illusion of the substance of experience – is to expose the observer to emptiness, pointlessness, and vanity within our good and normal world. Hence, creating spaces to be filled by each individual's acts of sympathy and reflection constitutes a major balancing mechanism to counter the overwhelming impressions that flood our awareness from the worlds of information and interpretation. Thus, institutions for remembering create space for study, self-inspection, silence, reflection on information and emotion, and for tears. At Ravensbrück, a vast area of concrete and dirt is tied together by ruins and trees, and is occasionally drawn into focus by huge portraits of some of the people who lived there. This arrangement invites meditation.

Discussion: about the language of the unspeakable

The continuation of relevant historical research, new reports, and juridical trials makes it clear that this is not a closed chapter in the history of medicine. As Ian Buruma has shown, different countries, most notably Japan and Germany, have established quite different policies and social practices in dealing with their history of medical war crimes (Buruma 1994; Sachse and Walker 2005). Others, such as the U.S., still find it difficult to develop responsible attitudes to their own contributions to medical crimes and related cover-ups. The recent Chinese outrage over the Japanese wartime atrocities in China, refueled by the school textbook controversy of 2006, is another reminder of the overwhelming depth of humanity's pain, inflicted and re-created through ignorance. The trauma caused cannot be ignored. To cite Dagan's poem, we need tongues and faces to prevent the planting and regrowth of systemic inhumanity. Dagan's poem seems to contradict Adorno's verdict that "writing poetry after Auschwitz is barbaric" (Adorno 1973: 362). He argued that the aesthetic self-referential nature of poetry pays homage to a cultural framework for humanity that failed to prevent the systematic atrocities of the Holocaust. However, Adorno later revoked this statement, observing that "Perennial suffering has as much right to expression as the tortured have to scream. . . . Hence it may have been wrong to say that no poem could be written after Auschwitz."

Although intellectuals and academic work play an important role in fostering this moral remembering, their contribution should not be overrated or glorified. In Germany, ever since "Group 47" began discussing the validity of language, arts, and culture "after the Holocaust," much attention has been paid to abstract ideas and the behavior of elites. Quite fundamentally, Auschwitz led Adorno to attack what he termed the "Western legacy of positivity," the innermost substance of traditional philosophy. Western culture had essentially failed in that it did not offer sufficient cultural and moral resistance to the Holocaust. Yet, what is the meaning of "after"? Is it all over? Can we stop here, when we continue to learn about the wrongs committed at the same time and in a similar fashion in other places, such as in East Asia? Such events raise disturbing questions about humanity itself, rather than just the inhabitants of particular regions and cultures. The prime task of philosophy and intellectual leadership in general remains to reflect on its own failure, its own complicity in these events.

Others have argued that the very absence of such moral commitment, caused by hubris, coercion, and seduction, would explain how moral degradation on such a scale was possible in the first place. In fact, the Constitution of postwar Germany may be understood as an attempt to learn from the half-hearted moral commitment that marked the founding of the Weimar Republic, by carving some of this substance into stone – such as the inalienability of human dignity and clear definitions of the limits of institutional power, including the power of the state, in the name of humanity. The containment of power by checks and balances at all levels, and the demarcation of a clearly defined area that is by definition inaccessible to authorities of any kind, is a major achievement that leaves room for citizens to engage with and raise the consciousness of individuals.

The establishment, and intellectuals in particular, have good reasons for being humble and regarding themselves as just one element amidst a host of interrelated social, economic, and cultural factors – that is, as humans among equals in the subjective terms of morality and action. The strong rejection by Adorno and other intellectuals of "positive" ethics and cultural norms indicates a turning away from an exaggerated expectation of the significance of the political and historical impact of academic philosophy and philosophical ideas (Weiss 1999).

Contemplating the faces and everyday lives of real people involved, as actors and as victims, can adjust our perspective on framing questions and seeking answers. This recontextualization of humanity serves to demythologize evil, accounting for its "banality" and confronting us, each person, with the task of doing things better, wherever we stand. In other words, we need a sophisticated universal framework for medical ethics that is equipped to counter exceptionalism in a constructive manner. At the same time, it should respect the fact that culture matters and that culture is not reducible to intellectual activity – it is to a significant extent a "normal" pursuit, which embraces the moral sensibilities of "ordinary" people. It is not a sound ethical argument to invoke "exceptional" intellectual, political, economic, or other powers in order to ride roughshod over the weak, as a way of building an "exceptional" ethics.

In sum, our reflection on remembering and learning from the past leads us to reject two forms of exceptionalism that amount to moral relativism and elitism. The trouble with positive exceptionalism such as is found in triage, selective killing, and human cloning is not that some people are confronted with dramatic or even tragic conflicts which demand responsible decisions, but that these decisions should be justified as ethical. Adorno's verdict, on the other hand, expresses a negative exceptionalism that is rooted in a frustrated sense of humanity in the face of the gross moral violations of which humans are capable. However, it lacks any confidence in the self-regenerating human capability for moral action, despite the absurdities of our existence, thereby adding a much deeper existential sense of vanity. In consequence, both forms of exceptionalism support each other, like hostile siblings arguing over the right way to save a burning house instead of simply going ahead and extinguishing the fire. I would encourage us all to trust the few general signposts we have in ethics and follow them patiently, as best as we can.

References and further reading

Adorno, Theodor W., *Negative Dialectics*, trans. E. B Ashton, New York: Seabury Press, 1973, 362.

Adorno, Theodor W., "Education after Auschwitz", in Helmut Schreier and Matthias Heyl (eds), *Never Again! The Holocaust's Challenge for Educators*, Hamburg: Krämer, 1997 (original 1966). Document taken from http://grace.evergreen.edu/~arunc/texts/frankfurt/auschwitz/AdornoEducation.pdf (accessed June 3, 2007).

Adorno, Theodor W., *Can One Live after Auschwitz? A Philosophical Reader*, trans. Rodney Livingstone, London: Stanford University Press, 2003.

Annas, G. and Grodin, M. (eds), *The Nazi Doctors and the Nuremberg Code: Human Rights in Human Experimentation*, New York: Oxford University Press, 1992.

Bradshaw, Leah, *Acting and Thinking: The Political Thought of Hannah Arendt*, Toronto: University of Toronto Press, 1989.

Buruma, Ian, *The Wages of Guilt*, New York: Farrar Straus Giroux, 1994.

Camus, Albert, *The Myth of Sisyphus*, New York: Vintage, 1955.

Döring, Ole, "Comments on Inhumanity in the Name of Medicine: Old Cases and New Voices for Responsible Medical Ethics from Japan and China," *Eubios Journal of Asian and International Bioethics* 11 (2), March 2001: 44–47.

Döring, Ole, "Moral Development and Education in Medical Ethics. An Attempt at a Confucian Aspiration," in Ole Döring and Renbiao Chen (eds), *Advances in Chinese Medical Ethics. Chinese and International Perspectives*, Hamburg (Mitteilungen des Instituts für Asienkunde No. 355), 2002: 178–194.

Döring, Ole, "Ethics Education in Medicine and Moral Preaching. Reflections on a Triangular Relationship and its Human Core," in Ole Döring (ed.), *Ethics in Medical Education in China. Distinguishing Education of Ethics from Moral Preaching*, Hamburg (Mitteilungen des Instituts für Asienkunde No. 358), 2002: 75–85.

Gottweis, Herbert and Triendl, Robert, "South Korean Policy Failure and the Hwang Debacle," *Nature Biotechnology* 24(2), February 2006: 141–143.

Gross, Michael L. *Bioethics and Armed Conflict. Moral Dilemmas of Medicine and War*, Cambridge, MA/London: MIT Press, 2006.

LaCapra, Dominick, "Trauma, Absence, Loss," in Dominick La Capra (ed.), *Writing History, Writing Trauma*, Baltimore, MD: Johns Hopkins University Press, 2000.

Levi, Primo, *Survival in Auschwitz: The Nazi Assault on Humanity*, trans. Stuart Woolf, New York: Simon & Schuster, 1996.

Lifton, Robert Jay, *The Nazi Doctors: Medical Killing and the Psychology of Genocide*, New York: Basic Books, 1986.

Mitscherlich, A. and Mielke, F. (eds), *Medizin ohne Menschlichkeit*, Frankfurt: Fischer Taschenbuch Verlag, 1978.

Morrisson, Jack G., *Ravensbrück. Das Leben in einem Konzentrationslager für Frauen*, Zürich and Munich: Pendo Verlag, 2005.

Muller-Hill, B., *Murderous Science*, Oxford: Oxford University Press, 1988.

Pember, Mieczyslaw (Mietek), *Der rettende Weg, Schindlers Liste – die wahre Geschichte* (2nd edn), Hamburg: Hoffmann und Campe, 2005.

Pross, C., "Schweigen bedeutet Komplizenschaft," *Deutsches Ärzteblatt* 1990, 41: A3104–3108.

Pross, C., "Nazi Doctors, German Medicine and Historical Truth," in G.J. Annas and M.A. Grodin (eds), *The Nazi Doctors and the Nuremberg Code – Human Rights in Human Experimentation*, New York and Oxford: Oxford University Press, 1992.

Roetz, Heiner, *Confucian Ethics of the Axial Age*, New York: SUNY Press, 1993.

Roth, John K., "Handle with Care: Some Ethical Implications of Interdisciplinary Holocaust Education." Document downloaded from http://www1.yadvashem.org/education/conference2004/roth.pdf (accessed June 2, 2007).

Sachse, Carola and Walker, Mark (eds), "Politics and Science in Wartime. Comparative International Perspectives on the Kaiser Wilhelm Institute," *Osiris* 20, 2005.

Saidel, Rochelle G., *The Jewish Women of Ravensbrueck Concentration Camp*, Madison: Terrace Books, 2004.

Sass, Hans-Martin, "Emergency Management in Public Health Ethics: Triage, Epidemics, Biomedical Terror and Warfare," *Eubios Journal of Asian and International Bioethics* 15, September 2005: 161–166.

Seidelman, W., "Mengele Medicus: Medicine's Nazi Heritage," *Milbank Quarterly* 66, 1988: 221–239.

Strebel, Bernhard, *Das Konzentrationslager Ravensbrueck*, Paderborn: Geschichte eines Lagerkomplexes, 2003.

Wegner, Gregory, "The Power of Selective Tradition: Buchenwald Concentration Camp and Holocaust Education for Youth in the New Germany," in Laura Hein and Mark Selden (eds), *Censoring History. Citizenship and Memory in Japan, Germany and the United States*, New York: M.E. Sharpe, 2000.

Wegner, Gregory, *Anti-Semitism and Schooling Under the Third Reich*, New York: RoutledgeFalmer, 2002.

Weiss, Sheila F., "Prelude to the Maelstrom: German Physicians as Custodians of the Nation's Health, 1870–1933 – A Cautionary Tale for Contemporary China?," in Ole Döring (ed.), *Chinese Scientists and Responsibility*, *Mitteilungen des Instituts für Asienkunde*, No. 314, Hamburg, 1999.

Wickert, Erwin, *John Rabe. Der gute Deutsche von Nanking*, Munich: Pantheon Verlag 2008.

8 Racial hygienist Otmar von Verschuer, the Confessing Church, and comparative reflections on postwar rehabilitation

Peter Degen

Introduction

It is commonly believed that the Nazi medical personnel were punished at Nuremberg, but the Japanese escaped prosecution. Here I provide an example of a German medical researcher who remained intact after the war despite his involvement in Nazi experimentation. His name is Otmar Freiherr von Verschuer. This scientist was involved in medical atrocities in Auschwitz through his assistant and collaborator Dr. Josef Mengele, but he was neither charged nor sentenced like other Nazi physicians who went on trial in Nuremberg nor sought as a criminal like Mengele. Instead, he rose again to scientific and social prominence after the war. One major factor that facilitated his rehabilitation was his membership in the Confessing Church, a Christian group opposed to Hitler's efforts to dominate the German Protestant Church. In this chapter, I offer a few glimpses of Verschuer's relationship with the Confessing Church, particularly through his relationship with pastors Otto Fricke and Herbert Mochalsky. Second, I discuss how these relationships helped his postwar efforts at rehabilitation. Finally, I briefly compare Verschuer's postwar career to those of the Japanese physicians of Unit 731.

Who was Otmar von Verschuer?

The German racial hygienist Otmar Freiherr von Verschuer (1896–1967) was a medical doctor, eugenicist, and anti-Semite. According to various sources, he was also a religious person with a Protestant background (Müller-Hill 1988, 116ff.). Verschuer's family was one of two "Patronatsfamilien" who owned the church building and church grounds of Solz in Northern Hesse that dated back to before the Reformation. It was not until 1969 that both were turned over to congregational ownership.

Verschuer was born in Northern Hesse in 1896. He began studying medicine in 1919. In 1922, he worked as an anthropological intern with Prof. Eugen Fischer, a famous eugenicist who patronized Verschuer. The textbook *Menschliche Erblehre und Rassenhygiene* [Human Heredity and Racial Hygiene], written by Erwin Bauer, Eugen Fischer, and Fritz Lenz, was published in the same year. This book not only provided Verschuer with an "exceptional spiritual experience," but also became his scientific "Bible" (Verschuer 2003, 152).

In 1922, Verschuer completed his medical studies, and in the following year he wrote his doctoral thesis. From 1923 to 1927 he collaborated at the medical polyclinic in Tübingen with Prof. Wilhelm Weitz, who encouraged him to undertake systematic research on human twins – a field in which Verschuer was to become a pioneer. In 1927, he gained the Habilitation in human genetics. Later that same year, following the establishment of the new Kaiser Wilhelm Institute of Anthropology, Human Heredity and Eugenics in Berlin, Verschuer was appointed Head of the Department of Human Heredity by Eugen Fischer, the founding director of the Institute. In 1934 Verschuer was called to the University of Frankfurt to head the newly founded University Institute of Racial Hygiene and Genetic Biology. He worked there until 1942, when he returned to the Kaiser Wilhelm Institute in Berlin as one of its two directors. He stayed on at the Institute until the end of the Second World War in 1945 (Zirlewagen 2006, 1437ff.).

Among Verschuer's students in Frankfurt was Josef Mengele, who earned his medical doctorate under his supervision. Mengele became very close to the Verschuer family and was known as "Uncle Josef." After joining Hitler's "Schutzstaffel" (SS), Mengele stayed on as Verschuer's assistant, an appointment that coincided with his tenure as doctor at the Auschwitz concentration camp. Mengele's human experiments in Auschwitz were supported by the Deutsche Forschungsgemeinschaft (DFG): the application for the research grant for his work was submitted by Verschuer (Hammerstein 1999, 423, 430–431).

One of Verschuer's most notable "achievements" as a scientist was to provide a scientific foundation for Nazi racial theory and to support its implementation through the practice of "racial hygiene." In many ways he helped turn the Nazi racial laws and policies into reality. His collaboration with Mengele involved him deeply in the medical atrocities committed during the War. Mengele frequently sent Verschuer blood specimens, eye samples, organs, and body parts taken from concentration camp inmates in Auschwitz after they had been killed (Weingart et al. 1988, 572ff.).

Verschuer's multiple personality

After the War, Verschuer was issued with an official "Berufsverbot" (job ban) that prohibited him from working as an academic teacher and scientific researcher. However, after undergoing a "denazification trial" and receiving a "whitewash" (Persilschein) from Nobel Laureate Prof. Adolph Butenandt in 1951, Verschuer was invited to take up a position at the University of Muenster as Professor of Human Genetics. At Muenster he established one of the largest institutes of human genetics in West Germany.

Verschuer, the teacher and scientific mentor of Mengele, claimed over and over again that his membership of the Confessing Church had precluded him from participating in any criminal or even unethical scientific activities during the Nazi era (Verschuer 1965, 9). This astonishing claim prompted me to look into his activities more closely.

According to various witnesses, Verschuer was a very "religious" man (see Müller-Hill 1988, 116), not in a dogmatic but rather in a general sense. During his first period in Berlin as Head of the Department of Human Heredity at the Kaiser Wilhelm Institute, Verschuer became a member of the village church in Dahlem, St. Anne's Church, where he met Pastor Martin Niemöller, a former U-Boot captain and a leader of the Confessing Church during the Nazi era. In 1933 Verschuer signed a public declaration promulgated by the "Jungreformatorische Bewegung" [Young Reformers' Movement] (Scharf 1977, 47–50), from which the Confessing Church emerged during the early 1930s. Its goal was to maintain Jesus Christ as its spiritual "Führer," and hence did not accept the leadership of a "superior Germanic race." According to one story, when Verschuer was preparing to move to Frankfurt, Niemöller suggested that he contact Pastor Otto Fricke, a member of the Confessing Church. Verschuer followed his advice (Verschuer, "Erbe-Umwelt-Führung," May 19, 1945, 4). During his time in Frankfurt (1934–1942), he was a regular member of Fricke's congregation (Fricke 1990, 124). Verschuer often had to make excuses to allow his son Helmuth to skip the Sunday morning gatherings of the "Jungvolk" [Young Folk], a junior branch of the Hitler Youth, in order to attend church with his father.

Verschuer and Fricke became lifelong friends. According to another account Verschuer joined Fricke's congregation because Verschuer's local pastor was a member of the "Deutsche Christen" [German Christians], who accepted the notion that the religion of the Germanic race should be the goal of the Protestant Church. As a member of the Confessing Church, Verschuer believed that the church should have only one leader, Jesus Christ, yet Hitler was to be accepted as leader of the government. Verschuer's son Helmuth remembers his father quoting Christ in the Gospels: "Render unto Caesar the things which are Caesar's, and unto God the things which are God's." He characterized his father's attitudes as steeped "in the Prussian-Protestant tradition of loyalty to authority" (Müller-Hill 1988, 117).

In 1936, Pastor Fricke was denounced and arrested as a result of a false report by a Gestapo agent. Verschuer invited Fricke's family to stay in his own home until Fricke was released from prison when the charges against him could not be substantiated. Following this event, the two families became closer and met weekly (Fricke 1990, 3). Fricke was a member of the governing board of the Confessing Church, the "Reichsbruderrat" [Brethren Council], and also of the provisional board of the provincial Hessian Church (Fricke 1990, 124). Fricke had once invited Verschuer to speak to his congregation on socio-ethical issues of eugenics because Fricke had taken an interest in this "scientific" field.

After returning to the Kaiser Wilhelm Institute in Berlin-Dahlem in 1942, Verschuer rejoined Niemöller's congregation at St. Anne's Church in Dahlem. However, by this time Niemöller was being held in a concentration camp as a "personal prisoner" of Adolf Hitler, having stated that he was a "better" national-socialist than the Nazis. Niemöller had voted for Hitler's party since 1924, when he first made this claim. In Dahlem now the pastor in charge was the young Herbert Mochalsky, also a member of the Confessing Church.

Pastor Fricke was conscripted into the army and based in Potsdam near Berlin. He often spent his leave breaks and holidays in Verschuer's villa in Dahlem and administered the rite of confirmation to Verschuer's daughter Sigrid on March 23, 1943. Fricke's closeness to Verschuer is also reflected in the fact that he had his own permanent room in Verschuer's Dahlem villa (Verschuer, May 19, 1945, 7).

Differences between the German Christians and the Confessing Church

After 1933, the clergy and laity of the Protestant Church in Germany felt the need to bring the church in line with the new ideology of national socialism. Intending to create a church devoted to a religion of the Germanic race, they called themselves "German Christians." On the other hand, a minority of pastors and Church members insisted on the ideological and institutional independence of the Protestant Church under the slogan "freies Bekenntnis" [free confession]. They argued that priority should be given unconditionally to the sole confession to Jesus Christ. In order to maintain this principle, the Church's independence had to be preserved and defended.

The chief bone of contention between these two groups lay in the "Aryan paragraph" inserted in 1935 into the church law entitled "Law for the Protection of German Blood and German Honour" that required dismissal of any pastor or church official who was non-Aryan by ethnic origin. Although the Confessing Church rejected the application of the law, few of its members had questioned the legislation when the Nazi state introduced it.

One member of the Confessing Church deserves a closer look at this point. Born into a family of pastors and professors, Dietrich Bonhoeffer became a seminal Protestant theologian and later took part in the July 20 plot to assassinate Hitler in 1944. The attempt failed, and Bonhoeffer was executed by the Nazis along with the others involved in the conspiracy. Bonhoeffer's unambiguous position stood in stark contrast to Verschuer's "multiple personality" – a man who could be a member of the Confessing Church while leading a professional life as a scientist supporting Nazi principles of eugenics and racial hygiene. As a matter of fact, Verschuer's nephew Adam von Trott zu Solz was involved in the assassination attempt of 1944 and was subsequently executed. As Verschuer's son points out, his father "did not show any understanding of this attitude" of resistance, due to his traditional Prussian-Protestant loyalty to authority (Müller-Hill 1988, 117).

After the War the mainstream German Christians in the Protestant Church fell into disrepute as a result of their support for Nazi ideology during the Third Reich. The German Protestant Church was re-established along the lines of the Confessing Church which was judged to have been in resistance during the Nazi era and therefore seen as morally intact and suitable to take up a responsible position in postwar democratic society. During the Nazi period, not only had Verschuer taken an active part in his congregation, but he was also involved with the "classes for pastors" of the "Evangelical Johannes Foundation" in Berlin-Spandau, where he lectured on the compatibility of racial hygiene and Christian ethics. Furthermore, he was a member of the "Centralausschuβ der Inneren Mission" [steering committee for home missions], which was in charge of the social work and outreach of the Protestant Church (Schleiermacher 1998, 29–30; Verschuer 2003, 16). In particular, he became the mentor of Dr. Hans Harmsen, who was also a member of the Centralausschuβ and was responsible for "public health." It was under Harmsen's leadership that the direction of the "Innere Mission" was changed from national-conservative to a "völkische" [community] orientation on questions of racial hygiene. The main impetus for this change was the advent of the new Nazi government in 1933. For Verschuer, this transformation was to demonstrate that national-socialist racial hygiene was compatible with Christian ethics (Verschuer 2003, 165). Hence the "Innere Mission" adopted the Nazi position on voluntary sterilization for people with serious genetic defects. However, whereas the Nazis argued that "voluntary sterilization" was to be regarded as a sacrifice for the "völkische Gemeinschaft" (German people's community), the "Innere Mission" argued that voluntary sterilization was a sacrifice to be carried out according to the Christian commandment of "love for neighbor" (Schleiermacher 1998, 180–276; Verschuer 2003, 165). Prior to 1933, Verschuer had already advocated such a policy at a church conference on eugenics in Treysa organized by the "Innere Mission." He clearly valued the ideology of the "völkisch" German community more than the rights of individuals. In 1931, the "Innere Mission" called for "eugenic laws," which were introduced by the Nazis after 1933 (Schleiermacher 1998, 180–276).

During the Nazi era Verschuer remained loyal to both his science – eugenics and racial hygiene – and to the Confessing Church. Reconciling these twin loyalties, science and church, was a basic tenet of "liberal-cultural Protestantism," which claimed, in contrast to Catholicism, compatibility with modern science. In fact, Protestant modernity meant the compatibility of science and Christian ethics. Clearly Verschuer had no problem with his synthesis of religion and science. However, Verschuer was unwilling to acknowledge the point at which he became personally involved in unethical and inhuman acts of scientific and medical research that culminated in his close collaboration with Mengele in Auschwitz (Winnacker 2000). Verschuer's scientific career is an excellent example of the "slippery slope" – the progressive process of "delimiting" science which culminated in Mengele's experiments and activities in Auschwitz (Markl 2001b; Sachse and Walker 2005: see the chapter "Science Without Moral Boundaries"; Weingart et al. 1988, 572–581).

Verschuer's exemption from conviction

Before the war came to an end, Verschuer transferred most of the collections and specimens housed in his Kaiser Wilhelm Institute to his residence at Solz, Northern Hesse. He intended to eventually bring all these materials to Frankfurt in order to use them as "Verhandlungsmasse" [negotiating material] to encourage the

University of Frankfurt to restore his former job or to re-establish the Kaiser Wilhelm Institute in Frankfurt.

After the War, Verschuer's plans encountered obstacles, and his prospects were not improved by an article in the *Frankfurter Neue Presse* that accused him of improper conduct during the Nazi era. The article was written by Prof. Robert Havemann, provisional president of the Kaiser Wilhelm Society, who was conducting an official investigation into Verschuer's activities during the Nazi period. Havemann came to the conclusion that Verschuer had acted contrary to "human and scientific ethics" and had made "concessions to the national socialist racial madness that went far beyond what was ethically and scientifically acceptable." Verschuer's collaboration with Mengele was the major factor in reaching this conclusion (Hammerstein 1989, 657–661).

In the end, however, Havemann's findings did not lead to prosecution (Weingart et al. 1988, 572ff.), but only to the imposition of a "Berufsverbot" (job ban). Verschuer was prohibited from working as a scientist or researcher, and therefore his chances of finding a job in Frankfurt evaporated. In this volatile situation, still facing official charges and at the urging of a friend, Verschuer decided to undergo a formal "denazification trial." The trial took place on November 7, 1946 in Frankfurt (Sachse 2004, 300). In an earlier note to Otto Hahn – President of the former Kaiser Wilhelm Society, now the Max Planck Society – Verschuer had admitted to what he considered to be the basic facts of his collaboration with Mengele in Auschwitz (Verschuer to Hahn, May 23, 1946). At the trial several factors played a decisive role in acquitting Verschuer, including a character reference by Pastor Fricke, who vouched for Verschuer's moral character and the integrity of his scientific work (Fricke 1946). He was fined 600 Reichsmarks and cleared of more serious charges, "although the connection of Verschuer with Mengele in Auschwitz was by now officially and publicly known in all of its gruesome details" (Hammerstein 1989, 658).

Verschuer's status as a "desk-murderer" may be compared to the case of Prof. Dr. Gerhard Rose, who was charged at the Nuremberg Trials and sentenced to life imprisonment, later commuted to 15 years. Rose was considered to be a "desk-murderer" as he did not personally commit any atrocities – they were carried out by an assistant or collaborator. Another view of Verschuer's exemption from conviction was suggested by Dr. Leo Alexander, who was in charge of Verschuer's case. Alexander noted that solid evidence proving Verschuer's collaboration with Mengele could not be established at the Nuremberg Trials (Alexander 1946).

On September 19, 1949, the Kaiser Wilhelm Society called for a final review of Verschuer's status. As we have seen, Prof. Adolph Butenandt's investigation vouched for Verschuer's integrity as a scientific teacher and researcher and testified to his "internal adversarial attitude," meaning that he had opposed Nazism based on his religious-ethical disposition. The references by Pastors Fricke and Mochalsky again helped to rescue Verschuer from accusations of being a Nazi racist. Both men certified his "anti-nationalsozialistische Haltung" [anti-national-socialist attitude] based on his membership of the Confessing Church (Denkschrift

1949, 2–3). Verschuer was cleared of all charges and became employable again, although not in Frankfurt.

It seems that Verschuer's denazification trial downplayed or ignored his Auschwitz connections as did the review conducted by Butenandt – no doubt in order to preserve his own reputation as well as that of the former Kaiser Wilhelm Society (now renamed the Max Planck Society). An additional question is whether the references by Pastors Fricke and Mochalsky were intended to preserve not only Verschuer's reputation but that of the Confessing Church. Fricke in particular went out of his way to prevent Verschuer from being charged with personal and scientific responsibility for committing unethical and criminal acts.

In 1951, Verschuer was appointed Professor of Human Genetics at the University of Münster in Northern Germany. His former superior at the Kaiser Wilhelm Institute, Eugen Fischer, helped him gain this position. In Münster, Verschuer established one of the largest institutes of human genetics of the German postwar era. Until the end of his life, Verschuer asserted repeatedly that his membership of the Confessing Church had precluded his involvement in Nazi medical atrocities (Kröner 1998, 236ff.; Verschuer 1965, 9).

Verschuer's self-defense in comparison with Japanese doctors of Unit 731

Why is it useful to compare Verschuer's case with the Japanese doctors of Unit 731 and its network? It seems to me that not just a few Far Eastern ethicists and historians of medicine seem to believe and applaud the fact that in the West because of their medical atrocities the Nazi doctors have been correctly treated by putting them on trial in Nuremberg and sentencing them. By contrast they deplore the fact that the Japanese doctors of Unit 731 and those of its network were not put on trial and even those who were sentenced got off sooner or later again. Neither had they even to confront a "Berufsverbot" [job ban] of any kind.

It seems to me that Verschuer who was not a minor among the Nazi doctors did not get charged in Nuremberg. Thus the picture of the Nazi doctors is more complicated. Furthermore, he managed to survive his denazification trial and a job ban based on an evaluation by Prof. Havemann, then President of the Kaiser Wilhelm Society and, though he was neither able to return to his former job at the Kaiser Wilhelm Society – shortly after the War converted into the Max Planck Society – nor to another former job at the University of Frankfurt/Main, he landed an appointment at the University of Münster with the help of the positive verdict of the Butenandt Commission, a second commission of the Kaiser Wilhelm (now the Max Planck) Society that examined Verschuer's case. The judgment of the members of the Commission in part relying on the character references of two pastors of the Confessing Church helped Verschuer to see his moral integrity as a researcher and teacher restored. This opened the road to his appointment in Münster. It seems that both Butenandt as a representative of the former Kaiser Wilhelm Society and pastors Fricke and Michalsky as representatives of the Confessing Church were interested in maintaining the reputation of their respective organizations which seemed to have remained unblemished during the Nazi era. Butenandt had a personal vested interest in a positive verdict because one of his collaborators was part of Verschuer's Auschwitz connection. The Kaiser Wilhelm Society and the University of Frankfurt/Main severed their relationship with Verschuer, but the Confessing Church never called Verschuer's membership of the Protestant Church into doubt. All concerned knew the basic facts about Verschuer, Mengele, and Auschwitz and firmly closed their eyes for obvious reasons, namely maintaining personal and organizational moral integrity.

While accusations continued to surface, Verschuer had little difficulty in putting them to rest by referring to his "denazification trial," the positive verdict of the Butenandt commission as well as his membership in the Confessing Church, which was widely regarded as having resisted the Nazis. He often used the image of a "deep trench" that separated him as a member of the Confessing Church from the real Nazi-racist scientists (Verschuer 1965, 9).

Meanwhile, Verschuer continued to be active in the Protestant Church as a lecturer to Protestant student congregations and as an advisor to the Home Mission. His major socio-ethical concern was the compatibility of what was now called "human genetics" – as opposed to "eugenics and racial hygiene" – with Christian ethics, and "bringing together the functions of physician (as human geneticist) and pastoral counselor" (Verschuer 1965, 10).

After retiring as a researcher and teacher in 1965, Verschuer continued to carry on his defense based on his membership of the Confessing Church, while remaining silent about his earlier activities as an advisor to the "Home Mission" and his peculiar blending of racial hygiene and Christian ethics. Nor did he ever express any remorse over his links with Mengele in Auschwitz. He evaded any concrete responsibility by simply admitting his complicity in "demonic times," mildly regretting his failure to a greater degree of resistance. In 1967, Verschuer was killed in a car accident.

First of all, we have seen that Verschuer's career is very similar to those of the Japanese doctors in that he averted legal consequences of his involvement with medical atrocities, though for different reasons. Verschuer escaped legal punishment for reasons we still cannot reconstruct. The worst he had to face was a temporary job ban, whereas the Japanese doctors went free owing to a deal between the U.S. and Japanese government to conceal the atrocities from the public and for exchange of the Japanese "scientific results."

Second, his postwar career, especially his postwar academic and social advancement, is very similar to that of many members of Unit 731 who rose to top positions in Japan's scientific, business, and academic circles in the postwar period, but again for different reasons. Whereas the Japanse doctors could without any serious interruption pursue their postwar careers, Verschuer could do so only after his job ban had been lifted after scientific colleagues and Protestant Church officials had helped whitewash him. Verschuer attained a senior position in the scientific and university establishment of the new Federal Republic, and he held a key position in the field of human genetics because many of his students would later occupy university chairs all over Germany. His membership in the new Protestant Church in postwar Germany was never contested.

Third, as in the case of the Japanese doctors, it took a long time for researchers to re-examine Verschuer's case. When German geneticist Benno Müller-Hill critically examined Verschuer in 1984 (see Müller-Hill 1984), it was Müller-Hill who faced legal challenges from the Max Planck Society, until his critique was finally accepted. Then in 1990 Verschuer's professional conduct during the Nazi era was officially investigated following pressures on the Max Planck Society to apologize to the surviving victims of scientists employed by the former Kaiser Wilhelm Society.

Even today it does not seem that the hierarchy of the Protestant Church of Germany sees any need to address this issue. Likewise, the provincial church of Hesse and Nassau does not take any related action. The careers of Pastors Niemöller, Fricke, and Mochalsky are still in need of further scrutiny with respect to their relations with Verschuer. His case demonstrates clearly that not all of those who were responsible for criminal human experimentation and medical atrocities during the Nazi era were indicted at the Nuremberg Tribunal. Verschuer was by no means a minor figure. The issue of the legal persecution of Nazi doctors is obviously more complicated.

Fourth, Verschuer's case is unique in the East as well as in the West with regard to the religious justification he deployed to distance himself from any professional misconduct. No Japanese doctor ever had to put up such a defense. Interestingly enough, as Nanyan Guo points out, at least two Japanese doctors are known who, owing to their Christian beliefs, refused to become involved in medical atrocities, though they knew of them and were part of the Unit 731 network. Interestingly enough, the daughter of Ishii Shiro spread the story that shortly before his death her father had been baptized and adopted the Christian name Joseph. So far no documentary evidence exists for her claim. It is the very symbolism of "being Christian," or for that matter, belonging to a group of faith, that stands to question, inasmuch as it builds upon claims of purity even under "evil" conditions. These cases make it clear that the degree of connectedness and mutual dependence between "harmless," opportunistic, and straightforward criminal members of a country's avant-garde can be as complex as the demarcations between good and bad can be blurred. We can never take such credit for granted.

Conclusion

During the Nazi era, Verschuer embraced twin loyalties: one to his vision of science (eugenics and racial hygiene), and one to Protestant religion and the Protestant Church, especially the Confessing Church. He was probably more motivated by anti-Semitism and anti-Judaism than by Nazi convictions. Verschuer was also a skillful opportunist who well knew how to avoid indictment at the Nuremberg Trials, survive a denazification trial, escape his "Berufsverbot" [job ban] with the help of pastors and scientists whom he had known, land a permanent significant academic position, and escape any serious legal challenge. He died with his reputation intact as a highly respected scientist in postwar Germany. To cover up his unethical and criminal behavior, and after the ideology was no longer an opportunistic asset, Verschuer conveniently separated science from national socialism and the national socialists as well as from an era characterized by "demonism." This strategy allowed him to blur his personal responsibility and accountability (Weingart et al. 1988, 575f.). He found peace of mind by accepting a generalized admission of guilt or complicity, a result, he insisted repeatedly, of his failure to engage in more active resistance. This was more a philosophical expression of the famous Lutheran dictum "simul iustus et peccator" [human beings are sinners before God and at the same time are saved only by God's grace through Jesus Christ]. Indeed, his membership of the Confessing Church served Verschuer well, helping him to free himself from his "Berufsverbot" and take up yet another academic position at the University of Münster where he again received research grants from the Deutsche Forschungsgemeinschaft (DFG), which supported his earlier collaboration with Mengele in Auschwitz.

Verschuer's case demonstrates clearly how religion and networks of the faithful may be used to protect a perpetrator from being exposed and charged, and even from coming to terms with the evil nature of his deeds. Instead of awakening a genuine sense of remorse, it provided Verschuer with a comfortable conscience. His case is an example of the dark side of humankind, which is not bound to any particular nationality, culture, or time. It offers a profound lesson demonstrating the massive human cost involved when humanity and respect for all individuals are no longer the core concerns of religion, but rather religion or religious affiliation is used as a means of concealment and obfuscation. Under conditions where bioethics tends to install abstract forms and instruments of governance it is not so easy but it is just as crucial to be aware of indicators of the patterns of "demonic times." This should be a topic in a cross-cultural dialogue between East Asia and the West.

References

Alexander, Leo, 1946 "Letter to his wife," cited in Paul Julian Weindling, *Nazi Medicine and the Nuremberg Trials*. Basingstoke: Palgrave Macmillan, 2006, pp. 245–246.

"Denkschrift betreffend Herrn Prof. Dr. med. Frhr. Von Verschuer," September 1949," III/86a/31, *Archiv für die Geschichte der Max Planck Gesellschaft*, Berlin.

Fricke, Otto, 1946, "Kirchliches Urteil über die Persönlichkeit und die wissenschaftliche Arbeit von Herr Professor Dr. Freiherr von Verschuer," III/86A/26, *Archiv für die Geschichte der Max Planck Gesellschaft*, Berlin.

Fricke, Otto, 1990, *Biographisch-Bibliographisches Kirchenlexikon*, Vol. II: p. 124.

Hammerstein, Notker, 1989, *Die Johann Wolfgang Goethe Universität Frankfurt am Main*. Neuwied/Frankfurt: Alfred Metzner Verlag.

Hammerstein, Notker, 1999, *Die Deutsche Forschungsgemeinschaft in der Weimarer Republik und im Dritten Reich*. Munich: Beck.

Kröner, Hans-Peter, 1998, *Von der Rassenhygiene zur Humangenetik. Das Kaiser Wilhelm-Institut für Anthropologie, menschliche Erblehre und Eugenik nach dem Krieg*. Stuttgart: Gustav Fischer.

Markl, Hubert, 2001a, "Symposium in Berlin: Biomedical Sciences and Human Experimentation at the Kaiser Wilhelm Institutes – The Auschwitz Connection," *Max Planck Research Supplement* 3.

Markl, Hubert, 2001b, "Entgrenzte Wissenschaft: Der Irrweg von Evolutionsbiologie und Genetik zu Rassimus und Mord." www.mpg.de/pdf/redenPraesidenten/011031emblMarkl.pdf.

Müller-Hill, Benno, 1984, *Tödliche Wissenschaft*. Reinbek, Hamburg: Rowohlt Verlag.

Müller-Hill, Benno, 1988, *Murderous Science*. Oxford: Oxford University Press.

Sachse, Carola, 2004, "Adolf von Butenandt und Otmar von Verschuer," in *Adolf Butenandt und die Kaiser-Wilhem Gesellschaft*, ed. Wolfgang Schieder und Achim Trunk. Göttingen: Wallstein.

Sachse, Carola and Walker, Mark, 2005, *Politics and Science in Wartime. Comparative International Perspectives on the Kaiser Wilhelm Institute*. Osiris No. 20.

Scharf, Kurt, 1977, *Brücken und Breschen*. Berlin: Furche.

Schleiermacher, Sabine, 1998, *Sozialethik im Spannungsfeld von Sozial-und Rassenhygiene*. Husum: Mathiessen.

Verschuer, Otmar, 1945, "Erbe-Umwelt-Führung" III/86A/3–1 (1–4), (May 19th), *Archiv für die Geschichte der Max Planck Gesellschaft*, Berlin.

Verschuer, Otmar, 1965, "Probleme der Eugenik-Aufgaben und Gefahren," III/86A/83, *Archiv für die Geschichte der Max Planck Gesellschaft*, Berlin.

Verschuer, Otmar, 2003, "Mein wissenschaftlicher Weg," in *Archivgespräche No. 9*, ed. *Archiv zur Geschichte der Max Planck Gesellschaft*, Berlin.

Verschuer to Hahn, 1946, II, 1A, PA Verschuer, No. 5, (May 23), *Archiv für die Geschichte der Max Planck Gesellschaft*, Berlin.

Weingart, Peter, Kroll, Jürgen and Bayertz, Kurt, 1988, *Rasse, Blut und Gene*. Frankfurt: Suhrkamp Verlag.

Winnacker, Ernste-Ludwig, 2000, "Rede von DFG-Präsident Ernst-Ludwig Winnacker anlässlich der Einweihung des Mahnmals zur Erinnerung an die Opfer nationalsozialistischer Euthanasieverbrechen in Berlin-Buch," October 14. http://www.dfg.de/aktuelles_presse/reden_stellungnahmen/2000/redstell/berlin_buch.html.

Zirlewagen, Marc, 2006, "Verschuer, Otmar," *Biographisch-Bibliographisches Kirchenlexikon*, Vol. XXVII: 1437–1447.

9   America's memory problems

Diaspora groups, civil society and
the perils of "chosen amnesia"

David B. MacDonald

Introduction

This chapter contextualizes America's decision to suppress knowledge of Japanese
war crimes within a larger framework of atrocity denial in American history. This
includes the government's denial of its own medical and other atrocities against
indigenous peoples and African-Americans and others. Its base has traditionally
been a strong adherence to the principles of realpolitik, but also the belief that as
most countries are founded on blood, a certain amount of "chosen amnesia" is
necessary in assessing the formation of the modern nation state. In this view,
dwelling too heavily on past crimes is unproductive for all concerned, especially
when perpetrators are allies. However, times are changing. The end of the Cold
War, the rise of identity politics, and the growing voices of minorities have led to
renewed calls for America to recognize its own historic atrocities and those of its
allies. This has been the case in commemoration of the Holocaust, the Armenian
genocide, and the wartime internment of Japanese-Americans, where promotion
of memory has come from diaspora organizations within the United States. More
vocal and confident Chinese-American and Korean-American communities have
made it possible for American civil society and government at times to raise
questions about Japanese war responsibility. Comfort women, who are not a focus
of this chapter, is the clearest instance.

In 1822, Ernest Renan famously observed that "the essential element of a nation
is that all its individuals must have many things in common but it must also have
forgotten many things" (Buckley-Zistel 2006, 132). More recently, Stanley Cohen
has noted how societies deliberately forget uncomfortable knowledge, which
then becomes a series of "open secrets" known by everyone but not discussed.
This becomes "social amnesia": "a mode of forgetting by which a whole society
separates itself from its discreditable past record." Alternatively, one can see this
as a practice of "chosen amnesia," when societies deliberately exclude unwanted
or unsavory aspects of their national past (Buckley-Zistel 2006, 133–4).

Jing-Bao Nie makes an impressive case for America to acknowledge and
compensate those whom it wronged by supporting Japanese medical experiments,
by suppressing this information from the public, and by refusing to prosecute
known war criminals, members of Units 731, 100, and others. Nie suggests that

America was an "accessory after the fact," aiding and abetting Japan's criminal activities by not bringing perpetrators to justice (Nie 2006, 24). Further, it is clear from a moral perspective that "This treatment of Japanese doctors by the USA can never be justified by the standards of moral traditions in any culture. Any government that supports and exploits such atrocities should apologise and compensate" (Nie 2002, S5).

Yet, America treads a fine line. It will not antagonize allies like Japan if the benefits (in terms of enhancing its international reputation) are perceived to be minimal. Reflecting a political science perspective I argue that the extent to which US policy will be "captured" by issue areas will depend on the strength of the support the electorate has for these issues. As Hansen and King argue persuasively:

> ideas are more likely to be translated into policy under three conditions: when there is a synergy between ideas and interests, when the actors possess the requisite enthusiasm and institutional position, and when timing contributes to a broad constellation of preferences that reinforce these ideas, rather than detracting from them.
>
> (Hansen and King 2001, 239)

America's larger and more influential diaspora groups operate at a time when identity politics has increasing salience. While ethnic groups in the United States are not able to dictate US policy per se, they can mold certain issue areas through organized and repeated pressure. Ironically, Chinese-Americans may gain an apology from the US if the crimes are presented in a way that scripts them as relatively unimportant in US history, but in a way that promotes the image of the US as a country committed to justice. This is perhaps not the argument other contributors to this volume will be making, but it is worth exploring further. The US is wont to ignore or suppress memories of the past when they are too painful – when their legacies might threaten to unravel the exceptionalist myths many Americans like to tell about their forefathers. Thus there have been no official apologies for the destruction of American indigenous peoples, nor for African-American slavery. Nor has any compensation for slavery been mooted publicly (Corlett 2001, 239; Howard-Hassmann 2004, 831). At the same time, in cases where there have been obvious injustices, but the injustices were not a central part of US narratives of the nation, the government has been willing to both acknowledge and compensate. The Reagan administration's apology for the internment of Japanese-Americans is an obvious example. President Reagan apologized to the 110,000 Japanese-Americans interned during World War II. In 1988 he followed a formal apology with US$20,000 for each person who was interned (Biondi 2003, 8).

In cases where the US has not been responsible for past atrocities like the Jewish Holocaust, efforts to commemorate, and secure apologies and compensation, are sometimes forthcoming. For example, the Holocaust has been enshrined as a key trope in American national identity. If American elites have rejected demands for compensation to the descendants of American slaves, they have certainly worked to secure reparations for Nazi-era slave laborers, Jews and others alike. The Clinton administration in particular helped pressure the German government to secure reparations, in part because it has promoted a feeling of the US promoting justice. America as a large and relatively fragmented democratic system also allows ethnic constituencies to promote their interests if they can deliver a block of votes or influence the general public.

I begin this chapter with a brief overview of Japanese atrocities, follow this with details of the cover-up, then offer some relevant context concerning America's own crimes. I then argue that Chinese-Americans may have a chance to gain acknowledgment of their suffering at an official level. They could even gain a Congressional Bill condemning Japanese denialism, and might even gain an apology for the American cover-up, amnesty for, and payment to ranking members of Unit 731. Whether this is a crucial issue around which Chinese-Americans will congregate is another matter, since there seems to be a stronger interest in mobilizing around the Nanjing massacre, as I have argued elsewhere (MacDonald 2005). In any case, acknowledgment of *America's* role in denying Japanese atrocities, and any potential compensation resulting from that denial, are unlikely to be forthcoming. This is doubly so in the current international climate. Contemporary ethical dilemmas like torture and permanent detention at Abu Ghraib and Guantanamo Bay, and the killing of civilians in US bombing in Iraq and Afghanistan, have drawn public attention in the US and globally.

Japanese atrocities and the US cover-up

Japan's biological experimentation was centered around Unit 731, a biological weapons program founded by Lieutenant General Ishii Shiro. Beginning with a biological experimental unit at the Tokyo Medical School, Ishii branched out into Japanese-controlled Manchukuo in 1932, establishing facilities in the city of Harbin, the town of Beiyinhe, followed by a larger facility at Pingfan in 1939. This sprawling facility of 70 buildings was soon known as "the secret of secrets" (Gold 2000, 29, 33, 39; Hicks 1998, 53–5).

America's collusion with the Japanese to cover up their medical crimes came soon after the Japanese surrender. Key members of Unit 731, like Ishii's second in command in Tokyo, Naito Ryoichi, approached American officials with information about the scientific achievements of the Unit. This was followed by a series of backroom deals, approved by President Truman and Supreme Allied Commander General MacArthur. In return for exclusive access to the experimental data, members of the Unit, from Ishii down, were granted immunity from prosecution. In so doing, America expeditiously gained 20 years'-worth of information at minimal financial cost (Gold 2000, 94–109).

Ishii died in 1959. Many former members went on to achieve high office in scientific and medical posts. Three of the most notorious members (involved in vivisections, frost-bite, and bacteriological research) founded the Green Cross, a Japan-based blood bank. Others became professors and deans of Japanese medical schools in Kyoto, Kinki, and Osaka. Many others remained in key positions within the health care sector (Gold 2000, 140–3).

The Tokyo Trials (convened from May 1946 to November 1948) enabled further denial, by excluding many Japanese crimes. Americans largely controlled the trials and their outcome, disproportionately punishing crimes against the United States (like Pearl Harbor) while down-playing other atrocities including Japanese medical crimes (Awaya 1998, 222–4; Eykholt 2000, 19; Finn 1992, 150; Hicks 1998, 7–8). Asian victims of sexual assault were also marginalized. While local B and C class trials investigated the sexual assault of Dutchwomen during the war, the "enslavement of Asian and Pacific Island women" was ignored (Yoneyama 1999, 11–12, 16). Further, Emperor Hirohito was neither charged nor called as a witness. His continuation as Emperor further buttressed official and popular denial (Nish 2000, 86).

In 1949, during the Soviet-led Khabarovsk Trial, many of the facts of Units 731 and 100 came to light. America's GHQ in Japan, on advice from the US State Department, denied that they had any information about Japanese medical experiments and accused the Soviets of propaganda (Hicks 1998, 51; Williams and Wallace 1989, 220–1).

Denial and America's ambiguous legacy in Japan

At an ideological level, America turned a blind eye to denialism, as Japan was rapidly converted from enemy to ally. Japan was on the front line of the Cold War, as it was on the front line of the Korean War and China's civil war. Denialism was promoted by the Japanese political and intellectual establishment, with American support. The ruling Liberal Democratic Party included many "die-hard nationalists" who traditionally viewed the Pacific war as a legitimate defense against communism's "Red Peril" and Western colonialism's "White Peril" in Asia (Dower 2002, 218–19).

Concerning Japanese crimes, a tacit understanding seems to have evolved. In return for maintaining Hirohito on the throne, and protecting many ranking military and government officials, the firebombing of Japanese cities in a strategy designed by General Curtis LeMay would be suppressed as an issue (Powers 1995). Lest we forget, over two million Japanese soldiers and sailors died in the War, alongside one million civilians. All major cities with the exception of Kyoto were razed, some 66 in total (Godemont 1997, 141). As Dower recalls: "It became commonplace to speak of the war dead themselves – and, indeed, of virtually all ordinary Japanese – as being 'victims' and 'sacrifices' " (Dower 2002, 218, 228). Orr similarly notes a "mythologizing of war victimhood" in the post-War peace movements "manifested in a tendency to privilege the facts of Japanese victimhood over considerations of what occasioned that victimhood" (Orr 2001, 3).

Japan also had a species of trump card – the legacy of Hiroshima and Nagasaki. Atomic devastation produced "victim consciousness" (*higaisha ishiki*) or "atomic victim exceptionalism" (Orr 2001, 7; Dower 1996, 123). As Dower describes the instrumental use of a bomb victim mentality: "Hiroshima and Nagasaki became icons of Japanese suffering . . . blotting out recollection of the Japanese victimization of others" (Dower 1996, 123). Certainly Japanese crimes were reasonably well known in Asia, but the atomic bomb was known throughout the world. These systematic bombings of civilians, in both the firebombing and atomic bombing of cities, constitute important atrocities. (Cohn 2006).

American crimes

As Barber has argued, myths of American "innocence" have functioned as a key binding force in US domestic and foreign policy. The belief that the US is both a good and unblemished actor in world politics is an important part of US exceptionalist narratives (Barber 1996, 49). However, the history of American expansion across the continent and beyond, and the history of slavery in the United States make such views difficult to sustain. America's indigenous peoples, for example, were subject to horrific treatment, making any founding myths of innocence highly contested in the present. Indeed, ethnocide, including widespread massacre, was a major part of early US expansionist policy (Hitchcock and Twedt 1997, 380). Between 1789 and 1898 there were an estimated 1,243 skirmishes between US troops and Indians, not to mention "hundreds of fights between bands of Indians and state troopers, posses, and Texas Rangers" (Hollon 1974, 133).

The use of disease as a primitive biological weapon is evident in many historic accounts. The "King Philip's War" (1675–76) appears to be the first case of conflict between indigenous peoples (the Wampanoag) and settlers prompted by a belief that colonists had deliberately spread disease among them (Stiffarm and Lane 1992, 32; Friedberg 2000, 339). Through a mixture of massacre, land theft, disease, forced marches, policies of starvation, a general declining birthrate, and a trail of broken treaties, the indigenous population of America had dropped from several million in the seventeenth century to just under 250,000 by 1920 (Stiffarm and Lane 1992, 37).

Further crimes were evident in the 14-year Philippines–American war and pacification. This conflict, which lasted from 1899 to 1913, saw conceptualizations of superior and inferior races and civilizations figuring prominently (Kramer 2006). Of a base population of seven million, between 600,000 and 900,000 Filipinos were killed, the great majority of them civilians. As Davis has observed, the main ports were closed during a major drought to deliberately starve the population into submission. Existing rice stores were destroyed, alongside cattle and other local food supplies. Such tactics presaged similar strategies in Vietnam (Davis 2001, 198–200).

American medical experimentation and the Cold War

The principles of the Nuremberg Code were first applied to medical research by four American judges during the Doctors' Trials at Nuremberg in 1946. Here, some 20 Nazi doctors were convicted on charges of war crimes and crimes against humanity, for conducting human experimentation at Auschwitz among other abuses (Childress 2000, 347; see also Katz 1992, 231–4). The resulting 10-point code enshrined such principles as informed consent, ensuring that research was socially important, using animal tests before human trials, and the right of human participants to end their involvement at any time. However, the code was a guide, and was conveniently set aside as the needs of governments required. As Childress argues: "For many years the Nuremberg Code played virtually no role in ethical discussions, public policies, and legal decisions in the United States" (Childress 2000, 350).

Indeed, during World War II and after, the United States, like many other countries including the Soviet Union, engaged in its own biological and chemical weapons research. In 1943, a BW research center was created at Camp Detrick (later Fort Detrick) near Frederick, Maryland, "[r]ivalled only by the Manhattan atom bomb project in secrecy" (Williams and Wallace 1989, 95). After 1945, research was expanded and it continues to the present. Williams and Wallace document the fact that the US continued the research of Unit 731 in post-War Japan, forming the "Tokyo Nutrition Research Centre" (code-named J2C 406) with the active involvement of Ishii Shiro. Animals and insects were bred *en masse* for medical experiments (Williams and Wallace 1989, 273–5).

In the 1950s, a $90 million biological mass production facility was constructed at Pine Bluff, Arkansas (Williams and Wallace 1989, 281–2). Camp Detrick was upgraded and BW research went into high gear. Special laboratories were built to breed *Aedes aegypti* mosquitoes, a vector for yellow fever. Scientists created facilities able to breed some 130 million mosquitoes per month, and "by the end of the decade [1950s] its laboratories were reported to contain mosquitoes infected with yellow and dengue fevers and malaria, as well as plague fleas, ticks contaminated with tularaemia and flies carrying cholera, anthrax and dysentery" (Williams and Wallace 1989, 283–4).

Consider another chapter in American history. As Welsome has documented in *The Plutonium Files*, and as Wang further documents in this volume (Chapter 2), thousands of Americans were subject to radiation experiments as the US created and tested atomic weaponry. As Welsome argues of the Atomic Energy Commission: "Thousands of human radiation experiments, many of them unethical and without therapeutic benefit, were funded by the AEC over the next three decades of the Cold War" (quoted in Markowitz 2000, 603). In the well-known case of the Vanderbilt University prenatal clinic, between 830 and 850 pregnant women were fed doses of radioactive iron to determine its rate of absorption into the body. The experiments were conducted between 1945 and 1949. A later follow-up study in 1969 was designed to "determine morbidity and mortality experiences in the children and mothers fed radioactive iron" (Rothman 2003, 28, 32).

Such experimentation was deliberately concealed, both to prevent lawsuits from victims and their families and to assure the availability of the subjects. Further, the AEC feared that too much public knowledge of nuclear radiation and its effects could dampen support for the Bomb (Markowitz 2000, 604–5). Despite guidelines and codes, the US government and medical establishment seem to have subordinated ethical considerations in the quest to best the Soviet Union. Despite the availability of large-scale data on the victims of Hiroshima and Nagasaki, the government sponsored detailed studies on humans charting the effects of radiation on body processes and its effects on the environment (Brandt and Freidenfelds 1996, 240).

To this we can add a number of Department of Defense and CIA-sponsored projects, performed at over 30 university campuses. A variety of experiments using hallucinogenic drugs and other controlled substances took place at Harvard and around the country. Prescott has documented the testing of potential "truth drugs" and a variety of other drugs which were used as mind-altering devices. This includes Wendt's Project CHATTER, based in the psychology department of the University of Rochester. Wendt was contracted by the Navy to study "the effects of a variety of drugs, including barbiturates, amphetamines, alcohol, and heroin." A wide variety of other studies followed, including the infamous project MKULTRA at the University of Minnesota and Missouri Institute of Psychiatry (Prescott 2002, 33–4; McCoy 2006).

As Moreno and Lederer reveal, there was little ethical oversight of human experimentation. Rather the reverse seems to have been true:

> [P]reviously classified transcripts of many of the Pentagon advisory bodies, such as the Committee on Medical Sciences, show that in 1951 and 1952 most members were definitely not in favor of devising new, rigorous protections for human research subjects. Not only did many members assert the necessity of human experiments for some of the work that needed to be done, some expressed grave doubts about the wisdom of creating any formal review mechanism at all.
>
> (Moreno and Lederer 1996, 231)

All of this tells us something about the climate of medical ethics in America during the Cold War, a climate in which individual human rights were sacrificed in order to defend the country against the Soviet Union. At base was the belief that the Soviets were a highly unscrupulous enemy who would stop at nothing to achieve world domination. This belief animated the desire to push science to its limits, where necessary with disregard for individual rights.

American medical experimentation and racism

The United States implemented extensive eugenic policies in the early twentieth century (Hansen and King 2001, 237–9). Eugenic and racial theories were popular among American elites, who disparaged not only African-Americans, Latinos, and indigenous peoples, but many immigrant groups as well. Women and the lower classes were also perceived to be biologically inferior. Modern birth control and family planning initiatives were premised largely on the higher reproduction rates among immigrants, versus the lower rates among white Americans. "Racial suicide" was commonly feared (Leonard 2003, 690–6).

Many indigenous women were subject to forced sterilizations during the twentieth century. While the Indian Health Service greatly improved medical care on reservations and dramatically lowered rates of tuberculosis and other diseases, it actively promoted "family planning" policies to counter the high indigenous birthrate (Lawrence 2000, 411). A report published in 1979 revealed that 60 percent of hospitals surveyed had "routinely sterilized women under the age of twenty-one," in violation of official guidelines established by the federal government (Udel 2001, 46). Ralstin-Lewis (2005, 71–2) reveals:

> Native women seeking treatment in Indian Health Service (IHS) hospitals and with IHS-contracted physicians were allowed neither the basic right of informed consent prior to sterilization nor the right to refuse the operation. . . . From 1970 to 1980, the birthrate for Indian women fell at a rate seven times greater than that of white women.

The situation continued until Congress passed the Indian Health Care Improvement Act in 1976, restoring tribal control over medical services. The levels of abuse dropped significantly thereafter (Lawrence 2000, 415).

Better known were the Tuskeegee experiments involving African-Americans. The US Public Health Service in tandem with several other organizations embarked on a lengthy study of the effects of untreated syphilis among uneducated black males. Patients were neither told they had the condition, nor informed of the methods available to treat it. The experiments were carried out in Macon County, Alabama, from the 1930s to the 1970s. Some 400 African-Americans were involved, and questions of informed consent were completely ignored. Residual effects remain, and African-Americans are still deeply distrustful of the medical profession, which many deem to be structurally racist (Harter et al. 2000, 21).

My point in presenting this partial catalogue of ethically questionable activities is to demonstrate that far from *merely* condoning and then covering up Japanese medical experiments, the United States continued Japan's biological research, and used its own citizens as human-guinea pigs on numerous now well-known occasions. This takes Nie's accusations a step further, effectively blurring the lines between perpetrator and accessory.

Change in the air

The end of the Cold War profoundly changed mainstream thinking about what lengths one needed to go to in order to tame the Soviet threat. What Nytagodien and Neal term "the age of apologies" (Nytagodien and Neal 2005, 465) or what Torpey calls "reparations politics" began in many Western countries in the wake of the collapse of the Soviet Union. Governments, churches, and private firms were increasingly held to account for past actions against indigenous peoples and other disadvantaged groups (Torpey 2001, 334). Olick's analysis of the "memory boom" which emerged following the Cold War is little different. Here too, national groups became caught up with "new versions of the past rather than the future"

(Olick 1998, 380). Marginalized groups asserted themselves, and more significantly, states were actually willing to listen.

With a conscientious objector from the Vietnam War in the White House, left-leaning Labor governments in Australia and Britain, and the decimation of Conservative rule in Canada, many Western societies now seemed more open to debating and discussing the past. Bill Clinton, Paul Keating, and Tony Blair all engaged in forms of "self-examination," apologizing to various wronged groups (native Hawaiians and Panamanians, Australian Aborigines, the Irish, and First Nation people) for the "gross historical crimes" committed in their own countries and against others (Olick and Coughlin 2003, 37). The Canadian government also apologized to First Nations, in 1998, although Prime Minister Chretien did not give an official apology (Nobles 2008, 74–5). In this climate, we see the rise of memory politics and activism on behalf of disadvantaged groups. Activism succeeds if it can tell a story about America that is palatable to the mainstream and that allows admission of some guilt without undermining the core national identity.

Ethnic groups certainly have the capacity to help shape foreign and domestic policy. First, if the majority is uninterested, apathetic, or generally ignorant about the specific issue, the group may exert a great deal of influence, especially if it can deliver blocks of votes in important constituencies or help fundraise for sympathetic candidates (Saideman 2002, 94). It is no accident that America's most vocal diasporas have proven to be the most successful. Armenian-Americans (nearly one million), Japanese-Americans (1.2 million), and Jewish-Americans (six million) have been successful in promoting several signature issues in Congress: recognition of the Armenian genocide, the incarceration of Japanese-Americans, and support for Israel. Indeed, during the 1990s, Armenia and Israel received the largest amount of US foreign aid per capita (Shain 2002, 116).

Armenian-Americans, in addition to pressing Turkey on the genocide question, were able to use their power during Armenia's war with Azerbaijan, and its annexation of Nagorno-Karabakh (which contained an Armenian majority). Due to Armenian-American pressure, Section 907 was added to the Freedom Support Act of 1992, which specifically prohibited American assistance to Azerbaijan. This effectively meant US rubber-stamping the invasion and annexation of part of another country (Saideman 2002, 99). Japanese-Americans won an apology and compensation from the Reagan administration for their imprisonment. Israeli lobby groups have secured long-term American support for the State of Israel and its policies, including the occupation of the West Bank and Gaza, the Israel nuclear weapons program, and the Gaza War. America has contributed more than $140 billion since 1948, roughly $3 billion annually in direct assistance (Mearsheimer and Walt 2006).

Other examples of diaspora success include Greek-American lobbying to have America only recognize the Yugoslav republic of Macedonia (now independent) as the "Former Yugoslav Republic of Macedonia" (FYROM). Further, diaspora pressure prompted the US to look the other way as Greece launched an economic blockade of FYROM, seriously weakening its economy (Saideman 2002, 98–9).

Continued US sanctions policy against Cuba further demonstrates the power of a small ethnic community to influence foreign policy at a national level (Moore 2002, 84).

Recognizing past atrocities: checks and balances

However, Congress, the Presidency, and other branches of government often perform a balancing role, acquiescing to some minority demands while refusing others that conflict with major US interests. Thus in the Armenian case, the diaspora has pressured Congress for decades to officially recognize the Armenian genocide, without success. Turkey as a key NATO ally continues to lobby successfully to prevent US official recognition of the genocide. When a non-binding Congressional resolution recognizing the genocide went before the House of Representatives in 2000, Turkey threatened to stop all American military flights from its Incirlik airbase, from where it was enforcing Iraq's no-fly zone (Shain 2002, 132). It also threatened to pull out of NATO. Clinton personally intervened to block the resolution (Auron 2003, 111–15). What is clear is that geopolitical exigencies have made America unable to recognize the facts of the genocide, although they submit to Armenian diaspora pressure in other ways.

America's indigenous peoples have lacked sufficient domestic political power to garner official recognition of the crimes committed against them, let alone apology or compensation. In 2000, the Department of Indian Affairs did accept "moral responsibility" for waging "war on Indian people . . . by threat, deceit and force," committing "acts so terrible that they infect, diminish and destroy the lives of Indian people decades later, generations later" (Kiernan 2002, 165). However, this stark admission failed to reflect official government or administration policy, and was consistent with the general thrust of American policies, which show a profound lack of remorse (Corlett 2001, 239).

The only prominent genocide that has achieved official recognition is the Holocaust. This is in part owing to the lobbying efforts of Jewish Americans to secure its recognition and continued US support for Israel. Integral to this effort is the fact that the Holocaust came into its own as a world-historical event during the 1960s and 1970s, especially after the Vietnam War (Ball 2000, 4). In a speech in 1978, President Carter recognized the central importance of the Holocaust in American life with powerful lessons to teach. Americans had helped liberate the camps, then functioned as a haven for many of the oppressed. Large numbers of survivors were granted asylum. Moreover, the Holocaust was presented as the embodiment of all that a democratic, pluralist, freedom-loving America was not. The Holocaust had other important moral lessons of another type to convey. As a bystander nation which did little to prevent the Holocaust, it was now America's special mission to spread democracy and freedom in the name of other victims of totalitarian systems (Young 1999, 73).

Many Jewish-American groups have responded by bringing the Holocaust directly into American life. In 1993, the United States Holocaust Memorial Museum opened its doors in central Washington, DC. The Museum Council made clear that "America is the enemy of racism and its ultimate expression, genocide. . . . in act and word the Nazis denied the deepest tenets of the American people" (Young 1999, 73). Another aspect of Holocaust Americanization was the campaign to compensate Jewish survivors and their families for slave labor they were forced to perform during the War. Another campaign focused on retrieving Holocaust-era assets from Swiss banks. In both cases, the US government pressured the German, Austrian, and Swiss governments, as well as banks and corporations within these countries, to compensate victims and their families (Barkan 2001, xv, 21).

Chinese diaspora politics in America

The US is now home to over one-third of overseas Chinese living outside of Asia. Approximately 70 percent of these are foreign born, the majority having immigrated since 1980. California and New York contain the largest numbers of Chinese-Americans, with 40 percent residing in California alone (Fan 2003, 261–2, 269–71). The *New York Times* has identified a "cottage industry" of remembrance, with "dozens of groups working the Internet to publicize it, as well as recent documentaries, novels and exhibits" (Marino 1998). While long divided between support for Taiwan and the People's Republic, in the 1990s, the diaspora began to speak with a more unified voice, joining together a "multiplicity of voices" (Maier 2000, 3).

A number of prominent Jewish-Americans have been active in promoting memory of Nanking and other Japanese crimes, especially in making common cause with Chinese scholars combating Japanese denialism (Shermer and Grobman 2000, 237). For example, Abraham Cooper, associate dean of the Wiesenthal Center, has argued that "In terms of cold, calculated cruelty, the people who operated Unit 731 would have been right at home with Josef Mengele and his associates" (quoted in Dobbs 2000, A1). Unlike the Armenian lobby's battles with the Turkish lobby, each promoting diametrically opposed positions, the situation vis-à-vis the crimes of Unit 731 is more nuanced.

The Japanese situation is different, for the simple reason that debate continues within Japan both at the societal and official levels about the atrocities. While the long-ruling LDP rejected compensation and was ambivalent about apology, as Jeans has noted, a number of "peace"-oriented museums, locally or privately operated, have been reviewing in quite a stark fashion the history of Japanese aggression in Asia, and a substantial scholarly literature has documented Japanese war atrocities. The Nagasaki Atomic Bomb Museum is a particularly fine example of a museum which has incorporated a section on Japan's expansionism accompanying the commemoration of atomic victims. Other progressive museums include the Osaka International Peace Center and the Kyoto Museum for World Peace. Of course, traditional "war" museums continue to promote denial, such as the Yasukuni Shrine War Museum, the Showa Hall, and the Chiran Peace Museum for Kamikaze Pilots (Jeans 2005, 151–82). In short, the issues of war crimes and atrocities remain deeply contested in Japan.

Further, Japanese courts have admitted that the crimes occurred, making any future American apology less dramatic. In 2002, 180 plaintiffs concluded a five-year-long civil case against the Japanese government for the crimes of Unit 731. The plaintiffs demanded US$83,500 each for the deaths of some 2,100 victims of medical experimentation. While the Tokyo court refused to award damages (claiming they have been settled by the Japanese government at the international level), they did admit that the crimes occurred, and that the Japanese army conducted experiments on civilians and used BW weaponry. The presiding judges described the crimes of Unit 731 as "inhumane," having caused "truly horrible and enormous" harm to their Chinese victims. Further, the judges upheld that both the Geneva and Hague Conventions had been broken by Japan during the war (Watts 2002, 857).

A further positive sign is the relative unity of Asian Americans as a lobbying force. The Congressional Asian Pacific American Caucus, chaired by Mike Honda, is bipartisan and claims to represent the interests of 11 million Asian Pacific Americans (APA). Honda describes the APA as a "community," which together has certain common interests, such as the elimination of racism in American society (Honda 2006). Prominent Congressional leaders like Norman Mineta, Patsy Mink, Robert A. Underwood, and David Wu have also had an important role to play. As a state congressman in California, Honda successfully passed AJR 27 through the California State Assembly, calling on Japan to apologize and pay compensation for its wartime atrocities (Chu Lin 2001). He has linked apologies and reparations for both groups as a "basic human rights issue. It took us 12 years to get our government to apologize to us. We are supporting these [Chinese-American] efforts because it is the right thing to do" (Dobbs 2000, A1). Yet we should be clear. While Congress might pass a resolution pushing for Japan to apologize, and might apologize for its own suppression of Japanese crimes, America will most likely not admit to further BW research in Japan or many of the details of its collusion with Ishii and his colleagues. Further, the road to compensation will be an extremely long one. This is doubly so since Japanese courts have already admitted guilt, thus in some respects absolving America as an accessory. As we have seen during the Clinton administration, apologies were heartfelt but often failed to go far enough to mollify victims of American-supported crimes.

Certainly Clinton did make numerous apologies for everything from the annexation of Hawaii to American support of right-wing Guatemalan military forces. Unfortunately many of these apologies never told the whole story. Clinton may have apologized for US support but did not apologize for any active involvement in Guatemala, for example. While Clinton *acknowledged* the evils of slavery during his state visit to Africa in 1998, he did not formally admit the US role or formally apologize. Monetary reparations were also off the agenda (Howard-Hassmann 2004, 831). For Gibney and Roxtrom, it was clear at the end of the Clinton years that most of these apologies were largely vacuous. They note rightly: "The biggest problem with state apologies is that the apologizing state wants it both ways: it wants credit for recognizing and acknowledging a wrong against others, but it also wants the world to remain exactly as it had been before the apology was issued" (Gibney and Roxtrom 2001, 936). Apologies had a strong feel-good factor, but when America was at fault, full and frank admissions that might imply costs for the American taxpayer were starkly limited.

Conclusions

Chinese-Americans might expect a limited apology, but the ideal of gaining compensation for atrocities the Japanese carried out on Chinese soil, while America was at war with Japan, is unlikely to transpire. What American history demonstrates time and again is that the government will champion the cause of justice (or appear to do so) when its own self-image is not threatened. However, as the American-Indian case demonstrates, the government is much less likely to do so when revelations about its past might cast doubt on US claims to an exceptional heritage. In addition, apologies require a president amenable to public displays of *mea culpa*. Bill Clinton was a master at such posturing; George W. Bush was not. It remains to be seen how President Obama will tackle such divisive and complicated issues.

In both Japan and the United States, recognition, apology, and just compensation to victims of atrocities will be difficult to achieve. The Japanese case is complicated by the persistence of the association of the Emperor and the former empire with purity. The American case is made difficult by its long-standing myths of exceptionalism, as well as its self-professed role in promoting global peace and stability, while championing democracy. In both countries there are social and political forces which, under appropriate conditions, can be mobilized to accept responsibility for past injustices. In both cases, social actors may help to pave the way for more harmonious future relations as the Reagan administration's apology and compensation for Japanese-Americans demonstrates. But this path is difficult. In the US, it is clear that society has changed in the wake of the 9/11 terrorist attacks and the wars in Afghanistan and Iraq. Yet while the Obama administration marks a departure from the past, it is yet too early to tell how far either Congress or the executive will be willing to reconceptualize America's past.

References and further reading

Auron, Y. (2003) *The Banality of Denial: Israel and the Armenian Genocide*, New York: Transaction Publishers.

Awaya, K. (1998) "Controversies Surrounding the Asia-Pacific War: The Tokyo War Crimes Trial", in P. West, S. Levine, and J. Hiltz (eds) *America's Wars in Asia: A Cultural Approach to History and Memory*, London: M.E. Sharpe.

Ball, K. (2000) "Introduction: Trauma and its Institutional Destinies", *Cultural Critique* 46.

Barber, B. R. (1996) *Jihad vs. McWorld*. New York: Ballantine Books.

Barenblatt, D. (2004) *A Plague Upon Humanity: The Secret Genocide of Axis Japan's Germ Warfare Operation*, London: HarperCollins.

Barkan, E. (2001) *The Guilt of Nations: Restitution and Negotiating Historical Injustices*, Baltimore, MD: Johns Hopkins University Press.

Biondi, M. (2003) "The Rise of the Reparations Movement", *Radical History Review* 87: 5–18.

Brandt, A. and L. Freidenfelds (1996), "Commentary: Research Ethics after World War II: The Insular Culture of Biomedicine", *Kennedy Institute of Ethics Journal* 6(3): 239–43.

Buckley-Zistel, S. (2006) "Remembering To Forget: Chosen Amnesia as a Strategy For Local Coexistence In Post-Genocide Rwanda", *Africa* 76(2): 131–50.

Cairns, A. (2003) "Coming to Terms with the Past", in J. Torpey (ed.) *Politics and the Past: On Repairing Historical Injustices*, Lanham, MD: Rowman & Littlefield.

Childress, J. (2000) "Nuremberg's Legacy: Some Ethical Reflections", *Perspectives in Biology and Medicine* 43(3): 347–61.

Chu Lin, S. (2001) "Congressman Mike Honda To Visit China", *Asia Week*, August 3–9, Available at http://www.asianweek.com/2001_08_03/news_honda.html.

Cohn, M. (2006) "War Crimes: Goose and Gander", *truthout*, 13 March. Available at http://www.truthout.org/docs_2006/031306J.shtml.

Corlett, J.A. (2001) "Reparations to Native Americans?", in A. Jokic (ed.) *War Crimes and Collective Wrongdoing: A Reader*, Oxford: Blackwell.

Davis, M. (2001) *Late Victorian Holocausts: El Nino Famines and the Making of the Third World*, London: Verso.

Dobbs, M. (2000) "Lawyers Target Japanese Abuses: WWII Compensation Effort Shifts From Europe to Asia", *Washington Post*, 5 March: A1.

Dower, J. (1996) "The Bombed: Hiroshimas and Nagasakis in Japanese Memory", in M. Hogan (ed.) *Hiroshima in History and Memory*, Cambridge: Cambridge University Press.

—— (2002) " 'An Aptitude for Being Unloved': War and Memory in Japan", in O. Bartov, A. Grossmann, and M. Nolan (eds) *Crimes of War: Guilt and Denial in the Twentieth Century*, New York: The New Press.

Eykholt, M. (2000) "Aggression, Victimization, and Chinese Historiography of the Nanjing Massacre", in J. Fogel (ed.) *The Nanjing Massacre in History and Historiography*, Berkeley, CA: University of California Press.

Fan, C. (2003) "Chinese Americans: Immigration, Settlement, and Social Geography", in L. Ma and C. Cartier (eds) *The Chinese Diaspora: Space, Place, Mobility, and Identity*, Lanham, MD: Rowman & Littlefield.

Federation of American Scientists (1998) "Biological Weapons: USA", October 19. Available at http://www.fas.org/nuke/guide/usa/cbw/bw.htm.

Finn, R. (1992) *Winners in Peace: MacArthur and Post War Japan*, Los Angeles: University of California Press.

Friedberg, L. (2000) "Dare to Compare: Americanizing the Holocaust", *American Indian Quarterly* 24(3).

Gibney, L. and E. Roxstrom (2001) "The Status of State Apologies", *Human Rights Quarterly* 23(4): 911–39.

Godemont, F. (1997) *The New Asian Renaissance: From Colonialism to the Post-Cold War*, London: Routledge.

Gold, H. (2000), *Unit 731 Testimony*, Singapore: Yen Books.

Hansen, R. and D. King (2001) "Eugenic Ideas, Political Interests, and Policy Variance: Immigration and Sterilization Policy in Britain and the U.S.", *World Politics* 53(2): 237–63.

Harter, L., R. Stephens and P. Japp (2000) "President Clinton's Apology for the Tuskegee Syphilis Experiment: A Narrative of Remembrance, Redefinition, and Reconciliation", *The Howard Journal of Communications* 11: 19–34.

Hicks, G. (1998) *Japan's War Memories: Amnesia or Concealment?* London: Ashgate.

Hitchcock, R. and T. Twedt (1997) "Physical and Cultural Genocides of Various Indigenous Peoples", in S. Totten, W. Parsons, and I. Charny (eds) *Century of Genocide: Eyewitness Accounts and Critical Views*, London: Garland Publishing.

Hollon, W.E. (1974) *Frontier Violence: Another Look*, New York: Oxford University Press.

Honda, M. (2006) "Chairman's Message". Available at http://www.honda.house.gov/CAPACwelcome.shtml.

Howard-Hassmann, R. (2004) "Getting to Reparations: Japanese Americans and African Americans", *Social Forces* 83(2): 823–40.

Jeans, R. (2005) "Victims or Victimizers? Museums, Textbooks, and the War Debate in Contemporary Japan", *The Journal of Military History* 69(1): 149–95.

Johnston, A. (2003) "Is China a Status Quo Power?", *International Security* 27(4): 5–56.

Katz, J. (1992) "The Consent Principle of the Nuremberg Code: Its Significance Now and Then", in G.J. Annas and M.A. Grodin (eds) *The Nazi Doctors and the Nuremberg Code: Human Rights in Human Experimentation*, New York: Oxford University Press.

Kiernan, B. (2002) "Cover-up and Denial of Genocide: Australia, the USA, East Timor, and the Aborigines", *Critical Asian Studies* 34(2): 163–92.

Kinzer, S. (2002) "Plans for Museum Buoy Armenians and Dismay Turks", *New York Times*, April 24: E1.

Kramer, P. (2006) "Race-making and Colonial Violence in the U.S. Empire: The Philippine–American War as Race War", *The Asia Pacific Journal: Japan Focus*. Available at http://japanfocus.org/-Paul_A_-Kramer/1745.

Lawrence, J. (2000) "The Indian Health Service and the Sterilization of Native American Women", *The American Indian Quarterly* 24(3): 400–19.

Leonard, T. (2003) " 'More Merciful and Not Less Effective': Eugenics and American Economics in the Progressive Era", *History of Political Economy* 35(4): 687–712.

Lombardo, P. and G. Dorr (2006) "Eugenics, Medical Education, and the Public Health Service: Another Perspective on the Tuskegee Syphilis Experiment", *Bulletin of the History of Medicine* 80(2): 291–316.

MacDonald, D. (2005) "Forgetting and Denying: Iris Chang, the Holocaust and the Challenge of Nanking", *International Politics* 42: 403–28.

McCoy, A.W. (2006) *A Question of Torture: CIA Interrogation, From the Cold War to the War on Terror*, New York: Metropolitan.

Maeda, D. (2002) "Achieving the Impossible Dream: How Japanese Americans Obtained Redress, and: Born in Seattle: The Campaign for Japanese American Redress (review)", *Journal of Asian American Studies* 5(1): 73–8.

Maier, C. (2000) "Introduction", in J. Fogel (ed.) *The Nanjing Massacre in History and Historiography*, Berkeley: University of California Press.

Marino, P. (1998) "Remember Nanking: With Global Alliance, Chang Recounts the Forgotten Holocaust of the Chinese People", *The Cupertino Courier*, August 26. Available at http://www.svcn.com/archives/cupertinocourier/08.26.98/CoverStory.html (accessed June 15, 2005).

Markowitz, G. (2000) " 'A Little of the Buchenwald Touch': America's Secret Radiation Experiments", *Reviews in American History* 28(4): 601–6.

Mearsheimer, J. and Walt, S. (2006) "The Israel Lobby", *London Review of Books* 28(6): 23.

Moeller, R. (2005) "Germans as Victims? Thoughts on a Post-Cold War History of World War II's Legacies", *History & Memory* 17(1/2): 147–94.

Moore, W. (2002) "Ethnic Minorities and Foreign Policy", *SAIS Review* 22(2): 77–91.

Moreno, J. and S. Lederer (1996) "Revising the History of Cold War Research Ethics", *Kennedy Institute of Ethics Journal* 6(3): 223–37.

Morris, C. (2001) "Bitter History of Armenian Genocide Row", *BBC News*, January 23.

Nie, J.B. (2002) "Japanese Doctors' Experimentation in Wartime China", *The Lancet* 360: S5–6.

Nie, L. (2006) "The United States Cover-up of Japanese Wartime Medical Atrocities: Complicity Committed in the National Interest and Two Proposals for Contemporary Action", *American Journal of Bioethics* 6(3): W21–W33.

Nish, I. (2000) "Nationalism in Japan", in M. Liefer (ed.) *Asian Nationalism*, London: Routledge.

Nobles, M. (2008) *The Politics of Official Apologies*, Cambridge: Cambridge University Press.

Novick, P. (1999) *The Holocaust and Collective Memory*, London: Bloomsbury.

Nytagodien, R.L. and A. Neal (2005) "Collective Trauma, Apologies, and the Politics of Memory", *Journal of Human Rights* 4: 465–75.

Olick, J. (1998) "Introduction: Memory and Nation – Continuities, Conflicts, and Transformations", *Social Science History* 22(4): 377–87.

Olick, J.K. and B. Coughlin (2003) "The Politics of Regret: Analytical Frames", in J. Torpey (ed.) *Politics and the Past*, Lanham, MD: Rowman & Littlefield.

Orr, J. (2001) *The Victim as Hero: Ideologies of Peace and National Identity in Postwar Japan*, Honolulu: University of Hawaii Press.

Powers, T. (1995) "Was It Right?", *The Atlantic Monthly*, July.

Prescott, H. (2002) "Using the Student Body: College and University Students as Research Subjects in the United States during the Twentieth Century", *Journal of the History of Medicine and Allied Sciences* 57(1): 3–38.

Ralstin-Lewis, D.M. (2005) "The Continuing Struggle against Genocide: Indigenous Women's Reproductive Rights", *Wicazo Sa Review* 20(1): 71–95.

Rothman, D. (2003) "Serving Clio and Client: The Historian as Expert Witness", *Bulletin of the History of Medicine* 77(1): 25–44.

Saideman, S. (2002) "The Power of the Small: The Impact of Ethnic Minorities on Foreign Policy", *SAIS Review* 22(2): 93–105.

Shain, Y. (2002) "The Role of Diasporas in Conflict Perpetuation or Resolution", *SAIS Review* 22(2): 115–44.

Shermer, M. and A. Grobman (2000) *Denying History: Who Says the Holocaust Never Happened and Why Do They Say It?* Berkeley: University of California Press.

Smith, R., E. Markusen, and R.J. Lifton (1995) "Professional Ethics and Denial of the Armenian Genocide", *Holocaust and Genocide Studies* 9(1): 1–22.

Stiffarm, L. and P. Lane (1992) "The Demography of Native North America: A Question of American Indian Survival", in M. Annette Jaimes (ed.) *The State of Native America*, Boston, MA: South End.

Torpey, J. (2001) " 'Making Whole What Has Been Smashed': Reflections on Reparations", *The Journal of Modern History* 73(2): 333–58.

Udel, L. (2001) "Revision and Resistance: The Politics of Native Women's Motherwork", *Frontiers: A Journal of Women Studies* 22(2): 43–62.

Vest, J. (2002) "Turkey, Israel and the US", *The Nation*, August 23. Available at http://www.thenation.com/doc/20020902/vest20020823 (accessed February 1, 2006).

Wang, G. (2000) *The Chinese Overseas: From Earthbound China to the Quest for Autonomy*, Cambridge, MA: Harvard University Press.

Watts, J. (2002) "Court Forces Japan to Admit to Dark Past of Bioweapons Programme", *The Lancet* 360(9336): 857.

Williams, P. and D. Wallace (1989) *Unit 731: Japan's Secret Biological Warfare in World War II*, New York: Free Press.

Yoneyama, L. (1999) *Hiroshima Traces: Time, Space, and the Dialectics of Memory*, Berkeley: University of California Press.

Young, J.E. (1999) "Inheriting the Holocaust: Jewish American Fiction and the Double Bind of the Second-Generation Survivor", in Hilene Flanzbaum (ed.) *The Americanization of The Holocaust*, Baltimore, MD: Johns Hopkins University Press.

Yu, H. (2001) *Thinking Orientals: Migration, Contact, and Exoticism in Modern America*, New York: Oxford University Press.

10 Japanese and American war atrocities, historical memory, and reconciliation

The Asia-Pacific War to today

Mark Selden

War crimes, atrocities, and state terrorism

The controversies that continue to swirl around the Nanjing Massacre, the military comfort women, Unit 731, and other Japanese military atrocities rooted in colonialism and the Asia-Pacific War are critical not only to understanding the dynamics of war, peace, and terror in the long twentieth century. They are also vital for understanding war memory and denial, with implications for peace and regional accommodation across the Asia-Pacific region and the US–Japan relationship.[1]

This chapter offers a comparative framework for understanding war atrocities and the ways in which they are remembered, forgotten, and memorialized. It examines a number of high-profile atrocities in an effort to understand their character and the reasons why recognizing and accepting responsibility for them has been so difficult. Neither committing atrocities nor suppressing their memories is the exclusive property of a single nation. The issues addressed here originated with atrocities committed by Japan and the United States during the Asia-Pacific War, but many continue in new forms to the present.

What explains the fact that Japanese denial and refusal to provide compensation to victims has long been the subject of sharp domestic and international contention, while there has been relatively little analysis of U.S. atrocities, less criticism or recrimination for that nation's commission and denial of atrocities, and still less demand for reparations? What are the consequences of this difference for the two nations and the contemporary international relations of the Asia-Pacific?

Among the major war crimes and atrocities committed in World War II, the Nanjing Massacre . . . or Rape of Nanjing, or Nankin Daigyakusatsu, or Nankin Jiken (Japanese) or Nanjing Datusha (Chinese) . . . remains the most controversial. These different names signal alternative Japanese, Chinese, and international perceptions of the event: as "incident," as "massacre," as "rape," as "massive butchery," or even, as Iris Chang styled it, "the forgotten Holocaust."

The Nanjing Massacre is controversial not because the most basic facts are in doubt, although historians continue to contest the number of deaths and the interpretation of certain events. Rather it is controversial owing to the shocking scale of the killing of Chinese civilians and prisoners of war in a single locale, because of the politics of denial relentlessly pursued by Japanese neonationalists, and because the relationship between the massacre and the character of the wider war remains little understood despite the outstanding research of Japanese and international scholars and journalists.[2]

It is not only that Japanese neonationalists deny the very existence of a massacre, but that they have sometimes been joined by post-Occupation Japanese governments in refusing to accept formal responsibility for either the massacre or the wider war of aggression in which between 10 and 30 million Chinese died. This explains why these issues remain contested and controversial among Japanese and across the Asia-Pacific. To understand why the Japanese government continues to fight this and other war memory battles in ways that have repeatedly poisoned its relations not only with its Asian neighbors but also with the United States and European nations requires reconsideration not only of contemporary Japanese nationalism, but of the international power structure that the U.S. set in place during the occupation and subsequently maintained.

The U.S. insulated Japan from war responsibility, first, by maintaining Hirohito on the throne and shielding him from war crimes charges; second, by protecting the Japanese state from war reparations claims from victims of colonialism, invasion, and atrocities, and finally by using its troops and bases to guarantee Japan's defense so as to assure its subordination within the orbit of U.S. power, and to isolate it from China, the Soviet Union, and other U.S. rivals.

As the authors of this volume reiterate, attempts to gauge war atrocities and to understand the ways in which they are remembered and suppressed require the application of universal standards as articulated during the Nuremberg and Tokyo Trials. In an age of nationalism, it is particularly important to apply such standards to the conduct of one's own nation. The German case, to which I return below, is particularly instructive. Germany, like Japan, was defeated by a U.S.-led coalition, and the U.S. played a key role in shaping institutions, war memories, and responses to war atrocities in both Germany and Japan.[3] Nevertheless, the outcomes in the two nations in the form of historical memory and reconciliation in the wake of war atrocities have differed sharply.

It is not the familiar terrain of the Japan–German comparison that I wish to emphasize here, however. To unravel the most contentious memory wars in the Asia-Pacific, I begin by offering a comparative framework for assessing Japanese and American war atrocities. Particular attention is paid to Japan's Nanjing Massacre and the American firebombing and atomic bombing of Japanese cities during World War II as each nation's signature atrocities. In each instance, I cast the issues in relation to the wider conduct of the War, and in the American case consider the legacy of the bombing for subsequent wars down to the present. At the center of the analysis is the assessment of these examples in light of principles of international law developed over many decades from the late nineteenth century, notably those enshrined in the Nuremberg and Tokyo Trials and the Geneva Convention of 1949, that identify as acts of terrorism and crimes against humanity the slaughter of civilians and non-combatants by states and their militaries.[4] It is only by considering crimes committed by the victors as well as the vanquished in the Asia-Pacific War and other wars that it is possible to lay to rest the ghosts of suppressed memories in order to build foundations for a peaceful cooperative order in the Asia-Pacific.

But first, Nanjing.

The Nanjing Massacre and structures of violence in the Sino-Japanese War

Substantial portions of the Nanjing Massacre literature in English and Chinese – both the scholarship and the public debate – treat the event as emblematic of the wartime conduct of the Japanese, thereby essentializing the massacre as the embodiment not only of the Japanese way of war in the years 1931 to 1945, but of the Japanese character. In the discussion that follows, I seek both to locate the unique and conjunctural features of the massacre and to understand its relationship to the character of Japan's protracted China war and the wider Asia-Pacific War.

Just as a small staged event by Japanese officers in 1931 provided the pretext for Japan's seizure of China's northeast and creation of the dependent state of Manchukuo, the minor clash between Japanese and Chinese troops at the Marco Polo Bridge on July 7, 1937 paved the way for full-scale invasion of China south of the Great Wall. By July 27, Japanese reinforcements from Korea and Manchuria as well as Naval Air Force units had joined the fight. The Army High Command dispatched three divisions from Japan and called up 209,000 men. With Japan's seizure of Beiping and Tianjin the next day followed by an attack on Shanghai in August, the (undeclared) war began in earnest. In October, a Shanghai Expeditionary Army (SEA) under Gen. Matsui Iwane with six divisions was ordered to destroy enemy forces in and around Shanghai. The Tenth Army commanded by Gen. Yanagawa Heisuke with four divisions soon joined in. Anticipating rapid surrender by Chiang Kai-shek's National Government, the Japanese military encountered stiff resistance: 9185 Japanese were killed and 31,125 wounded at Shanghai. However, after landing at Hangzhou Bay, Japanese forces quickly gained control of Shanghai. By November 7, the two Japanese armies combined to form a Central China Area Army (CCAA) with an estimated 160,000 to 200,000 men.[5]

With Chinese forces in flight, Matsui's CCAA, having received no orders from Tokyo, set out to capture the Chinese capital Nanjing. Each unit competed for the honor of being the first to enter the capital. Historians such as Fujiwara Akira and Yoshida Yutaka sensibly date the start of the Nanjing Massacre to the atrocities committed against civilians en route to Nanjing. "Thus began," Fujiwara wrote, "the most enormous, expensive, and deadly war in modern Japanese history – one waged without just cause or cogent reason." And one that paved the way to the Asia-Pacific War that followed.

Japan's behavior at Nanjing departed dramatically from that in the capture of cities in earlier Japanese military engagements from the Russo-Japanese War of 1905 forward as well as from subsequent campaigns. One reason for the barbarity at Nanjing and subsequently was that, counting on the "shock and awe" of the

November attack on Shanghai to produce surrender, Japanese troops were unprepared for the fierce resistance and heavy casualties that they encountered, prompting a desire for revenge. Indeed, throughout the war, like the Americans in Vietnam decades later, the Japanese displayed a profound inability to grasp the roots and strength of the nationalist resistance in the face of invading forces who enjoyed overwhelming weapons and logistical superiority. A second reason for the atrocities was that, as the two armies raced to capture Nanjing, the high command lost control, resulting in a volatile and violent situation.

The contempt felt by the Japanese military for Chinese military forces and the Chinese people set in motion a dynamic that led to the massacre. In the absence of a declaration of war, as Utsumi Aiko documents, the Japanese high command held that it was under no obligation to treat captured Chinese soldiers as POWs or observe other international protocols of warfare that Japan had scrupulously adhered to in the 1904 to 1905 Russo-Japanese War, such as the protection of the rights of civilians. Later, Japan would recognize captured U.S. and Allied forces as POWs, although they too were treated badly.[6]

As Yoshida Yutaka notes, Japanese soldiers were subjected to extreme physical and mental abuse by their superiors. Regularly sent on forced marches carrying 30 to 60 kilograms of equipment, they also faced ruthless military discipline. Perhaps most important for understanding the pattern of atrocities that emerged in 1937, in the absence of food provisions, as the troops raced toward Nanjing, they plundered villages and slaughtered their inhabitants in order to feed themselves.[7]

Chinese forces were belatedly ordered to retreat from Nanjing on the evening of December 12, but Japanese troops had already surrounded the city and many were captured. Other Chinese troops discarded weapons and uniforms, and sought to blend in with the civilian population or surrender. Using diaries, battle reports, press accounts, and interviews, Fujiwara Akira documents the slaughter of tens of thousands of POWs, including 14,777 by the Yamada Detachment of the 13th Division. Daqing Yang points out that Gen. Yamada had his troops execute the prisoners after twice being told by Shanghai Expeditionary Army headquarters to "kill them all."[8]

Major Gen. Sasaki Toichi confided to his diary on December 13:

> our detachment alone must have taken care of over 20,000. Later, the enemy surrendered in the thousands. Frenzied troops – rebuffing efforts by superiors to restrain them – finished off these POWs one after another . . . men would yell, "Kill the whole damn lot!" after recalling the past ten days of bloody fighting in which so many buddies had shed so much blood.

The killing at Nanjing was not limited to captured Chinese soldiers. Large numbers of civilians were raped and/or killed. Lt. Gen. Okamura Yasuji, who in 1938 became commander of the Tenth Army, recalled "that tens of thousands of acts of violence, such as looting and rape, took place against civilians during the assault on Nanjing. Second, front-line troops indulged in the evil practice of executing POWs on the pretext of [lacking] rations."

Chinese and foreigners in Nanjing comprehensively documented the crimes committed in the immediate aftermath of Japanese capture of the city. Nevertheless, the most important and telling evidence of the massacre is that provided by Japanese troops who participated in the capture of the city. What should have been a fatal blow to "Nanjing denial" occurred when the Kaikosha, a fraternal order of former military officers and neonationalist revisionists, issued a call to soldiers who had fought in Nanjing to describe their experience. Publishing the responses in a March 1985 "Summing Up," editor Katogawa Kotaro cited reports by Unemoto Masami that he saw 3 to 6000 victims, and by Itakura Masaaki, 13,000 deaths. Katogawa concluded: "No matter what the conditions of battle were, and no matter how that affected the hearts of men, such large-scale illegal killings cannot be justified. As someone affiliated with the former Japanese army, I can only apologize deeply to the Chinese people."

A fatal blow . . . except that incontrovertible evidence provided by unimpeachable sources has never stayed the hands of incorrigible deniers. I have highlighted the direct testimony of Japanese generals and enlisted men who documented the range and scale of atrocities committed during the Nanjing Massacre in order to show how difficult it is, even in the face of such compelling evidence, to overcome denial.

Two other points emerge clearly from this discussion. The first is that the atrocities at Nanjing – just as with the comfort women and Unit 731 – have been the subject of fierce public controversy. This controversy has erupted again and again over the textbook content and the statements of leaders ever since Japan's surrender, and particularly since the 1990s. The second is that, unlike their leaders, many Japanese citizens have consistently recognized and deeply regretted Japanese atrocities. Many have also supported reparations for victims.

The massacre had consequences far beyond Nanjing. The Japanese high command, up to Emperor Hirohito, the commander-in-chief, while closely monitoring events at Nanjing, issued no reprimand and meted out no punishment to the officers and men who perpetrated these crimes. Instead, the leadership and the press celebrated the victory at the Chinese capital in ways that invite comparison with the elation of an American president as U.S. forces seized Baghdad within weeks of the 2003 invasion.[9] In both cases, the "victory" initiated what proved to be the beginning and not the end of a war that could neither be won nor terminated for years to come, and which would soon be extended to new territories and new enemies. In both instances, we will show, it was followed by atrocities that intensified and were extended from the capital to the entire country.

Following the Nanjing Massacre, the Japanese high command did move determinedly to rein in troops to prevent further anarchic violence, particularly violence played out in front of the Chinese and international press. Leaders feared that such wanton acts could undermine efforts to win over, or at least neutralize, the Chinese population and lead to Japan's international isolation.

A measure of the success of the leadership's response to the Nanjing Massacre is that no incident of comparable proportions occurred during the capture of a major Chinese city over the next eight years of war. Japan succeeded in capturing and pacifying major Chinese cities, not least by winning the accommodation of significant elites in Manchukuo and in the Nanjing government of Wang Jingwei, as well as in cities directly ruled by Japanese forces and administrators.[10]

This was not, however, the end of the slaughter of Chinese civilians and captives. Far from it. Throughout the War, Japan continued to rain destruction from the air on Chongqing, Chiang Kai-shek's wartime capital, and in the final years of the war, as the authors of this volume document, it deployed chemical and biological bombs against Ningbo and throughout Zhejiang and Hunan provinces.[11]

Above all, the systematic slaughter of civilians that characterized the Nanjing Massacre was subsequently enacted throughout the rural areas where resistance stalemated Japanese forces in the course of eight years of war. This is illustrated by the *sanko sakusen* or three-all policies implemented throughout rural North China by Japanese forces seeking to crush both the communist-led resistance in guerrilla base areas behind Japanese lines and in areas dominated by Guomindang and warlord troops.[12] Other measures implemented at Nanjing would exact a heavy toll on the countryside: military units regularly relied on plunder to secure provisions, conducted systematic slaughter of villagers in contested areas, and denied POW status to Chinese captives, often killing all prisoners. Above all, where Japanese forces encountered resistance, they adopted scorched-earth policies that deprived villagers of subsistence.

One leadership response to the adverse public relations effects of the Nanjing Massacre was the establishment of the comfort women system. This represented an effort to control and channel the sexual energies of Japanese soldiers, curb venereal disease, and prevent rape that could stoke anti-Japanese sentiment.[13] Imperial armies everywhere, then and now, are accompanied by prostitution systems serving their forces. Still, the comfort women system offers a compelling example of the institutionalized character of atrocities associated with Japan's China invasion and subsequently with the Asia-Pacific War.

In short, the anarchic violence displayed at Nanjing paved the way for more systematic policies of slaughter carried out by the Japanese military throughout the countryside. The comfort women system, the testing practices of biowarfare Unit 731, and the three-all policies reveal some of the diverse ways in which systematic oppression was orchestrated by the military high command in Tokyo and applied throughout the war.

Nanjing then is less a typical atrocity than a seminal event that shaped the everyday structure of Japanese war making over eight years of war. The Nanjing Massacre was a signature atrocity of twentieth-century warfare. But war atrocities were hardly unique to Japan.

American war atrocities: civilian bombing, state terror, and international law

Throughout the long twentieth century, and particularly since World War II, the inexorable advance of weapons technology has gone hand-in-hand with international efforts to place limits on killing and the barbarism associated with war, notably indiscriminate bombing raids and other attacks directed against civilians. Advances in international law have provided important points of reference for establishing international governance norms, and for inspiring and guiding social movements seeking to control the ravages of war and advance the cause of world peace.

In the following sections I consider the conduct of U.S. warfare from the perspective of the emerging norms. In light of these norms, international criticism has long centered on German and Japanese atrocities, notably the Holocaust and specific atrocities including the Nanjing Massacre, the comfort women and the biowarfare conducted by Unit 731. U.S. military actions, notably the atomic bombing of Hiroshima and Nagasaki and its conduct of the Korean, Indochina, and subsequent wars, have repeatedly prompted international controversy and criticism.[14] However, the U.S. has been largely free of formal sanction by international authorities, and above all, in striking contrast with Japan and Germany, it has never been required to change the fundamental character of the succession of wars it has waged since 1939, to engage in self-criticism at the level of state or people, or to pay reparations to other nations or victims of war atrocities.

While the strategic impact and ethical implications of the nuclear bombing of Hiroshima and Nagasaki have generated a vast contentious literature, U.S. air war leading to the destruction of more than 60 Japanese cities prior to Hiroshima has until recently been slighted both in the scholarly literatures in English and Japanese, and in popular consciousness in Japan, the U.S., and globally.[15]

Germany, England, and Japan led the way in what is euphemistically known as "area bombing," the targeting for destruction of entire cities with conventional weapons. From 1932 to the early years of World War II, the United States repeatedly criticized the bombing of cities. President Franklin Roosevelt appealed to the warring nations in 1939 on the first day of World War II, "under no circumstances [to] undertake the bombardment from the air of civilian populations or of unfortified cities."[16] After Pearl Harbor, the U.S. continued to claim the moral high ground by abjuring civilian bombing. This stance was consistent with the prevailing Air Force doctrine that the most efficient bombing strategies were those that pinpointed destruction of enemy forces and strategic installations, not those designed to terrorize or kill non-combatants.

Nevertheless, the U.S. collaborated with Britain in indiscriminate bombing at Casablanca in 1943. While the British sought to destroy entire cities, the Americans continued to target military and industrial sites. On February 13–14, 1945, British bombers followed by U.S. planes destroyed Dresden, a historic cultural center with no significant military industry or bases. By conservative estimate, 35,000 people were incinerated in that raid.[17]

But it was in Japan, in the final six months of the war, that the U.S. deployed air power in a campaign to burn whole cities to the ground and terrorize, incapacitate, and kill their largely defenseless residents, in order to force surrender. In those months the American way of war, with the bombing of cities at its center, was set in place.

Maj. Gen. Curtis LeMay, appointed Commander of the 21st Bomber Command in the Pacific on January 20, 1945, became the primary architect, a strategic innovator, and most quotable spokesman for the U.S. policy of putting enemy cities to the torch. The full fury of firebombing was first unleashed on the night of March 9–10, 1945, when LeMay sent 334 B-29s low over Tokyo, unloading 496,000 incendiaries in that single raid. Their mission was to reduce the city to rubble, kill its citizens, and instill terror in the survivors. The attack on an area that the U.S. Strategic Bombing Survey estimated to be 84.7 percent residential succeeded beyond the planners' wildest dreams. Whipped up by fierce winds, flames detonated by the bombs leaped across a 15-square-mile area of Tokyo, generating immense firestorms.

How many people died on the night of March 9–10, in what Flight Commander Gen. Thomas Power termed "the greatest single disaster incurred by any enemy in military history"? The figure of roughly 100,000 deaths and one million homes destroyed, provided by Japanese and American authorities, may understate the destruction, given the population density, wind conditions, and survivors' accounts.[18] An estimated 1.5 million people lived in the burned-out areas. Given a near total inability to fight fires of the magnitude and speed produced by the bombs, casualties could have been several times higher than these estimates. The figure of 100,000 deaths in Tokyo may be compared with total U.S. casualties in the four years of the Pacific War – 103,000 – and Japanese war casualties of more than three million.

Following the Tokyo raid of March 9–10, the U.S. extended firebombing nationwide. In the ten-day period beginning on March 9, 9373 tons of bombs destroyed 31 square miles of Tokyo, Nagoya, Osaka, and Kobe. Overall, bombing strikes pulverized 40 percent of the 66 Japanese cities targeted.[19]

Many more (primarily civilians) died in the firebombing of Japanese cities than in Hiroshima (140,000 by the end of 1945) and Nagasaki (70,000), although deaths and suffering from injury and radiation from the atomic bombing would continue over the years and decades to come. The bombing was driven not only by a belief that it could end the War but also, as Max Hastings shows, by the attempt by the Air Force to claim credit for the U.S. victory, and to redeem the enormous costs of developing and producing thousands of B-29s and the $2 billion cost of the atomic bomb. It was also intended to send a powerful signal to potential enemies, notably the Soviet Union, of the invincibility of American power.[20]

The single most important way in which World War II shaped the moral climate and the tenor of mass destruction was the erosion of the stigma associated with the targeting of civilian populations from the air. If area bombing remained controversial throughout much of World War II, something to be concealed or denied by its practitioners, by the end of the war, with the enormous increase in the destructive power of bombing, it had become the centerpiece of US war making, and therefore the international norm.[21] This approach to the destruction of cities, which was perfected in 1944 to 1945, melded technological predominance with minimization of U.S. casualties to produce overwhelming "kill ratios."

The USAAF offered this ecstatic assessment of LeMay's missions, claiming that the firebombing and atomic bombing secured U.S. victory and averted a costly land battle:

> In its climactic five months of jellied fire attacks, the vaunted Twentieth killed outright 310,000 Japanese, injured 412,000 more, and rendered 9,200,000 homeless. . . . Never in the history of war had such colossal devastation been visited on an enemy at so slight a cost to the conqueror. . . . The 1945 application of American Power, so destructive and concentrated as to cremate 65 Japanese cities in five months, forced an enemy's surrender without land invasion for the first time in military history. . . . Very long range air power gained victory, decisive and complete.[22]

This triumphalist (and flawed) account, which exaggerated the efficacy of air power and ignored the critical importance of sea power, the Soviet attack on Japan, and U.S. softening of the terms of the Potsdam Declaration to guarantee the security of Hirohito, all crucial to the Japanese decision to surrender, would not only deeply inflect American remembrance of victory in the Pacific War, it would profoundly shape the conduct of all subsequent American wars.

How should we compare the Nanjing Massacre and U.S. bombing of cities? The Nanjing Massacre involved face-to-face slaughter of civilians and captured soldiers. By contrast, in U.S. (likewise Japanese) bombing of cities, technological annihilation from the air distanced victim from assailant.[23] Yet it is worth reflecting on the common elements, most notably mass slaughter of civilians in violation of international law and humanitarian ethics.

Why have only the atrocities of Japan at Nanjing and elsewhere drawn consistent international condemnation and vigorous debate, despite the fact that the U.S. likewise engaged – and continues to engage – in mass slaughter of civilians in violation both of international law and ethics?

American war crimes and the problem of impunity

Victory in World War II propelled the U.S. to a hegemonic position globally, allowing it to substantially shape the parameters and dominate the structures of central institutions of the international order: notably the United Nations, the International Monetary Fund, and the World Bank. It also gave it, together with its allies, authority to define and punish war crimes committed by vanquished nations. This privileged position was and remains a major obstacle to a thorough-going reassessment of the American and Allied conduct of World War II and subsequent wars.

The logical starting point for such an investigation is a re-examination of the systematic bombing of civilians in Japanese cities. Only by engaging the issues raised by such a re-examination – from which Americans were explicitly shielded by judges during the Tokyo Tribunals – is it possible to begin to approach the Nuremberg ideal, which holds victors as well as vanquished to the same standard with respect to crimes against humanity, or the yardstick of the 1949 Geneva Accord, which mandates the protection of all civilians in time of war. This is the principle of universality proclaimed at Nuremberg and systematically violated in practice by the U.S. ever since. The centrality of air power to target civilians runs like a red line from the U.S. bombings of Germany and Japan in 1944 to 1945 through the Korean and Indochinese wars to the Persian Gulf, Afghanistan, and Iraq wars.[24]

In the course of three years, U.S./U.N. forces in Korea flew 1,040,708 sorties and dropped 386,037 tons of bombs and 32,357 tons of napalm. Counting all types of airborne ordnance, including rockets and machine-gun ammunition, the total comes to 698,000 tons. Using U.N. data, Marilyn Young estimates the death-toll in Korea, mostly non-combatants, at two to four million.[25]

Three examples from the Indochina War illustrate the nature of U.S. bombing of civilians. In a burst of anger on December 9, 1970, President Richard M. Nixon railed at what he saw as the Air Force's lackluster bombing campaign in Cambodia. "I want them to hit everything. I want them to use the big planes, the small planes, everything they can that will help out there, and let's start giving them a little shock." Kissinger relayed the order: "A massive bombing campaign in Cambodia. Anything that flies on anything that moves."[26] In the course of the Vietnam War, the U.S. also embraced cluster bombs and chemical and biological weapons of mass destruction as integral parts of its arsenal.

An important U.S. strategic development of the Indochina War was the extension of the arc of civilian bombing from cities to the countryside. In addition to firebombs and cluster bombs, the U.S. introduced Agent Orange (dioxin), a chemical defoliant, which not only eliminated the forest cover, but also exacted a heavy long-term toll on the local population including large-scale intergenerational damage in the form of birth defects. Between 1962 and 1971, the U.S. sprayed 20 million gallons of the herbicide across wide areas of Vietnam. Vietnam's Ministry of Foreign Affairs estimates that 4.8 million Vietnamese were exposed to the poison gas, resulting in death or injury to 400,000 and producing 500,000 birth defects.[27]

In Iraq, the U.S. military, while continuing to pursue massive bombing of neighborhoods in Fallujah, Baghdad, and elsewhere, has thrown a cloak of silence over the air war. While the media has averted its eyes and cameras, air power remains among the major causes of death, destruction, dislocation, and division in contemporary Iraq.[28] The war had taken approximately 655,000 lives by the summer of 2006 and close to twice that number by the fall of 2007, according to the most authoritative study to date, that of the *Lancet*. Air war has also played a major part in creating the world's most acute refugee problem. By early 2006, the United Nations High Commissioner for Refugees estimated that 1.7 million Iraqis had fled the country while approximately the same number were internal refugees, with the total number of refugees rising to well over four million by 2009.[29] Nearly all of the dead and displaced are civilians.

Both the plight of refugees and the intensification of aerial bombing of 2007 to 2009 have been largely invisible in the U.S. mainstream press. This is the central reality of American state terror in Iraq and Afghanistan. Nevertheless, despite America's unchallenged air supremacy in Iraq since 1991, despite the creation of an array of military bases to permanently occupy Iraq and anchor American power in the Middle East's second largest oil supplier, with the war in its sixth year, there is no end in sight, and indeed, with the shift in priority to the war in Afghanistan and Pakistan, war now rages throughout the region.[30] Indeed, with the U.S. high command actively debating the dispatch of 40,000 more troops to Afghanistan, there is little prospect of exit from the region. It is of course a region in which the geopolitical stakes far exceed those in either Korea or Vietnam.

Historical memory and the future of the Asia-Pacific

I began by considering the Nanjing Massacre's relationship to structural and ideological foundations of Japanese colonialism and war making, to U.S. bombing of Japanese civilians in the Pacific War in 1945, and subsequently to U.S. bombing of Korean, Indochinese, and Iraqi civilians. In each instance the primary focus has not been the headlined atrocity – Nanjing, Unit 731, Hiroshima, Nogunri, Mylai, Abu Ghraib – but the foundational practices that systematically violate international law provisions designed to protect civilians.

In both the Japanese and U.S. cases, nationalism and national pride in the service of war and empire have eased the path for war crimes perpetrated against civilian populations. In both countries, nationalism has obfuscated, even eradicated, memories of the war crimes and atrocities committed by one's own nation, while privileging memories of the atrocities committed by adversaries. Consider, for example, American memories of the killing of 2800 mainly Americans on September 11, 2001 compared with more than one million Iraqi deaths, millions more injured, and more than four million refugees. Heroic virtue reigns supreme in official memory and in representations such as museums, monuments, and textbooks, and often, but not always, in popular memory.

Striking differences distinguish Japanese and U.S. responses to their respective war atrocities and war crimes. Occupied Japan looked back at the War from the midst of bombed-out cities and an economy in ruins, grieving the loss of three million compatriots but also, buoyed by postwar hopes for recovery and democracy, significant numbers of Japanese reflected on and criticized imperial Japan's war crimes. Reflecting on the disastrous war that Japan had embarked on, many Japanese embraced and continue to embrace the peace provision of the Constitution, which renounced war-making capacity for Japan. If the Japanese state under Liberal Democratic Party rule between 1955 and September 2009 failed to come to terms with Japan's war atrocities, we should not minimize the significance of the fact that a Japan that was perpetually at war between 1895 and 1945 has not gone to war for more than six decades. It is fair to attribute this transformation in part to the widespread aversion to war and embracement of the principles enshrined in Article 9 of the peace constitution, though it is equally necessary to factor in Japan's financial and logistical support for every U.S. war since Korea and Japan's subordinate position to American power.

In the decades since 1945, the issues of war have remained alive and contentious in public memory and in the actions of the Japanese state. After the formal independence promulgated by the 1951 San Francisco Treaty, with Hirohito still on the throne, Japanese governments reaffirmed the aims of colonialism and war of the Greater East Asia Co-prosperity Sphere of the 1931 to 1945 era. They released from prison and restored the reputations of former war criminals, making possible the election of Kishi Nobusuke as Prime Minister (and subsequently his grandson Abe Shinzo). In 1955, when the Liberal Democratic Party inaugurated its nearly 40-year grip on power, the Ministry of Education pressed authors of textbooks to downplay or omit altogether reference to the Nanjing Massacre, the comfort women, Unit 731, and military-coerced suicides of Okinawan citizens during the Battle of Okinawa. Yet these official efforts, then and since, have never gone unchallenged by the victims, by historians, or by peace activists.

From the early 1980s, in the wake of the Ienaga Saburo legal challenge to Ministry of Education textbook censorship, memory controversies over textbook treatments of colonialism and war precipitated international disputes with China and Korea, as well as domestic disputes over the Battle of Okinawa. In Japan, conservative governments backed by neonationalist groups clashed with citizens and scholars who embraced criticism of Japan's war crimes and supported the peace constitution.[31]

In contrast to this half-century debate both within Japan and between Japan and victims of colonialism and war, notably China and Korea, not only the U.S. government but also most Americans remain oblivious to the war atrocities committed by U.S. forces as outlined above. The exceptions are important. Investigative reporting revealing atrocities such as the massacres at Nogunri in Korea and My Lai in Vietnam, and torture at Abu Ghraib Prison in Iraq and Guantanamo Bay, Cuba, have convinced most Americans that these events took place. Yet, precisely as presented in the official story and reiterated in the press, most see these as aberrant crimes committed by a handful of low-ranking officers and enlisted men. In each case, prosecution and sentencing burnished the image of American justice: meting out punishment to low-ranking military personnel while the responsible authorities – the generals, the Secretary of Defense, and the President – remain free to go about their business while making cosmetic changes in laws and regulations. The embedded structure of violence, the strategic thinking that lay behind the specific incidents, and the responsibility for the atrocities committed up the chain of command, were silenced or ignored. As in wartime Japan, so in wartime America from the Asia-Pacific War to the present. . . .

Apologies are difficult for the leaders and people of any nation regardless of political system. Two exceptions to the lack of reflection and resistance to apology provide perspective on American complacency about its conduct of wars. President Ronald Reagan signed the Civil Liberties Act of 1988, which offered apologies and $20,000 in compensation to survivors among the 110,000 Japanese and Japanese Americans who had been interned by the U.S. government in the years 1942 to 1945. Then, in 1993 on the 100th anniversary of the U.S. overthrow of the Hawaiian monarchy, President Bill Clinton offered an apology (but no recompense) to native Hawaiians. In both cases, the crucial fact is that the victims' descendants are American citizens and not foreign nationals.[32]

One additional quasi-apology bears mention. In March 1999, Clinton, speaking in Guatemala City of the U.S. role in the killing of 200,000 Guatemalans over previous decades, made this statement: "For the United States, it is important that I state clearly that support for military forces and intelligence units which engaged in violence and widespread repression was wrong, and the United States must not repeat that mistake." The remarks had a certain political significance at the time, yet they had more of the weight of a feather than of Mt. Tai. No word of apology was included. No remuneration was made to victims. Above all, the United States did not act to end its violent interventions in scores of countries in Latin America, Asia, or elsewhere.[33]

There have of course been no apologies or reparations for U.S. firebombing or atomic bombing of Japan, or for killing millions and creating vast numbers of refugees in Korea, Vietnam, Iraq, and Afghanistan, nor for U.S. interventions in scores of other ongoing conflicts in the Americas and Asia. Such is the prerogative of impunity of the world's most powerful nation.[34]

However, there has been one important act of recognition of the systemic character of American atrocities in Vietnam, and subsequently in Iraq and Afghanistan. Just as Japanese troops provided the most compelling testimony on Japanese wartime atrocities, it is American veterans whose testimony most effectively unmasked the deep structure of the American way of war in Vietnam and Iraq.

In the Winter Soldier investigation in Detroit on January 31 to February 2, 1971, Vietnam Veterans Against the War organized testimony by 109 discharged veterans and 16 civilians. John Kerry, later a U.S. Senator and presidential candidate, testified two months afterward in hearings at the Senate Foreign Relations Committee as representative of the Winter Soldier event. Kerry summed up the testimony:

> They had personally raped, cut off ears, cut off heads, taped wires from port-able telephones to human genitals and turned up the power, cut off limbs, blown up bodies, randomly shot at civilians, razed villages in fashion remi-niscent of Genghis Khan, shot cattle and dogs for fun, poisoned food stocks, and generally ravaged the countryside of South Vietnam.[35]

Kerry continued: "We rationalized destroying villages in order to save them. . . . We learned the meaning of free fire zones, shooting anything that moves, and we watched while America placed a cheapness on the lives of orientals."

On March 13–16, 2008 a second Winter Soldier gathering took place in Washington, D.C., with hundreds of Iraq War veterans providing testimony, photographs, and videos documenting brutality, torture, and murder in cases such as the Haditha Massacre and the Abu Ghraib torture.[36] As in the first Winter Soldier, the mainstream media ignored the event organized by Iraq Veterans Against War. Again, however, the voices of these veterans have reached out to some through films and new electronic and broadcast media such as YouTube.

The importance of apology and reparations lies in the fact that through processes of recognition of wrongdoing and efforts to make amends (however belated or inadequate) to victims, where such apologies are enshrined in the textbooks, monuments, and official stories of the nation's past, the poisonous legacies of war and colonialism may be alleviated or overcome and foundations laid for a harmonious future. In Germany, this involved renunciation of Nazism, the formation of a new government distinctive from and critical of the former government; consensus expressed in the nation's textbooks and curricula critical of Nazi genocide and aggression; monuments and museums commemorating the victims; and payment of substantial reparations to individual victims (albeit under U.S. pressure). These actions paved the way for Germany's re-emergence at the center of the European Union, and contributed to a healing process among opposing sides in World War II.

In contrast to their German counterparts, Japanese and American leaders have strongly resisted meaningful and lasting apology and reparations. While many Japanese people have reflected deeply on their nation's war atrocities, Japan's long-ruling Liberal Democratic Party leaders, sheltered from Asia by the U.S.–Japan security relationship, had little incentive to reflect deeply on the nation's wartime record in China, Korea, or elsewhere. Americans, for their part, have felt little pressure (either domestic or international) to recognize, apologize, or provide reparations to victims from other nations.

It has been widely recognized that a major obstacle to the emergence of a harmonious order in the Asia-Pacific is the politics of denial of atrocities associated with war and empire. China, Korea, and other former victims of Japanese invasion and colonization have repeatedly criticized Japan. Largely ignored in debates over the future of the Asia-Pacific has been the responsibility of the U.S. to recognize and provide reparations for its own numerous war atrocities as detailed above, notably in the bombing of Japanese, Korean, Vietnamese, and Iraqi civilians. Ultimately, what is important is that citizens of perpetrator nations, in this instance Japan and the United States, recognize the acts committed by their compatriots and seek to make amends in the interest of a common future.

Perhaps in the end it is the United States that holds the key to outcomes larger than itself. Responsible actions by the world's most powerful nation would make it possible to bring closure to unresolved war issues both for the many individual victims of U.S. bombing and other atrocities, and the continued hostilities between states, above all the U.S.–North Korea conflict and the division of the two Koreas. It would also pave the way for a Japan which remains within the American embrace to acknowledge and recompense victims of its own war crimes. Might it not also help pave the way for an end to U.S. wars across the Asia-Pacific and beyond?

Acknowledgments

I am indebted to Herbert Bix, Richard Falk, and especially Laura Hein for criticism and suggestions on earlier drafts of this chapter. This is a revised and expanded version of a talk delivered on December 15, 2007 at the Tokyo International Symposium to Commemorate the Seventieth Anniversary of the Nanjing Massacre.

Notes

1   Most discussion of historical memory issues has centered on the Japan–China and the Japan–Korea relationships. However, the controversy that erupted in 2007 over the U.S. congressional resolution calling on Japan to formally apologize to and provide compensation for the former comfort women illustrates the ways in which the U.S.–Japan relationship is also at stake. Kinue Tokudome, "Passage of H.Res. 121 on 'Comfort Women', the US Congress and Historical Memory in Japan," *The Asia-Pacific Journal*, http://japanfocus.org/-Kinue-TOKUDOME/2510. Tessa Morris-Suzuki, "Japan's 'Comfort Women': It's Time for The Truth (in the Ordinary, Everyday Sense of the Word)," *The Asia-Pacific Journal*, http://japanfocus.org/-Tessa-Morris_Suzuki/237.

2   Fierce debate continues among historians, activists, and nations over the number of victims during the Nanjing Massacre. The issue involves differences over both the temporal and spatial definition of the massacre. The official Chinese claim inscribed on the Nanjing Massacre Memorial is that 300,000 were killed. The most careful attempts to record the numbers by Japanese historians, which include deaths of civilians and soldiers during the march from Shanghai to Nanjing as well as deaths following the capture of the capital, suggest numbers in the 80,000 to 200,000 range. In recent years, the first serious Chinese research examining the massacre, built on 55 volumes of documents, has begun to appear. See Kasahara Tokushi, *Nankin Jiken Ronsoshi. Nihonjin wa shijitsu o do ninshiki shite kita ka?* [*The Nanjing Incident Debate. How Have Japanese Understood the Historical Evidence?*] (Tokyo: Heibonsha, 2007) for the changing contours of the Japanese debate over the decades. Kasahara Tokushi and Daqing Yang explore "The Nanjing Incident in World History" [Sekaishi no naka no Nankin Jiken] in a discussion in *Ronza*, January 2008, 184–195, ranging widely across international and joint research and the importance of new documentation from the 1970s to the present.

3   I first addressed these issues in Laura Hein and Mark Selden, eds, *Censoring History: Citizenship and Memory in Japan, China and the United States* (Armonk: M.E. Sharpe, 2000).

4   For discussion of the international legal issues and definition of state terrorism see the Introduction and Chapter 2 of Mark Selden and Alvin So, eds, *War and State Terrorism: The United States, Japan and the Asia-Pacific in the Long Twentieth Century* (Lanham: Rowman & Littlefield, 2004), pp. 1–40. See also Richard Falk's chapter in that volume, "State Terror versus Humanitarian Law," pp. 41–62.

5   The following discussion of the Nanjing Massacre and its antecedents draws heavily on the diverse contributions to Bob Tadashi Wakabayashi, ed., *The Nanking Atrocity 1937–38: Complicating the Picture* (New York and London: Berghahn Books, 2007) and particularly the chapter by the late Fujiwara Akira, "The Nanking Atrocity: An Interpretive Overview," available in a revised version at *The Asia-Pacific Journal*, http://japanfocus.org/-Fujiwara-Akira/2553. Chapters in the Wakabayashi volume closely examine and refute the exaggerated claims not only of official Chinese historiography and Japanese deniers, but also of progressive critics of the massacre. While recognizing legitimate points in the arguments of all of these, the work is devastating toward the deniers who hew to their mantra in the face of overwhelming evidence (see, e.g., p. 143).

6   Utsumi Aiko, "Japanese Racism, War, and the POW Experience," in Mark Selden and Alvin So, eds, *War and State Terrorism*, pp. 119–142.

7 Presentation at the Tokyo International Symposium to Commemorate the Seventieth Anniversary of the Nanjing Massacre, December 15, 2007.

8 Daqing Yang, "Atrocities in Nanjing: Searching for Explanations," in Diana Lary and Stephen MacKinnon, eds, *Scars of War. The Impact of Warfare on Modern China* (Vancouver: UBC Press, 2001), pp. 76–97.

9 The signature statement was that of George W. Bush on March 19, 2003:

> My fellow citizens, at this hour, American and coalition forces are in the early stages of military operations to disarm Iraq, to free its people and to defend the world from grave danger . . . the dangers to our country and the world will be overcome. . . . We will defend our freedom. We will bring freedom to others and we will prevail.

10 Timothy Brook, *Collaboration: Japanese Agents and Local Elites in Wartime China* (Cambridge, MA: Harvard University Press. 2005).

11 Tsuneishi Keiichi, "Unit 731 and the Japanese Imperial Army's Biological Warfare Program," trans. John Junkerman, *The Asia-Pacific Journal*, http://japanfocus.org/-Tsuneishi-Keiichi/2194.

12 Mark Selden, *China in Revolution: The Yenan Way Revisited* (Armonk: M.E. Sharpe, 1995); Chen Yung-fa, *Making Revolution: The Chinese Communist Revolution in Eastern and Central China, 1937–1945* (Berkeley: University of California Press, 1986); Edward Friedman, Paul G. Pickowicz and Mark Selden, *Chinese Village, Socialist State* (New Haven: Yale University Press, 1991); Chalmers Johnson, *Peasant Nationalism and Communist Power: The Emergence of Revolutionary China* (Stanford: Stanford University Press, 1962). In carrying out a reign of terror in resistance base areas, Japanese forces anticipated many of the strategic approaches that the U.S. and its Korean allies would later apply in Vietnam. For example, Japanese forces pioneered in constructing "strategic hamlets" involving relocation of rural people, torching of entire resistance villages, terrorizing the local population, and imposing heavy taxation and labor burdens. Equally important is the direct line from the biowar activities of Japan in China to the massive U.S. application of the defoliant dioxin (Agent Orange) to denude the forests and kill and injure villagers in Vietnam. This legacy continues to take a toll on Vietnamese more than three decades after the end of the war. As James Dao observed in a *New York Times* story of October 12, 2009, the Pentagon is investigating extending benefits to U.S. soldiers who may have been affected by Agent Orange: "Door Opens to Health Claims Tied to Agent Orange." The United States has never formally accepted responsibility, apologized for, or provided compensation to, Vietnamese victims for this, the most flagrant use of biological warfare undertaken anywhere in the course of modern warfare.

13 Yuki Tanaka, *Japan's Comfort Women: Sexual Slavery and Prostitution during World War II and the US Occupation* (London: Routledge, 2002). This systematic atrocity against women has haunted Japan since the 1980s when the first former comfort women broke silence and began public testimony. The Japanese government eventually responded to international protest by recognizing the atrocities committed under the comfort women system, while denying official and military responsibility. It established a government-supported but ostensibly private Asian Women's Fund to apologize and pay reparations to former comfort women, many of whom rejected the terms of a private settlement. See Alexis Dudden and Kozo Yamaguchi, "Abe's Violent Denial: Japan's Prime Minister and the 'Comfort Women,' " *The Asia-Pacific Journal*, http://japanfocus.org/-Alexis-Dudden/2368. See Wada Haruki for a defense of the fund for Japanese and English discussion and documents archived at the website: "The Comfort Women, the Asian Women's Fund and the Digital Museum," *The Asia-Pacific Journal*, http://japanfocus.org/-Wada-Haruki/2653.

14 Peter J. Kuznick, "The Decision to Risk the Future: Harry Truman, the Atomic Bomb and the Apocalyptic Narrative," *The Asia-Pacific Journal*, http://japanfocus.org/

-Peter_J_–Kuznick/2479. The International War Crimes Tribunal, organized by Bertrand Russell and representatives from 18 countries, subjected the U.S.-Indochina War to scrutiny in 1966 and 1967. J. Duffett, ed., *Against The Crime of Silence: Proceedings of The Russell International War Crimes Tribunal* (New York: O'Hare Books, 1968). See "The Russell Tribunal," http://en.wikipedia.org/wiki/Russell_Tribunal for discussion of the controversy.

15 Early works that drew attention to U.S. war atrocities, often centered on the torture, killing, and desecration of the remains of captured Japanese soldiers are Peter Schrijvers, *The GI War Against Japan. American Soldiers in Asia and the Pacific During World War II* (New York: New York University Press, 2002) and John W. Dower, *War Without Mercy: Race and Power in the Pacific War* (New York: Pantheon, 1986); see also *The Wartime Journals of Charles Lindbergh* (New York: Harcourt Brace Jovanovich, 1970). A growing literature has begun to examine U.S. bombing policies. A. C. Grayling, *Among the Dead Cities*, provides a thorough assessment of U.S. and British strategic bombing (including atomic bombing) through the lenses of ethics and international law. Grayling concludes that the U.S. and British killing of non-combatants "did in fact involve the commission of wrongs" on a very large scale (pp. 5–6; 276–277). See Herbert P. Bix, "War Crimes Law and American Wars in 20th Century Asia," *Hitotsubashi Journal of Social Studies*, 33, 1 (July 2001), pp. 119–132.

16 Quoted in Sven Lindqvist, *A History of Bombing* (New York: New Press, 2000), p. 81. The U.S. debate over the bombing of cities is detailed in Michael Sherry, *The Rise of American Air Power: The Creation of Armageddon* (New Haven: Yale University Press, 1987), pp. 23–28, pp. 57–59; Ronald Schaffer, *Wings of Judgment: American Bombing in World War II* (New York: Oxford University Press, 1985), pp. 20–30, 108–109; and Sahr Conway-Lanz, *Collateral Damage, Americans, Noncombatant Immunity, and Atrocity After World War II* (London: Routledge, 2006), p. 10. See Mark Selden, "A Forgotten Holocaust: US Bombing Strategy, the Destruction of Japanese Cities and the American Way of War from the Pacific War to Iraq," *The Asia-Pacific Journal*, http://japanfocus.org/-Mark-Selden/2414.

17 Sherry, *Air Power*, p. 260. With much U.S. bombing already relying on radar, the distinction between tactical and strategic bombing had long been violated in practice. The top brass, from George Marshall to Air Force Chief Henry Arnold to Dwight Eisenhower, had all earlier given tacit approval for area bombing, yet no orders from on high spelled out a new bombing strategy.

18 The Committee for the Compilation of Materials on Damage Caused by the Atomic bombs in Hiroshima and Nagasaki, *Hiroshima and Nagasaki: The Physical, Medical and Social Effects of the Atomic Bombing* (New York: Basic Books, 1991), pp. 420–421; Cf. U.S. Strategic Bombing Survey, Field Report Covering Air Raid Protection and Allied Subjects Tokyo (n.p. 1946), pp. 3, 79; *The U.S. Strategic Bombing Survey Study of Effects of Air Attack on Urban Complex Tokyo-Kawasaki-Yokohama* (n.p. 1947). In contrast to the vast survivor testimony on Hiroshima and Nagasaki, in addition to poems, short stories, novels, manga, anime, and film documenting the atomic bombing, the testimony for the firebombing of Tokyo and other cities is sparse. Max Hastings provides valuable first-person accounts of the Tokyo bombing based on survivor recollection in *Retribution. The Battle for Japan 1944–45* (New York: Knopf, 2008), pp. 297–306.

19 All but five cities of any size were destroyed. Of these cities, four were designated atomic bomb targets, while Kyoto was spared. John W. Dower, "Sensational Rumors, Seditious Graffiti, and the Nightmares of the Thought Police," in *Japan in War and Peace* (New York: The New Press, 1993), p. 117; United States Strategic Bombing Survey, *Summary Report*, Vol I, pp. 16–20.

20 *Retribution*, pp. 296–297. Hastings (p. 318) makes a compelling case that the Japanese surrender owed most to the naval blockade which isolated Japan and denied it access

to the oil, steel, and much more in severing the links to the empire. Gar Alperovitz, *Atomic Diplomacy* (New York: Simon & Schuster, 1965 [1985])) is the classic study linking the atomic decision to the origins of the Soviet–American conflict to follow. See also Mark Selden, "Introduction," *The Atomic Bomb: Voices From Hiroshima and Nagasaki* (Armonk: M.E. Sharpe, 1989), pp. xi–xxxvi.

21   The horror felt around the world at the German bombing at Guernica, the Japanese bombing of Shanghai and Chongqing, and the British bombing of Dresden would not be felt so intensely and universally ever again, regardless of the scale of bombing and the deaths of victims at Hiroshima and Nagasaki, in Korea, Vietnam, or Iraq . . . with the possible exception of the outpouring of sympathy for the 2800 victims of the 9/11 bombing of the New York World Trade Center when the term "terror bombing" would come into vogue, not, of course, to be applied to the United States.

22   "Postwar Narrative," quoted in Hastings, *Retribution*, p. 317.

23   There were, of course, important differences in the character of the wars fought by Japan and the U.S. Japan's invasion of China involved very different dynamics from the U.S.–Japan conflict between two expansionist powers. This chapter does not explore this issue.

24   In practice. Sahr Conway-Lanz provides the definitive study of the "collateral damage" argument that has been repeatedly used to deny the deliberate killing of civilians in U.S. bombing: *Collateral Damage, Americans, Noncombatant Immunity, and Atrocity After World War II*.

25   Marilyn Young, "Total War," in Marilyn Young and Yuki Tanaka, eds, *Bombing Civilians*. (New York: The New Press, 2009).

26   Elizabeth Becker, "Kissinger Tapes Describe Crises, War and Stark Photos of Abuse," *New York Times*, May 27, 2004.

27   Seymour Hersh, *Chemical and Biological Warfare* (New York: Anchor Books,1969), pp. 131–133. Hersh notes that the $60 million worth of defoliants and herbicides in the 1967 Pentagon budget would have been sufficient to defoliate 3.6 million acres if all were used optimally. Agent Orange was introduced first in Korea, but it was in Vietnam that it was used on a vast scale. "Agent Orange," Wikipedia, http://en.wikipedia.org/wiki/Agent_Orange.

28   In contrast to the Vietnam War in particular, in which critical journalism in major media eventually played a powerful role in fueling and reinforcing the anti-war movement, the major print and broadcasting media in the Iraq War have dutifully averted their eyes from the air war in deference to the Bush administration's wishes. On the air war, see, for example, Seymour Hersh, "Up in the Air. Where is the Iraq War Headed Next?," *The New Yorker*, December 5, 2005; Dahr Jamail, "Living Under the Bombs," *TomDispatch*, February 2, 2005; Michael Schwartz, "A Formula for Slaughter. The American Rules of Engagement from the Air," *TomDispatch*, January 14, 2005; Nick Turse, "America's Secret Air War in Iraq," *TomDispatch*, February 7, 2007; Tom Engelhardt, "9 Propositions on the U.S. Air War for Terror," *TomDispatch*, April 8, 2008. The invisibility of the air war is nicely revealed in conducting a Google search for "Iraq War" and "Air War in Iraq." The former produces numerous references to the *New York Times*, the *Washington Post*, CNN, Wikipedia, and a wide range of powerful media. The latter produces references almost exclusively to blogs and critical sources such as those cited in this note.

29   Sabrina Tavernese, "For Iraqis, Exodus to Syria, Jordan Continues," *New York Times*, June 14, 2006; Michael Schwartz, "Iraq's Tidal Wave of Misery. The First History of the Planet's Worst Refugee Crisis," *TomDispatch*, February 10, 2008. The U.N. estimates that there are 1.25 million Iraqi refugees in Syria and 500,000 in Jordan, 200,000 throughout the Gulf states, and 100,000 more in Europe. The United States accepted 463 refugees between the start of the war in 2003 and mid-2007. The International Organization for Migration estimated the displacement rate throughout 2006 to 2007 at 60,000 per month, and with the American "surge" accelerating

displacement, already more than one in seven Iraqis in a nation of 28 million people have been displaced.

30   Anthony Arnove, "Four Years Later . . . And Counting. Billboarding the Iraqi Disaster," *TomDispatch*, March 18, 2007; Seymour Hersh, "The Redirection. Is the Administration's New Policy Benefiting our Enemies in the War on Terrorism?," *The New Yorker*, March 3, 2007; Michael Schwartz, "Baghdad Surges into Hell. First Results from the President's Offensive," *TomDispatch*, February 12, 2007; Tom Engelhardt, "Will Today's U.S.-armed Ally Be Tomorrow's Enemy?," *TomDispatch*, October 18, 2009.

31   Mark Selden, "Nationalism, Historical Memory and Contemporary Conflicts in the Asia Pacific: The Yasukuni Phenomenon, Japan, and the United States," *The Asia-Pacific Journal*, http://japanfocus.org/-Mark-Selden/2204; Yoshiko Nozaki and Mark Selden, "Historical Memory, International Conflict and Japanese Textbook Controversies in Three Epochs," *The Journal of Educational Media, Memory, and Society*, I, 1; Takashi Yoshida, "Revising the Past, Complicating the Future: The Yushukan War Museum in Modern Japanese History," *The Asia-Pacific Journal*, http://japanfocus.org/-Takashi-YOSHIDA/2594; Laura Hein and Akiko Takenaka, "Exhibiting World War II in Japan and the United States," *The Asia-Pacific Journal*, http://japanfocus.org/-Laura-Hein/2477; Aniya Masaaki, "Compulsory Mass Suicide, the Battle of Okinawa, and Japan's Textbook Controversy," *The Asia-Pacific Journal*, http://japanfocus.org/-Aniya-Masaaki/2629.

32   Thanks to Laura Hein for suggesting the framing of this issue. On the Reagan decision, reparations, and the Civil Liberties Act of 1988, see Mitchell T. Maki, Harry H. Kitano, and S. Megan Berthold, *Achieving the Impossible Dream: How Japanese Americans Obtained Redress* (Champaign: University of Illinois Press, 1999); http://en.wikipedia.org/wiki/Civil_Liberties_Act_of_1988. Clinton's apology to Hawaiians took the form of Public Law 103–150, http://www.hawaii-nation.org/publawsum.html. The formal apology recognized the devastating effects of subsequent social changes for the Hawaiian people and looked to reconciliation, but offered no reparations or other specific measures to alleviate the sufferings caused by U.S. actions.

33   Emily Rosenberg drew my attention to the Guatemala quasi-apology. Clinton's remarks were prompted by the February 1999 publication of the findings of the independent Historical Clarification Commission which concluded that the U.S. was responsible for most of the human rights abuses committed during the 36-year war in which 200,000 died. See Martin Kettle and Jeremy Lennard, "Clinton Apology to Guatemala," *Guardian*, March 12, 1999, http://www.guardian.co.uk/world/1999/mar/12/jeremylennard.martinkettle; Mark Weisbrot, "Clinton's Apology to Guatemala is a Necessary First Step," March 15, 1999, Knight-Ridder/Tribune Media Services, http://www.cepr.net/index.php/op-eds-columns/op-eds-columns/clinton-s-apology-to-guatemala-is-a-necessary-first-step/. Clinton was perhaps the most apologetic of presidents, making several apologies during his tenure. None carried the weight of an official government apology, and none was accompanied by compensation to victims. These included apologies to the survivors of the Tuskegee syphilis study (http://www.cdc.gov/tuskegee/clintonp.htm), and another apology to interned Japanese-Americans (http://www.pbs.org/childofcamp/history/clinton.html).

34   How are we to define power? If no nation remotely rivals American military power, particularly in the wake of the demise of the Soviet Union, if the United States military budget in 2008 and 2009 is larger than that of all other nations combined – before counting the special appropriations for the wars in Iraq and Afghanistan – the striking fact is that the U.S. has fought to stalemate or defeat in each of the major wars it has entered since World War II.

35   Kerry's testimony, ignored by the mass media but made available through film and other media, is available at http://www.c-span.org/vote2004/jkerrytestimony.asp.

36   See the testimony and the historical record at http://www.zcommunications.org/zvideo/25776 and at http://www.zcommunications.org/zvideo/2577.

Part IV

Annotated bibliography and appendices

11 Annotated bibliography

Primary sources and secondary
liaturature in Japanese, Chinese,
and English

Nanyan Guo and Jing-Bao Nie

Introduction

A great deal of literature – both primary materials and secondary studies – has been produced on Japan's wartime medical atrocities and their aftermath. This bibliography consists of works published in Japanese, Chinese, and English on the subject – essential, original, significant, and representative – with some entries annotated. It indicates the areas that have so far been covered by scholars and journalists as well as what remains to be done from an intellectual and political perspective.

The bibliography is arranged in alphabetical order of names of authors. Where appropriate, entries are given in the original Japanese and Chinese.

For some related Russian and German works on the subject see the lists of references at the end of chapters 3, 4, 7 and 8 (this volume).

This bibliography excludes original publications by Japanese medical researchers that are evidently based on human experimentation, or suspected of being so. Nevertheless, Chapter 4 discusses some of these studies and lists them as references.

However, we have not excluded works which express doubt or skepticism about the activities of Unit 731 and other war crimes laid at the feet of Japan (see Hata 1998; Nakagawa 2002; Nakata 1983; Yoshimura 1970).

For the convenience of readers, in the discussion below we have grouped entries according to subject, under the authors' surnames. However, many works cover more than one subject and grouping them into a single category may be misleading to some extent.

The primary sources listed include archival material, court records, reports of investigators, accounts by victims, participants' confessions, eye-witness reports, and interviews with victims, perpetrators, and witnesses. See Asaeda, Awaya & Yoshimi, Cheng, Fell, Foreign Languages Publishing House, Fu, Han 1985, Han and Xin, Hill, Hong, Inaba, Jiang, JJCA, Kiku no bokyu iinkai, King, Kitajima, Kobayashi and Kojima, Kondo, Liaoningsheng danganguan, Liu, H., Matsumura 1985, Matsumura and Kanehira, Miyatake, Mori et al., Nikkan kankei o kirokusuru kai, Pollitzer, Quzhoushi weishengzhi bangongshi, Rikugun Guni gakko boekigaku kyoshitu, Rong, Sanders, Takahashi, M., Tan, X., Tanaka and Matsumura,

Thompson, Wang, G., Wang, S., Wang, Z., Xinhua shishi congkanshe, Xu, W., Yang et al., Yoshimi and Matsuno, Zhongguo Heilongjiangshen danganguan, Zhongguo Jilinshen danganguan, Zhongyang danganguan et al.

A number of perpetrators and accessory witnesses have produced confessions of their activities. See Akiyama et al., Chugoku kikansha renrakukai, Chugoku kikansha renrakukai kanko iinkai, Endo, S., Gold, Gunji 1982a, 1982b, Han and Jin, Hoshi, Ishida, Kochi shimbunsha henshukyoku shakaibu, Koga, Koshi, Mitomo, Mizutani 1995, Morimura 1990, Nanasanichi kenkyukai, Nihon chugoku yuko kyokai and Chugoku kikansha renrakukai, Shinozuka and Takayanagi, Takana, Takasugi, I., Takehana, Takidani, Tamura, Wada, Yoshifusa, Yoshikai, Zhongyang Danganguan et al.

One major focus of research is Unit 731 and the activities of the Ishii network. See Aki 1984, Aoki, Asano and Tsuneishi, Chaen, Ban, Dongbei renmin zhengfu weishengbu, Han 1993, Harris, Hatakeyama, Honda, Fujii, Han and Yin, Hata 1990, 1993, Ienaga, Inoue and Hiroshima, Kasukawa, Kinoshita, Kyokasho kentei sosho o shiensuru zenkoku renrakukai 1991, 1997, Matsumura 1991, 1996a, 1996b, 1996c, 1997a, 1997b, 1997c, 1998, 2001a, 2001b, 2002, Matsumura and Yano, Mima, Minamoto, Mineo, Mizutani 1997, Monma, Mori 1990, 1998, Nezu, Nihon no senso sekinin siryo senta, Nishino, Nishizato 1996b, Oga, Omata, Osanai, Saito, Seki, Shimamura, Shimozato, Takasugi 1984, Tanaka and Eda, Tsuneishi 1981, 1984a, 1985, 1994a, 1995, 2002b, Williams and Wallace 1985, 1989, Watanabe, Xu, J., Zhang and Zhao, Yoshinaga 1976a, 1976b, 1982, 2001.

A large number of historical studies and journalistic investigations have been published on Japan's biological warfare program. See Bao, Barenblatt, Behr, Bu, Bu and Gao, Bu et al., Cao, Chen, X., Chu, Gao, Gao and Zhao, Guo and Liao, Han 2003, Harris and Paxman, Honda and Naganuma, Huang, Huang and Wu, Huang et al., Hunan wenli xueyuan xijunzhan zuixing yanjiusuo, Ivanov and Bogachi, Kyodo tsushinsha shakaibu, Ji, Li, Lishi buneng wangji chongshu bianweihui, Liu, Q., Liu, Y. and Gong, Matsumura 1994a, 1994b, 1996a, 1996b, 1996v. 1997a, 1997b, 1997c, 1998, 2001a, 2001b, 2002, Matsumura and Xie, Matsuno, Minguo dangan, Mori 1995, Mori and Kasukawa, Nanasanichi butai kokusai symposium jikko iinkai, Nanasanichi butai shinso chosa zenkoku renraku kyogikai, Nanasanichi saikinsen saiban kyanpein iinkai, Newman, Nie, L. 2006a, 2006b, Nihongun ni yoru saikinsen no rekishi jijitsu o akirakani suru kai, Niki, Ozaki, Qinhua rijun xijun 731 budui zuizheng chenlieguan, Qiu, Ran, Renmin ribao, Seki et al., Sha, Sun and Ni, Takasugi 1982b, Tan, Y., Takeda, Tanaka, T., Tanaka, Y., Tatsumi, Tong, Tsuneishi 2005b, Wu, Wu and Xie, Xie et al., Xing and Chen, Yang and Xin, Yoshimi and Iko, Zhang, L.

A few studies are devoted to the wartime vivisections at Kyushu Imperial University: see Hirako, Kamisaka, Senba, Tono.

Some studies have focused on the exemption from prosecution of Japanese war criminals and on compensation for victims: Arai, A. et al., Awaya, Awaya et al., Brackman, Chugokujin senso higai baisho seikyu jiken bengodan, Daya wenhua, *East Asia*, Iwakawa, Koshida, Nishizato 1996a, 1996c, 2002, Ota 1999, 2001, Powell, Torii, Zhang, S.

Some literary representations – documentary novels – have appeared as well: Biokai, Hiraoka, Hiyama, Jin, Kindai senshi kenkyukai, Morimura 1981, 1982a, 1982b, 1983, 1984, Nakazono, Tsuneishi and Asano, Ura, Yamada 1973, 1974.

A series of crimes and scandals in postwar Japan have been linked with Unit 731 and Japan's other wartime medical atrocities. For the connection between the Ishii network and the Imperial Bank incident in which 12 people were poisoned to death on January 26, 1948, see Endo, M., Morikawa, Tsuneishi 2002a, Utsumi. For the connection between the Ishii network and the former Military Medical College, see Guni gakko atochi de hakkensareta jinkotsu mondai o kyumeisuru kai, Tsuneishi 1992. On the connection between the Ishii network and the Green Cross scandal, see Hirokiawa 1992, Matsushita 1996.

For more than half a century, some attention has been paid to these atrocities by specialists in either international or East Asian medical ethics. With the outstanding exception of a handful of Japanese scholars, the subject has been treated as if it had minimal relevance to contemporary science, medicine, and medical ethics, even in Japan and China. For relevant ethical studies, see Aki 1994, Akimoto, Azami, Baader et al., Chen, R., Dickinson, Doering, Kanagawa daigaku hyoronshu senmon iinkai, Kenmochi, LaFleur et al., Leavitt 2002, 2003a, 2003b, Morioka, Nie, J. 2001, 2002, 2003, 2004, 2005, 2006, Nie et al. 2008, Nie et al. 2003, Nishiyama, Noda, Sass, Shen, Shibata 1997, 1998, Takahashi, Takasugi 1973, 1974, 1982a, Thomas 2003a, 2003b, Tsuchiya, T. 2001, 2003a, 2003b, 2008, Tsuneishi 1990, 1994b, 1998, 2007, Yamaguchi. For an overview, see Nie et al. 2008.

This bibliography is largely indebted to the bibliography compiled by Kondo Shoji which was added to his translation of Harris' *Factories of Death* (1994) published in 1999 in Tokyo.

Annotated bibliography

Aki, Motoo 安芸基雄 1984, Education about Infectious Diseases and the Kwantung Army's Unit for Epidemic Prevention and Water Supply 伝染病補備教育と関東軍防疫給水部, in Aki's *Those Who Make Peace* 平和を作る人たち. Tokyo: Misuzu shobo, pp. 65–75.
—— 1994, *Working as a Clinical Doctor: Questioning Medical Treatment in Modern Japan* 一臨床医として生きて: 現代日本の医療を問う, Tokyo: Iwanami shoten.
Akimoto, Sueo 秋元寿恵夫 1983, *Questioning Medical Ethics: My Experiences with Unit 731* 医の倫理を問う: 第七三一部隊での体験から, Tokyo: Keiso shobo.
Akiyama, Hiroshi 秋山浩 (pseudonym) 1956, *Special Army Unit 731* 特殊 部隊七三一, Kyoto: Sanichi shobo.
[With the exception of those indicted at the Khabarovsk Trial, this book is the first full confessional account of the atrocities carried out at Unit 731 by a member of the Unit.]
Aoki, Fukiko 青木富貴子 2005 (reprint 2008), *731*, Tokyo: Shinchosha.
[Based on a notebook by Ishii Shiro recording his daily life after the war, other documents, and visits to places associated with Ishii, the author paints a detailed picture of Ishii's life and his role in Unit 731, as well as American efforts to gain Japanese experimental data and exempt the Ishii network from criminal charges.]

Arai, Akira 新井章 et al. (eds) 1997, *Seeking the Truth from History, the Media and the Courts* 「事実」をつかむ—歴史・報道・裁判の場から考える, Tokyo: Kochi shobo.

[Analyzes the reasons behind the Japanese Court's ruling against Ienaga Saburo, a historian who took out several lawsuits against the Japanese Education Ministry which ordered him to erase reference to Unit 731 in his school textbook, despite overwhelming evidence of the activities of Unit 731.]

Arai, Toshio and Fujiwara, Akira 新井利男, 藤原彰 1999, *Testimonies of Invasion: Written by Japanese Prisoners of War in China* 侵略の証言：中国における日本人戦犯自筆供述書, Iwanami shoten.

Asaeda, Shigeharu 朝枝繁春 1997, *Reminiscences of 52 Years Ago* 追憶五二年以前, published by the author, pp. 11–16.

[The author was a staff officer in the Kwantung Army who ordered the destruction of all evidence of the work of Unit 731 as the Soviet Army advanced.]

Asano, Tomizo and Tsuneishi, Keiichi 浅野富三, 常石敬一 1985, *A Mysterious Disease: Epidemic Hemorrhagic Fever* 奇病流行性出血熱, Tokyo: Shinchosha.

Awaya, Kentaro 粟屋憲太郎 1994, *Unresolved Issues of War Responsibility* 未決の戦争責任, Tokyo: Kashiwa shobo.

[Includes chapters on legal exemption from responsibility for biological and poison gas warfare.]

Awaya, Kentaro and Yoshimi, Yoshiaki 粟屋憲太郎, 吉見義明 (eds) 1989, *Documents on Poison Gas Warfare* 毒ガス戦関係資料, Tokyo: Fuji shuppan.

Awaya, Kentaro 粟屋憲太郎 et al. 1994, *War Responsibility, Post-war Responsibility: How Japan Differs from Germany* 戦争責任・戦後責任 日本とドイツとどう違うか, Tokyo: Asahi shimbunsha.

Azami, Shozo 莇昭三 2000, *War and Medical Treatment: The Doctors' 15-Year War* 戦争と医療：医師たちの十五年戦争, Kyoto: Kamogawa shuppan.

Baader, G., Lederer, S.E., Low, M., Schmaltz, F., and Von. Schwerin, A. 2005, Pathways to Human Experimentation, 1933–1945: Germany, Japan, and the United States. *Osiris*, 20: 205–231.

Ban, Shigeo 伴繁雄 2001, *The Truth about the Army's Noborito Research Institute* 陸軍登戸研究所の真実, Tokyo: Fuyo shobo shuppan.

[Reflects the author's experiences of participation in human experiments in Nanjing.]

Bao, Xiaofeng 包晓峰 2005, A Review of Research on the Japanese Army's Bacteriological Warfare Crimes in Zhejiang Province 日军对浙江实施细菌战的罪行综述, *Dangshi yanjiu yu jiaoxue*, 4.

Barenblatt, Daniel 2004, *A Plague upon Humanity: The Secret Genocide of Axis Japan's Germ Warfare Operation*, New York: Harper Collins.

Behr, Edward 1989, *Hirohito: Behind the Myth*, New York: Villard Books.

[A Japanese version was translated by the editorial department at Chubunkan Shoten, 裕仁天皇：神話に包まれて (上), Okayama: Chubunkan, 1992.]

Biokai 美鴨会, ed. 1972, *Ah, Burma! A Record of the 26th Division of the Open Field Epidemic Prevention and Water Supply Unit* あゝビルマ：第二六野戦防疫給水部記録, Kyoto: Mitsumura suiko shoin.

Brackman, Arnold C. 1987, *The Other Nuremberg: The Untold Story of the Tokyo War Crimes Trials*, New York: Morrow. Translated into Japanese by Y. Higurashi, 東京裁判：もう一つのニュルンベルク, Tokyo: Jijitsushinsha, 1995, pp. 211–222.

Bu, Ping 步平 1995, trans. Y. Yamabe and K. Miyazaki, *Japan's Invasion of China and Poison Gas Warfare* 日本の中国侵略と毒ガス兵器, Tokyo: Akashi shoten, pp. 146–147, 165–182, 260–263.

Bu, Ping and Gao, Xiaoyan 步平, 高晓燕 1999, *Crimes Revealed: Documents from Japanese Army's Biological Warfare Programme* 阳光下的罪恶——侵华日军毒气战实录, Harbin: Heilongjiang renmin chubanshe.

[Details the kinds of poison gas used by Japanese forces in various regions of China.]

Bu, Ping, Gao, Xiaoyan and Da, Zhigang 步平, 高晓燕, 笪志刚 2004, *The Chemical War Waged by Japan during its Invasion of China* 日本侵华时期的化学战, Beijing: Shehui kexue wenxian chubanshe.

Cao, Yuan 草原 1951, *The Crime of Japanese Bacteriological Warfare* 日寇細菌戰暴行, Shanghai: Tonglian shudian.

Chaen, Yoshio 茶園義男 1985, The Personnel of the Kwantung Army's Epidemic Prevention and Water Supply Unit 関東軍防疫給水部の人びと, in *Shikoku during the Wars of the Showa Period* 昭和戦史の四国, Tokushima: Kyoiku shuppan senta, pp. 79–88.

Chen, Rongxia 2002, Why Bring up the Past Tragedy Again? *Eubios Journal of Asian and International Bioethics*, 11: 107.

Chen, Xianchu 陈先初 2004, *The Overturn of Humanity: A Study of Japanese Atrocities in Hunan* 人道的颠覆：日军侵湘暴行研究, Beijing: Shehui kexue wenxian chubanshe.

[Chapter 3 describes bacteriological warfare carried out by the Japanese Army in Changde, Hunan Province.]

Cheng, Jisi 程吉思 1986, The Hailin Branch of Unit 731 of the Japanese Army in China 侵华日军第七三一部队・海林支队, in Zhengxie Heilongjiangshen weiyuanhui 政协黑龙江省委员会, ed. *Historical Documents of Heilongjiang, Volume 22*, 黑龙江文史资料第二十二辑, Harbin: Heilongjiang renmin chubanshe.

Chu, Hua 儲華, ed. 1951, *The Crimes of the Japanese Army, Including its Inhumane Bacteriological Warfare Campaign* 日寇的滔天罪行 慘無人道的細菌戰爭, Shanghai: Dadong shudianju chupan.

Chugoku kikansha renrakukai (Association of Returned Prisoners of War from China) 中国帰還者連絡会 1998, *Chukiren* 中帰連, December.

[This journal issue comprises a series of papers on Unit 731, its impact, and suggestions for accepting responsibility and the need for reconciliation.]

Chugoku kikansha renrakukai kanko iinkai 中国帰還者連絡会刊行委員会 2000, *A Journey in Acknowledgement of Crime: Unit 731 and the Records of Mio Yutaka* 認罪の旅：７３１部隊と三尾豊の記録, Tokyo: the author.

Chugokujin senso higai baisho seikyu jiken bengodan (Defense for Demanding for Compensation for Chinese War Victims)中国人戦争被害賠償請求事件弁護団, ed. 2005, *Barriers of Sand: Ten Years of Litigating Compensation for Chinese Victims* 砂上の障壁：中国人戦後補償裁判10年の軌跡, Tokyo: Nihon hyoronsha.

Daya wenhua 大雅文化, ed., 2005, *Litigation in Search of Justice* 正义之诉, Shijiazhuang: Huashan wenyi chubansha.

Dickinson, Frederick R. 2007, Biohazard: Unit 731 in Postwar Japanese Politics of National "Forgetfulness", in William R. LaFleur, et al., eds, *Dark Medicine: Rationalizing Unethical Medical Research*, Bloomington: Indiana University Press.

Döring, Ole 2001, Comments on Inhumanity in the Name of Medicine: Old Cases and New Voices for Responsible Medical Ethics from Japan and China. *Eubios Journal of Asian and International Bioethics*, 11: 44–47.

Dongbei renmin zhengfu weishengbu (Department of Public Health, Northeast People's Goverment) 東北人民政府衛生部 1952, *A Report on the Criminal Activities of Biological Warfare Unit 731 and Unit 100* 関於調査七三一和一〇〇細菌部隊罪悪活動的報告.

[The first systematic Chinese report on Unit 731 and Unit 100, with 34 photos. Translated and included in Kojima 1995. Also available in Liaoningshen danganguan 1995.]

East Asia: An International Quarterly 2000, 2001, A special issue on Japanese wartime atrocities and questions of reparation, Parts I and II.

Endo, Makoto 遠藤誠 1986, New Evidence from America アメリカからやって来た新証拠, in *The Mystery of the Imperial Bank Incident Trial: From the GHQ's Secret Archives* 帝銀事件裁判の謎—GHQ 秘密公文書は語る, Tokyo: Aoyamakan.

[Describes the American cover-up of the real criminal behind the Incident owing to its links with Unit 731 (pp. 3–14). A new edition was published in 1990 by Gendai shokan (Tokyo).]

Endo, Saburo 遠藤三郎 1974, *My Part in the Fifteen-year War between Japan and China: Branded a Traitor and "Red General"* 日中十五年戦争と私：国賊・赤の将軍と人はいう, Tokyo: Nicchu shorin, pp. 162–164, 442–443.

[A former army general describes Ishii's experiments and biological warfare.]

Fell, H. Norbert 1947, "Report by Norbert H. Fell". Available in Kondo 2003.

[The first report from the U.S. to document the human experiments conducted by Unit 731.]

Fu, Yang 佛洋 ed. 1997, *The Khabarovsk Trials: Confessions of 12 Japanese Biological Warfare Criminals* 伯力審判—12名前日本細菌战犯自供词, Changchun: Jilin renmin chubanshe.

[A reprint of the Chinese version of Foreign Languages Publishing House 1950, with a Preface by the editor.]

Fujii, Shizue 藤井志津枝 1997, *Unit 731: Horrors of the Japanese Biological Warfare Campaign* 七三一部隊：日本魔鬼生化戦的恐怖, Taipei: Wenyingtang.

Gao, Fanfu and Zhao Deqin 高凡夫, 赵徳芹 2005, Japan's Emperor Hirohito and Biological Warfare 日本天皇裕仁与細菌戦, *Hunan wenli xueyuan xuebao (shehui kexue ban)*, 2.

Gao, Xiaoyan 高暁燕 1996, trans. Y. Yamabe and K. Miyazaki, *Poison Gas Weapons Discarded by the Japanese Army* 日本軍遺棄毒ガス兵器, Tokyo: Akashi shoten.

Gold, Hal 1996, *Unit 731: Testimony*, Rutland, VT: Charles E. Tuttle.

[An outline of the activities of Unit 731 followed by a series of confessions by participants from the Ishii Network. The Japanese version was translated by Hamada T. 証言・731部隊の真相：生体実験の全貌と戦後謀略の軌跡 (Tokyo: Kosaido shuppan, 1997) and reprinted in 2002.]

Guni gakko atochi de hakkensareta jinkotsu mondai o kyumeisuru kai (Association of Investigation of Military Medical School Site) 軍医学校跡地で発見された人骨問題を究明する会 ed. 1991–1999, *Kyumeisuru kai News*.

[These newsletters focus on tracing the origins of the human bones found in the ruins of the former Military Medical School, and their links with Unit 731.]

Gunji, Yoko 郡司陽子 1982a, *My Testimony on Unit 731: Revelations of a Female Member* 証言 七三一石井部隊：今、初めて明かす女子隊員の記録, Tokyo: Tokuma shoten.

—— ed. 1982b, *The Truth about Ishii's Germ Troops: Testimonies from Participants in Top-secret Tasks* 真相石井細菌戦部隊：極秘任務を遂行した隊員たちの証言, Tokyo: Tokuma shoten.

Guo, Chengzhou and Liao, Yingchang 郭成周, 廖应昌, 1997, *The Hidden Story of the Japanese Army's Biological Warfare Campaign* 侵华日军细菌战纪实—历史上被隐藏的篇章, Beijing: Yanshan chubanshe.

[A major historical study in Chinese which includes the extensive use of primary materials.]

Han, Xiao 韩晓 1986, Collection of the Fascist Atrocities of Unit 731 of the Japanese Army 日军七三一部队法西斯暴行辑录, in Zhengxie Heilongjiangshen weiyuanhui, ed., *Historical Documents of Heilongjiang, Volume 19: The History We Must Not Forget* 黑龙江文史资料第十九辑： 不能忘记的历史, Harbin: Heilongjiang renmin chubanshe.

—— 1993, trans. Y. Yamabe, *The Crimes of Unit 731* 七三一部隊の犯罪, Tokyo: Sanichi shobo.

[A collection of research papers published in China, based on testimony by laborers, victims' relatives, and members of Unit 731, as well as on documents relating to Unit 731 in local public security bureaus in Northeastern China and the Central Archives Bureau.]

—— 2003, Research into Japanese Biological Warfare in China 关于侵华日軍细菌战罪行的研究, *Changde shifan xueyuan xuebao (shehui kexue ban)*, 3.

Han, Xiao and Jin, Chengmin 韩晓, 金成民, 1997, trans. M. Nakano, *Telling the Truth before Dying: Testimonies from Chinese on the Crimes of Unit 731 of the Japanese Army* 死ぬまえに真実を——侵略日本軍七三一部隊の犯罪中国人の証言, two vols. Chofu, Tokyo: Seinen shuppansha.

[Volume 1 comprises testimonies by Chinese, and Volume 2 those by Japanese participants.]

Han, Xiao and Xin, Peilin 韩晓, 辛培林, 1991, *Historical Documents of Heilongjiang, Volume 31, A History of the Crimes of Unit 731 of the Japanese Army* 黑龙江文史资料第三十一辑： 日军七三一部队罪恶史, Harbin: Heilongjian renmin chubanshe.

Han, Xiao and Yin, Qingfang 韩晓, 尹庆芳, 1986, The Use of Chinese Labour in Unit 731 of the Japanese Army 侵华日军第七三一部队里的劳工, Heilongjiangsheng weiyuanhui wenshiziliao yanjiuweiyuanhui, ed. *Historical Documents of Heilongjiang, Volume 22*, 黑龙江文史资料第二十二辑, Harbin: Heilongjiang renmin chubanshe.

Harris, Robert and Paxman, Jeremy 1982, *A Higher Form of Killing: the Secret Story of Gas and Germ Warfare*, London: Chatto & Windus. Translated into Japanese by Oshima K., and published as 化学兵器:その恐怖と悲劇, Tokyo: Kinda bungeisha, pp. 108–116, 194–195, 209–211. Translated into Chinese by Lu Mingjun and published by Qunzhong chubanshe (Beijing) in 1988.

Harris, Sheldon H. 2002 (revised edn; 1st edn 1994), *Factories of Death: Japanese Biological Warfare 1932–1945 and the American Cover-up,* New York: Routledge. The 1994 edition was translated into Japanese by Kondo S. as 死の工場—隠蔽された七三一部隊, and published in 1999 by Kashiwa shobo (Tokyo).

[Kondo added a comprehensive bibliography of publications on the Ishii network. The 1994 edition was also translated into Chinese by X. Wang et al. as 死亡工厂：美国掩盖的日本细菌战犯罪 and published in 2000 by Shanghai renmin chubanshe (Shanghai).]

Hata, Ikuhiko 秦郁彦 1990, In Search of the Secrets of the Showa Period: Japanese Biological Warfare, Unit 731 and Ishii Shiro 昭和史の謎を追う—日本の細菌戦—七三一部隊と石井四郎—, Part 1, Part 2, *Seiron*, March, April.

—— 1993, Japan's Biological Warfare Programme 日本の細菌戦, *In Search of the Secrets of the Showa Period, Vol. 1* 昭和史の謎を追う(上), Tokyo: Bungei shunju, pp. 316–395.

—— 1998, "Linking the Comfort Women with Unit 731" 「慰安婦と七三一部隊」合体の仕掛人, in *Controversial Issues in Modern History* 現代史の争点, revised version 2001, Tokyo: Bungei shunju, pp. 55–73.

Hatakeyama, Kiyoyuki 畠山清行 1966, *The Army's Nakano School* 陸軍中野学校, Tokyo: Sankei shimbun shuppansha, pp. 90–91, 100–101, 115, 195–202. Reprinted in 1972 by Bancho shobo (Tokyo).

Hill, Edwin V. and Victor, Joseph 1947, *Summary Report on BW Investigation*, December 12.

[This was the second report to document human experimentation in Unit 731. Available in Kondo 2003. This report is also included in Matsumura 1994a.]

Hirako, Goichi 平光吾一 1957, Military Medicine in the Dirt: The Story behind the Vivisection Incident 戦争医学の汚辱にふれて――生体解剖事件始末記, *Bungei shunju*, December: 204–214.

[An account By one of the participants in the vivisection of eight American pilots at Kyushu Imperial University.]

Hiraoka, Masaaki 平岡正明 1972, Rabbit-catching and Chinese Monkeys: The Double Face of Ishii Unit うさぎ狩りとチャイナモンキー 石井部隊の二つの顔; Unit 731 of the Kwantung Army in Manchuria 関東軍満州七三一部隊, in *What the Japanese Did in China: A Record of Holocaust* 日本人は中国で何をしたか: 中国人大虐殺の記録, Tokyo: Shio shuppansha. Reprinted in 1985 by Shio shuppansha.

Hiyama, Yoshiaki 檜山良昭 1980, *Chasing the Doctors of the Germ Troops* 細菌部隊の医師を追え, Tokyo: Kodansha.

Honda, Katsuichi 本多勝一 1972, Human Experiments Involving Bacteria and Vivisection 人間の細菌実験と生体解剖, in Honda's *A Journey to China* 中国の旅, Tokyo: Asahi Shimbunsha.

[Based on the earlier studies published in Japan and China. The book was reprinted in 1981.]

Honda, Katsuichi and Naganuma Setsuo 本多勝一, 長沼節夫 1991, *The Emperor's Army* 天皇の軍隊, Tokyo: Asahi shimbunsha.

Hong, Guiji 洪桂己 ed. 1985, *A Record of Japanese Atrocities in China: 1928–1945* 日本在華暴行録: 民國十七年至三十四年 1928–1945, Taipei: Guoshiguan.

Hoshi, Toru 星徹 2002 (revised edn 2006), *What We Did in China: Testimonies from the Association of Returned Prisoners of War from China* 私たちが中国でしたこと:中国帰還者連絡会の人びと Tokyo: Ryokufu shuppan.

[Among the former POWs interviewed by the author, Watanabe Nobuichi, Mio Yutaka, Shinotsuka (Tamura) Yoshio, and Yuasa Ken detail their involvement in medical atrocities.]

Huang, Jialai 黄加来 2005, Revealing the Secrets of the Japanese Army's Bacteriological Warfare Campaign in Changde 日军常德细菌战揭秘. *Dangan shikong*, 3.

Huang, Ketai and Wu, Yuanzhang 黄可泰, 吴元章 eds 1994, *The Unimaginable Cruelty of Bacteriological Warfare: Historical Facts about the 1940 Plague in Ningbo* 惨绝人寰的细菌战一九四〇年宁波鼠疫史实, Nanjing: Dongnan daxue chubanshe.

Huang, Ketai, Qiu, Huashi and Xia, Suqin 黄可泰, 邱華士, 夏素琴 eds 1999, *The Plague in Ningbo: Proof of the Japanese Army's Biological Warfare Campaign* 宁波鼠疫史实——侵华日军细菌战罪证, Beijing: Zhongguo wenlian chubanshe.

Hunan wenli xueyuan xijunzhan zuixing yanjiusuo (Research Institute of Biological Warfare Crimes, Hunan University of Arts and Science) 湖南文理学院细菌战罪行研究所 ed. 2003, *Revealing the Darkest Secret: Collected Papers from an International Conference on Biological Warfare Held in Changde, China, in 2002* 揭开黑幕：二〇〇二中国常德细菌战罪行国际学术研讨会论文集, Beijing: Zhongguo wenshi chubanshe.

Ienaga, Saburo 家永三郎 1968, *The Pacific War* 太平洋戦争, Tokyo: Iwanami shoten, pp. 216–217.

[Translated into English and published by Pantheon Books (New York) in 1978. It includes material on the activities of Unit 731 and describes the vivisection carried out at Kyushu Imperial University on captured American airmen (pp.188–190). A second edition was published in 1986; see pp. 233–235, 369–371.]

Inaba, Masao 稲葉正夫 ed. 1970, Appendix: Ishii's Top-secret Institute 付録：石井極秘機関, in Inaba's *Materials Relating to General Okamura Yasuji, Volume 1, Reminiscences of the Battlefield* 岡村寧次大将資料（上）戦場回想編, Tokyo: Hara shobo, pp. 387–390.

Inoue Kiyoshi and Hiroshima, Tadashi 井上清、廣島正 1994, *What Did the Japanese Army Do in China?* 日本軍は中国で何をしたのか, Kumamoto: Kumamoto shuppan bunka kaikan.

[Includes a chapter on poison gas warfare and Ishii's germ troops (pp. 273–303).]

Ishida, Shinsaku 石田新作 1982, *Dedicated to Evil – The Japanese Military Doctors* 悪魔の日本軍医, Tokyo: Yamate shobo.

[The author, a former military surgeon in the Japanese Army, describes medical atrocities committed both inside and outside the Ishii network.]

Ivanov, N. and Bogachi, V. 1991, trans K. Nakanishi Оружиевнезакона, *The Horrors of Biological Warfare: Unit 731 of the Kwantung Army on Trial* 恐怖の細菌戦―裁かれた関東軍第七三一部隊, Tokyo: Kobunsha.

Iwakawa, Takashi 岩川隆 1995, "The Soviet Trial" ソ連裁判, *Like the Soil of a Remote Island: The Trial of B and C-Class War Criminals* 孤島の土となるとも：BC 級戦犯裁判, Tokyo: Kodansha, pp. 617–646.

Jiang, Li 姜力 ed. 2005, *1949: The Khabarovsk Trial* 1949: 伯利大审判―侵华日军使用细菌武器案庭审实录, Beijing: Jiefangjun wenxue chubanshe.

[A reprint of the 1950 Chinese edition.]

Ji, Xueren 紀学仁 1996, trans. T. Murata, *Chemical Warfare Waged by the Japanese Army: Poison Gas Operations in China* 日本軍の化学戦 ：中国戦場における毒ガス作戦, Tokyo: Otsuki shoten.

Jin, He 金河 1998, *Devils' Nest: Germ Troops of Unit 731 of the Japanese Army in Pingfang* 平房魔窟：侵华日军 731 细菌部队, Shijiazhuang: Huashan chubanshe.

JJCA CHINA REPORT 1945, Subject: Japanese Use of BW at CHANGTEH, Hunan Province, from J. R. Giddes to Harold Pride, June 28, Kunming, R-731-CH-45, Secret, copy 4 of 5, Public Record Office (London).

[This report is based on an investigation in Changde conducted by J. R. Giddes, who confirmed the possibility of Japan's use of plague bacteria in Changde. Available in Kondo 2003; see also Matsumura 1997a.]

Kamisaka, Fuyuko 上坂冬子 1979, *Vivisection: The Incident at Kyushu University's Medical School* 生体解剖　九州大学医学部事件, Tokyo: Mainichi shimbunsha.

[This documentary novel has been frequently reprinted since 1979.]

Kanagawa daigaku hyoronshu senmon iinkai 神奈川大学評論編集専門委員会 ed. 1994, *Medical Science and War: Japan and Germany* 医学と戦争 ：日本とドイツ, Tokyo: Ochanomizu shobo.

Kasukawa, Yoshiya 糟川良谷 1986 (revised edn 1995), Horrific Vivisection and Bacteriological Experiment 悪魔の生体・細菌実験, in Masataka Mori, ed., *China Will Not Forget: The Untold Story of [Japan's] War of Aggression* 中国の大地は忘れない：侵略・語られなかった戦争, Tokyo: Shakai hyoronsha, pp. 73–112, 177–194.

Kenmochi, Kazumi 剣持一巳 1970, Exposing War Crimes 戦争犯罪の告発, in Kenmochi's *Bearing Death for Humanity – Crimes of Modern Science* 現代科学の犯罪：人間を死に追いやるもの Tokyo: Shinsensha, pp. 255–290.

The Khabarovsk Trial 1950, *Materials on the Trial of Former Servicemen of the Japanese Army Charged with Manufacturing and Employing Biological Weapons*, Moscow: Foreign Language Publishing House.

[This is the primary publication by the Soviet Union on the trial conducted in Khabarovsk in 1949. It was originally translated and published in Russian, Chinese, English, and Japanese in 1950. The Japanese version was reprinted in 1982 by Fuji shuppan (Tokyo) and kaien shobo (Tokyo). The Chinese version was reprinted in Xinhua shishi congkanshe 1950, Fu 1997 and Jiang 2005.]

Kiku no bokyu iinkai 「菊の防給」委員会 ed. 1980, *The Imperial Epidemic Prevention and Water Supply Unit: The Development of the 11th Division of the Epidemic Prevention and Water Supply Unit* 菊の防給：第十一防給のあゆみ, Tokyo: Kyusuikai.

Kindai senshi kenkyukai 近代戦史研究会 ed. 1966, *Women's War Records, No.11, The Horrors of Human Experimentation: Memoirs of a Female Civilian Employee of the Kwantung Army, by Yoshinaga Reiko* 女の戦記　第11、人体実験の恐怖——ある関東軍女子軍属の手記(吉永玲子), Tokyo: Naniwa shobo.

[A semi-fictional account of a woman who worked at Unit 731. Reprinted in 1970.]

King, P. Z. 金宝善 1942, Japanese Attempt at Biological Warfare in China, March 31, 1942, Public Record Office (London), WO 188/680.

[The first report which documents the spreading of plague bacteria by Japanese aircraft over Quxian, Ningbo, and Jinhua in Zhejiang Province in October and November 1940, and Changde in Hunan Province in November 1941. Available in Kondo 2003.]

Kinoshita, Kenzo 木下健蔵 1994, *Removing all Traces of the Research Institute for Clandestine Warfare* 消された秘密戦研究所, Nagano: Shinao Mainichi shimbun sha.

[Contains chapters on balloon bombs, biochemical weapons, and the Army's Noborito Research Institute.]

Kitajima, Kikuro 北島規矩朗 ed. 1936, *Fifty Years of the Military College* 陸軍軍医学校五十年史, Tokyo: Military College. pp.187–192, 364–367.

[Deals with the research conducted by the Ishii network from 1933 to 1934. Reprinted in 1988 by Fuji shuppansha (Tokyo).]

Kobayashi, Hideo 小林英夫 and Kojima Toshiro 児嶋俊郎 eds 1995, *Germ Troops Unit 731: New Material from China* 七三一細菌戦部隊・中国新資料, Tokyo: Fuji shuppan.

[A translation by M. Hayashi of historical documents held by the Liaoning Province Archival Bureau. See also Liaoningsheng danganguan 1995.]

Kochi shimbunsha henshukyoku shakaibu 高知新聞社編集局社会部 ed. 1998, *The Ever-changing State: Who Will Make Reparation for the Crime?* 流転：その罪だれが償うか, Kochi: Kochi shimbunsha.

[Records conversations between journalist Amano Hiromiki and a former Unit 731 member who has been tormented by memories of the atrocities.]

Koga, Katsuhiko 古賀勝彦 1992, The Truth about Unit 731 七三一部隊の真実, in *The Battlefield Journal of a Secret Service Member: A Memoir of My Years Devoted to "Special Projects" in China* 諜報機関員の戦場：中国大陸で特殊任務に明け暮れた青春の回想録, Musashino, Tokyo: Reika chugokugo kaiwa kyoshitsu, pp. 89–181.

Kondo, Shoji 近藤昭二 ed. 2003, *Unit 731 and Biological Warfare – A CD-ROM Collection* ＜CD-ROM 版＞七三一部隊・細菌戦資料集成, Tokyo: Kashiwa shobo.

[These eight CD-ROMs contain original English-language documents relating to the attempts by Naito Ryoichi to obtain virulent strains of the yellow fever virus; the plague epidemic incidents in Changde; postwar investigations of Japan's biological warfare program and human experimentation by the Soviet Union and the U.S.; the exemption from prosecution granted to the Ishii network by the U.S. at the Tokyo Trials; research reports by members of the Ishii network; and investigations into bacteriological warfare during the Korean War.]

Koshi, Sadao 越定男 1983, *The Japanese Flag is Soaked in Red Tears: A Confession by a Member of Unit 731* 日の丸は紅い泪に：第七三一部隊員告白記, Tokyo: Kyoiku shiryo shuppankai.

[As a driver in Unit 731, the author witnessed the mass killing of prisoners at the end of the War, and transported human ashes for deposition in Songhua River. He recalls Ishii's order which required all members to keep the secrets, and mentions that important data were taken to Kanazawa City and later concealed.]

Koshida, Takashi 越田稜 1998, The War Responsibiliy of Unit 731 七三一部隊の戦争責任, in Ajia ni taisuru Nihon no senso sekinin o tou minshu hotei junbikai アジアに対する日本の戦争責任を問う民衆法廷準備, ed., *War Responsibility: From the Past to the Future* 戦争責任：過去から未来へ, Tokyo: Ryokufu shuppan, pp. 330–350.

Kyodo tsushinsha shakaibu 共同通信社社会部 ed. 1996, The Emperor's Army: Erasing the Evidence, Human Experimentation, and the anger of Tojo Hideki 天皇の軍隊　遠泳に証拠を隠滅せよ／生体実験／東条英機の怒り, in *Silent Documents* 沈黙のファイル, Tokyo: Kyodo tsushinsha, pp. 119–138. Reprinted in 1999 by Shinchosha (Tokyo).

Kyokasho kentei sosho o shiensuru zenkoku renrakukai (National Network for Supporting Textbook Trials) 教科書検定訴訟を支援する全国連絡会 ed. 1991, *The Ienaga Textbook Trials: The 3rd Lawsuit at District Court, No. 4, regarding Nanjing Massacre and Unit 731* 家永・教科書裁判　第3次訴訟　地裁編4　南京大虐殺・七三一部隊, Tokyo: Rongu shuppan. Reprinted in 1995.

—— ed. 1997, *The Ienaga Textbook Trials: The 3rd Lawsuit at the High Court, No. 2, regarding Nanjing Massacre, Korean Resistance and Unit 731* 家永・教科書裁判　第3 次訴訟　高裁編 2　南京大虐殺 ・ 朝鮮人民の抵抗 ・ 731部隊, Tokyo: Minshusha, pp. 219–325, 338–343, 345, 362–368.

Lafleur, William R., Böhme, Gernot, and Shimozono, Susumu eds 2007, *Dark Medicine: Rationalizing Unethical Medical Research*, Bloomington: Indiana University Press.

Leavitt, Frank 2002, Is Asian Bioethics at Fault? Commentary on Tsuchiya, Morioka, and Nie. *Eubios Journal of Asian and International Bioethics*, 11: 7–8.

Leavitt, Frank J. 2003a, Let's Stop Bashing Japan: Commentary on Tsuchiya, Sass, Thomas, Nie & Tsuneishi. *Eubios Journal of Asian and International Bioethics*, 13: 134–135.

Leavitt, Frank J. 2003b, Commentary: Bash Evil in Every Generation, But Don't Bash Innocent Children and Grandchildren. *Eubios Journal of Asian and International Bioethics*, 13: 168.

Li, Xiaofang 李晓方 ed. 2005, *Blood-sweeping Indictment: Records of Anthrax Victims* 泣血控诉—侵华日军细菌战炭疽、鼻疽受害者幸存者实录, Beijing: Zhongyang wenxian chubanshe.

Liaoningsheng danganguan (Liaoning Prefecture Archive) 辽宁省档案馆 ed. 1995, *Corps of Evil: Units 731 and 100* 罪恶的「七三一」「一〇〇」, Shenyang: Liaoning minzu chubanshe.

[Includes documents (dated 1945) and reports from the early 1950s from the northeastern region of China outlining the activities of the Ishii network and their impact on Chinese victims.]

Lishi buneng wangji chongshu bianweihui (Editing Board for Series of Unforgettable History) 历史不能忘记丛书编委会 ed. 1999, *Crimes of Japan's Biological Warfare Troops* 日本细菌战部队罪行录, Beijing: Zhongguo minzhu fazhi chubanshe.

Liu, Haitao 劉海涛 1936, *Report on the Situation in Manchuria* (満州の情況に関する報告).

[Reports the escape of Chinese prisoners from the "Epidemic Prevention Unit" in Beiyinhe. Available in Central Archives et al. 1991.]

Liu, Qi-an 刘启安 2005, *Calling Back the Spirits of the Dead: Exposing the Secrets of Biological Warfare Carried out by the Japanese Army in Changde* 叫魂—侵华日军常德细菌战首次独家揭秘, Nanchang: Ershiyi shiji chubanshe.

Liu, Yaling and Gong, Jigang 刘雅玲、龚积刚 2004, *Litigation by Victims of Biological Warfare* 细菌战受害大诉讼, Changsha: Hunan renmin chuban.

[Discusses Japanese biological warfare and the progress of lawsuits taken by Chinese victims.]

Matsumura, Takao 松村高夫 1985, "Two Reports of Experiments from Unit 731" 「七三一部隊」の実験報告書, *Rekishigaku kenkyu*. 538, February.

[Quotes two newly discovered reports on Unit 731's experiments with poison gas bombs and tetanus inoculation 「きい弾射撃ニ因ル皮膚傷害並一般臨床的症状観察」「破傷風毒素並芽胞接種時ニ於ケル筋『クロナキシー』ニ就テ」, pp. 56–64.]

—— 1991, The Meaning of Proof in the Historical Sciences: Considering Unit 731 歴史学における実証とは何か：七三一部隊を考える. *Rodoshi kenkyu*, 5『労働史研究』論創社、5号、1991年。

—— ed. 1994a, *The Debate on Unit 731* ＜論争＞七三一部隊, Tokyo: Banseisha.

[A collection of testimonials given during the "Ienaga Textbook Lawsuit" filed in 1984 by Ienaga Saburo 家永三郎 following the order by the Japanese Ministry of Education in 1983 to erase the references to Unit 731 from his textbook. Matsumura's book was revised, with new information on Japanese biological warfare in Changde in 1941, and republished in 1997 as 「[増補版]＜論争＞七三一部隊」. Matsumura acted as a witness for Ienaga, and Hata Ikuhiko was a witness for the Ministry. Matsumura's research on Unit 731 confirmed the accuracy of Ienaga's textbook.]

—— 1994b, Unit 731 and the Third Textbook Lawsuit 七三一部隊と第三次教科書訴訟. *Rekishi hyoron*, 528, April.

—— 1996a, Unit 731 is not a Thing of the Past 七三一部隊は過去のできごとか. *Sanshokuki*, April, 577.

[Gives a complete picture of Unit 731's activities and the suffering of victims' families.]

—— 1996b, Unit 731 and the Prison Camp in Fengtian 七三一部隊と奉天俘虜収容所. *Senso sekinin kenkyu*, 13: 74–76.

—— 1996c, Unit 731 and Human Experimentation 七三一部隊と人体実験, in ICJ Kokusai Seminar Tokyo Iinkai 国際セミナー東京委員会 ed., *Japan under*

Judgement: The Japanese Army's Comfort Women and Forced Labour 裁かれるニッポン：日本軍「慰安婦」・強制労働をめぐって, Tokyo: Nihon hyoronsha.

—— 1997a, Unit 731 七三一部隊, in Tokushi Kasahara 笠原十九司 et al., eds, *How to Identify and Teach Historical Facts: Unit 731, Nanjing Massacre and Military Comfort Women* 歴史の事実をどう認定しどう教えるか——検証731部隊・南京虐殺事件・「従軍慰安婦」, Tokyo: Kyoiku shiryo shuppankai.

—— 1997b, Biological Warfare in Changde, Hunan Prefecture, in 1941, 1941 年湖南常徳的細菌作戦. *Zhejiang Xuekan*, April.

—— 1997c, The Devil's Gluttony: The Black Marks Left by Unit 731「悪魔の飽食　七三一部隊の黒い爪痕」. *Shukan kinyobi*, September 5, 189: 28–31.

[A record of a round-table discussion with John W. Powell and Shimozato Masaki.]

—— 1998, Unit 731 and Biological Warfare: A Black Spot on Japan's Modern History 七三一部隊と細菌戦——日本現代史の汚点. *Mita gakkai zasshi*, 91, 2, July.

[This is the author's "Verification Report" presented to the Tokyo District Court for the lawsuit pursued from 1995 by families of victims of Unit 731.]

—— 2001a, Understanding Unit 731 through Documents from Japan, the US, China and the Soviet Union 日・米・中・ソの資料による七三一部隊の解明, in Nanasanichi Saikinsen saiban campaign iinkai et al. 七三一・細菌戦裁判キャンペーン委員会 他 eds, *Biological Warfare under Judgment: Series No. 6* 裁かれる細菌戦——資料シリーズ No.6, pp.11–124.

[This is the author's "Verification Report" presented to the Tokyo District Court for the lawsuit pursued from 1997 by 180 relatives of victims of Japanese biological warfare.]

—— 2001b, The 20th Century as the Century of War: Unit 731 and Biological Warfare 戦争の世紀としての二〇世紀——七三一部隊と細菌戦, in Yokohama, Kawasaki heiwa no tame no sensoten jikko iinkai, 横浜・川崎平和のための戦争展実行委員会, ed. *The Universities and the Military during the Asia-Pacific War* アジア太平洋戦争の大学と軍隊.

—— 2002, Research on Unit 731 in Japan 日本における七三一部隊の解明, Akira Tanaka 田中明, ed., *Reconsidering Modern Japan–China Relations* 近代日中関係史再考, Tokyo: Nihon keizai hyoronsha.

Matsumura, Takao and Kanehira, Shigenori 松村高夫, 金平茂紀 1991, The Hill Report: an Investigative Report from America on the Human Experiments Carried out by Unit 731, No. 1 ヒル・レポート——七三一部隊の人体実験に関するアメリカ側調査報告（上）. *Mita gakkai zasshi*, 84 2, July.

Matsumura, Takao and Xie, Xueshi 松村高夫, 謝学詩 et al. 1997, *Unit 731 – Herald of War and Plague* 戦争と疫病——七三一部隊のもたらしたもの, Tokyo: Honnotomo sha.

[A study of Unit 731 with materials from China, the U.K., the U.S., and Japan. It includes bacteriological bombing operations in Zhejiang and Jingxi provinces, and Xinjing (today's Changchun). Translated into Chinese as 战争与恶疫——七三一部队罪行考, and published by Renmin chubanshe (Beijing) in 1998.]

Matsumura, Takao and Yano, Hisashi 松村高夫, 矢野久 eds 2007, *Justice and the Historical Sciences: Unit 731 as Seen from the Courtroom* 裁判と歴史学——七三一細菌戦部隊を法廷からみる, Tokyo: Gendai shokan.

[Examines Matsumura's quest for the historical facts of Unit 731's activities and the Japanese biological warfare program in order to support Ienaga Saburo's lawsuit against the Ministry of Education, which had instructed Ienaga to delete references to Unit 731 in his history textbook. As a result of efforts by Matsumura and others, Ienaga eventually won his lawsuit in 1997 and the Ministry's ruling was rescinded.]

Matsuno, Seiya 松野誠也 2005, *The Japanese Army's Poison Gas Weapons* 日本軍の毒ガス兵器, Tokyo: Gaifusha.

Matsushita, Kazunari 松下一成 1996, *The Green Cross and Unit 731* ミドリ十字と 731 部隊, Tokyo: Sanichi shobo.

Mima, Satoaki 美馬聡昭 1998, Prevention of Tuberculosis Established by Vivisection 生体解剖による結核予防法の確立. *Senso sekinin kenkyu*, 20: 76–85.

Minamoto, Shokyu 源昌久 2002, Unit 731 and the Study of Military Geography in Japan: a Bibliographical Survey 石井(第七三一)部隊と兵要地誌に関する一考察：書誌学的研究, *Bulletin of the College of Sociology, Shukutoku University*, 36: 1–17.

Mineo, Kyudai 三根生久大 1992, *A Roughneck in the General Staff Office: Army Staff Officer Asaeda Shigeharu* 参謀本部の暴れ者：陸軍参謀朝枝繁春, Tokyo: Bungei shunju, pp. 313–339.

Minguo dangan 民国檔案 1995, Archival Records of the Investigation into the Japanese Army's Biological Warfare Campaign in China 有関調査侵華日軍細菌戦部隊的檔案資料. *Minguo dangan*, 3.

Mitomo, Kazuo 三友一男 1987, *The Crime of Biological Warfare: My Days in the Officers' Prison at Ivanovo* 細菌戦の罪：イワノボ将官収容所虜囚記, Tokyo: Tairyusha.

[The author, who was sentenced to 15 years' imprisonment at the Khabarovsk Trial, describes his time in prison and his experiences with Unit 100.]

Miyatake, Go 宮武剛 1986, Chilling Footprints 戦慄の足跡, in *A General's Will: Endo Saburo's Diary* 将軍の遺言：遠藤三郎日記, Tokyo: Mainichi shimbunsha, pp. 75–91.

Mizutani, Naoko 水谷尚子 1995, Testimony of a Former Member of Unit 1644: Army Illustrator Ishida Jintaro 元一六四四部隊員の証言：軍画兵、石田 甚太郎の体験から *Senso sekinin kenkyu*, 10: 56–65.

—— 1997, The Organization and Activities of Unit 1644, 一六四四部隊の組織と活動 (1) and (2), *Senso sekinin kenkyu*, 15: 50–59, and 16: 66–71.

Monma, Takashi 門間貴志 1995, The Japanese in Hong Kong Cinema: Unit 731 and Army Comfort Women 香港映画の日本人　七三一部隊と従軍慰安婦, *The Portrayal of Japan in Asian Film, Vol. 1, China, Hong Kong, Taiwan* アジア映画にみる日本1 (中国・香港・台湾編), Tokyo: Shakai hyoronsha, pp. 148–154.

Mori, Masataka 森正孝 1990, War Crimes of the Germ Troops: Unit 1644 in Nanjing 細菌戦部隊　南京「栄」一六四四部隊の戦争犯罪, in Ajia minshu hotei junbikai, ed., *The Unforgivable War Guilt Carried by the Emperor and Japan* 時効なき戦争責任裁かれる天皇と日本, Tokyo: Ryokufu shuppan, pp. 217–254.

—— 1995, Victims of Biological Warfare 細菌戦被害の人々, in Haboho kenkyukai, ed., *Fifty Years of War Responsibility* 50 年目の戦争責任, Tokyo: Seiunsha, pp. 77–93.

—— 1998, *The Truth about Biological Warfare Must Be Revealed Now* いま伝えたい, 細菌戦のはなし：隠された歴史を照らす, Tokyo: Akashi shoten.

Mori, Masataka 森正孝 et al. eds 1991, *Materials from China: The Japanese Invasion of China* 中国側資料　日本の中国侵略, Tokyo: Akashi shoten.

[Contains documents about Unit 1644 which conducted human experiments in Nanjing, and attacks on Ningbo and Changde using biological bombs.]

Mori, Masataka and Kasukawa Yoshiya 森正孝, 糟川良谷 eds 1995, *Materials from China: The Invasion of China and Unit 731's Biological Warfare Campaign – What Japanese Army's Biological Weaponry Inflicted on the Chinese People* 中国側史

料 中国侵略と七三一部隊の細菌戦──日本軍の細菌攻撃は中国人民に何をもたらしたか Tokyo: Akashi shoten.
[Based on investigations carried out by Mori and others from 1991 to determine the facts about biological warfare in Zhejiang and Jiangsu provinces.]

Morikawa, Tetsuro 森川哲郎 1978, The Imperial Bank Incident and Unit 731, in *Unsolved Mysteries of Japan* 日本迷宮入事件, Tokyo: Sanichi shobo, pp. 120–171.

Morimura, Seiichi 森村誠一 1981, *The Devil's Gluttony: A Complete Picture of the Horrors of the Germ Warfare Troops of the Kwantung Army, Volume One* 悪魔の飽食：「関東軍細菌戦部隊」恐怖の全貌！ 第1部, Tokyo: Kobunsha.
[This book makes Unit 731 widely known in Japan. It is based on Morimura and Shimozato's interviews with more than 30 former members of Unit 731, research reports written by Unit 731 members, and the Khabarovsk Trial documents. A new edition was published in 1983 by Kadokawa shoten (Tokyo). This was translated into Chinese by B. Zu and Y. Tang as 食人魔窟：日本关东军细菌战部队的恐怖内幕, and was published by Qunzhong chubanshe (Beijing) in 1982. A second Chinese translation was made by C. Guan and M. Xu as 魔鬼的乐园：关东军细菌战部队恐怖的真相, and was published by Heilongjiang renmin chubanshe (Harbin) in 1983.]

—— 1982a, *Notes on The Devil's Gluttony* 悪魔の飽食ノート, Tokyo: Banseisha.
[Translates major sections of Powell 1981.]

—— 1982b, *The Devil's Gluttony, Part 2: The Riddle of Kwantung Army's Germ Warfare Troops* 続悪魔の飽食：「関東軍細菌戦部隊」謎の戦後史, Tokyo: Kobunsha.
[A revised edition 新版続悪魔の飽食：第七三一部隊の戦慄の全貌 was published in 1983 by Kadokawa shoten (Tokyo), and a further revision in pocketbook form in 1991. This was translated into Chinese by C. Guan and M. Xu as 魔鬼的乐园：续篇关东军细菌战部队战后秘史, and was published by Heilongjiang renmin chubanshe (Harbin) in 1984.]

—— 1983, *The Devil's Gluttony, Part 3* 悪魔の飽食 第三部, Tokyo: Kadokawa shoten.
[Based on the author's investigations of Unit 731's locations at Harbin, Pingfang, and Changchun. The three volumes provide perspectives from Japan, the U.S. and China on Unit 731, and fill a gap in modern Japanese history. All were printed in pocketbook form in 1985. Translated into Chinese by W. Luo and N. Chen as 恶魔的饱食：日本细菌战部队揭秘, and published by Xueyuan chubanshe (Beijing) in 2003.]

—— 1984, *Enough of The Devil's Gluttony* ノーモア＜悪魔の飽食＞, Tokyo: Banseisha.

—— ed. 1990 (new edn 1995), *Unit 731 on Trial* 裁かれた七三一部隊, Tokyo: Banseisha.
[A collection of testimonials prepared for the "Ienaga Textbook Trials" in 1987.]

Morioka, Masahiro 2001, Commentary on Tsuchiya. *Eubios Journal of Asian and International Bioethics*, 10: 280–281.

Nakagawa, Yatsuhiro 中川八洋 2002, *The Devil's Gluttony* is Propaganda by the Former Soviet Union 「悪魔の飽食」は旧ソ連のプロパガンダだった, *Seiron*, November, 363: 276–287.

Nakata, Takeo 中田建夫 1983, Assessing the Fake Photographs in Part 2 of *The Devil's Gluttony*: Who is the Glutton? 「続・悪魔の飽食」ニセ写真事件を考える"飽食"したのは誰だ, *Bungei shunjiu*, February, 61, 2: 362–386.

Nakazono, Eisuke 中薗英助 1968, *An Incubator in the Night* 夜の培養者, Tokyo: Yomiuri shimbunsha.
[Reprinted in 1972 by Kodansha (Tokyo), in 1981 by Tokuma shoten (Tokyo), and in 1996 by Shakai shisosha (Tokyo).]

Nanasanichi butai kokusai symposium jikko iinkai (Committee for International Symposium on Unit 731) 七三一部隊国際シンポジウム実行委員会 ed. 1996, *The Japanese Army's Biological Warfare and Poison Gas Campaigns: Japan's Invasion of China and Japanese War Crimes* 日本軍の細菌戦・毒ガス戦：日本の中国侵略と戦争犯罪, Tokyo: Akashi shoten.

[A collection of papers presented at the 731 International Symposium in August 1995 in Harbin, attended by Chinese and Japanese researchers.]

Nanasanichi butai shinso chosa zenkoku renraku kyogikai (National Network for Investigation of Unit 731) 部隊真相調査全国連絡協議会 ed. 1997, *Unit 731 and Discarded Poison Gas Weapons: Investigation and Testimonies* 731 部隊・遺棄毒ガス問題—検証と証言—, Tokyo: privately published.

Nanasanichi kenkyukai (Society of Research on 731) 七三一研究会 ed. 1996, *The Germ Troops* 細菌戦部隊, Tokyo: Banseisha.

[A collection of testimonies by 24 former members of Unit 731, Unit 100, Unit 1855, Unit 1644, Unit 8604, Unit 9420, and units from other regions of China. A bibliography of works related to Unit 731, prepared by Kondo Shoji, is included.]

Nanasanichi saikinsen saiban campaign iinkai 七三一・細菌戦裁判キャンペーン委員会 et al. ed. 2001–2002, *Biological Warfare under Judgement: Collected Documents* 裁かれる細菌戦—資料シリーズ, Vol. 1, 2, 3, 4, 5, 6, 7, 8, Urawa: the editor.

Newman, Barclay 1944, *Japan's Secret Weapon*, ed. Peter Greenleaf, New York: Current Publishing.

Nezu, Masashi ねず・まさし 1993, The Formation of Germ Troops was Ordered by the Emperor 天皇細菌部隊の設置を命ず, in *A Cross-section of Modern History: The Invasion of China* 現代史の断面・中国侵略, Tokyo: Azekura shobo, pp. 85–114.

Nie, Jing-Bao 2001, Challenges of Japanese Doctors' Human Experimentation in China for East-Asian and Chinese Bioethics. *Eubios Journal of Asian and International Bioethics*, 11: 3–7.

—— 2002, Japanese Doctors' Experimentation in Wartime China. *The Lancet*, 360: s5–s6.

—— 2003, Let's Never Stop Bashing Inhumanity: A Reply to Frank Leavitt and a Call for Further Ethical Studies on Japanese Doctors' Wartime Experimentation. *Eubios Journal of Asian and International Bioethics*, 13: 106–107.

—— 2004, The West's Dismissal of the Khabarovsk Trial as "Communist Propaganda": Ideology, Evidence and International Bioethics. *Journal of Bioethics Inquiry*, 1, 1: 32–42.

—— 2005, State Violence in Twentieth-century China: Some Shared Features of the Japanese Army's Atrocities and the Cultural Revolution's Terror, in Ludger Kühnhardt and Mamoru Takayama, eds, *Menchenrechte, Kulturen und Gewalt: Ansaetze einer Interkulturellen Ethik* [*Human Rights, Cultures, and Violence: Perspectives of Intercultural Ethics*], Baden-Baden: Nomos, pp. 161–176, with a Commentary by Ole Döring, pp. 177–181.

—— 2006, The United States Cover-up of Japanese Wartime Medical Atrocities: Complicity Committed in the National Interest and Two Proposals for Contemporary Action. *American Journal of Bioethics*, 6, 3: W21–W33.

Nie, Jing-Bao, Tsuchiya, Takashi, and Li, Lun 2009, Japanese Doctors' Experimentation in China, 1932–1945, and Medical Ethics, in Robert B. Baker and Laurence B. McCullough, eds, *The Cambridge World History of Medical Ethics*, Cambridge: Cambridge University Press, pp. 589–594. A modified Chinese version, trans. J. Li and X. Chen, was published as 侵华日军的人体实验及其对当代医学伦理的挑战, *Yixue yu zhexue*, 25, 6: 35–38.

Nie, Jing-Bao, Tsuchiya, Takashi, Sass, Hans-Martin, and Tsuneishi, Keiichi 2003, A Call for Further Studies on the Ethical Lessons of Japanese Doctors' Experimentation in Wartime China for Asian and International Bioethics Today. *Eubios Journal of Asian and International Bioethics*, 13: 106–107.

Nie, Lili (Jo, Riri) 聶莉莉 2006a, *Chinese People's Memory of War: The Scars Left by Japanese Army's Biological Warfare Campaign* 中国民衆の戦争記憶—日本軍の細菌戦による傷跡, Tokyo: Akashi shoten.

[Details the damage done to Changde by biological warfare.]

—— 2006b, An Anthropological Study of Victims' Memories of Japanese Army's Biological Warfare Campaign in Changde 日軍細菌戦常特德民衆受害記憶的文化人類学研究, *Hunan wenli xueyuan xuebao (shehui kexue ban)*, 6.

Nihon chugoku yuko kyokai (Japan–China Friendship Association) and Chugoku kikansha renrakukai 日本中国友好協会, 中国帰還者連絡会 eds 1970, *My Experience of Aggressive Warfare: Soldiers' Testimonies* 私の戦争体験記　侵略：従軍兵士の証言, Tokyo: Nihon seinen shuppansha.

[Includes three soldiers' confessions: "Learning from Vivisection," "Participating in Poison Gas Operations," and "Against Humanity: The Horror of Germ Bombs." Revised and reprinted in 1975 and 1982 by Nicchu shuppan (Tokyo).]

Nihon no senso sekinin siryo center (Centre for Research and Documentation on Japan's War Responsibilities) 日本の戦争責任資料センター 1993, *Senso sekinin kenkyu [Research on Japan's War Responsibility]*, No. 2. "Special Edition, The Truth behind Unit 731: The Shocking Germ Troops who Spread out across Asia 特集　731部隊の実相に迫る：全アジアに展開された戦慄の細菌戦部隊".

Nihongun ni yoru saikinsen no rekishi jijitsu o akirakani suru kai (Association of Investigation of Japanese Army's Biological Warfare) 日本軍による細菌戦の歴史事実を明らかにする会 ed. 1998, *Ningbo, 1940: Biological Warfare in China's Back Yard* 細菌戦が中国人民にもたらしたもの—1940年の寧波—, Tokyo: Akashi shoten.

[Provides rich sources on biological warfare in Ningbo.]

Niki, Fumiko 仁木ふみ子 1995, Regarding Unit 731, in *The Holocaust that Created a No-man's Land beside the Great Wall: The Tragedy of Xinglong Province* 無人区長城のホロコースト：興隆の悲劇, Tokyo: Aoki shoten, pp. 167–226.

Nikkan kankei o kirokusuru kai (Association of Documentation on Japan–Korean Relations) 日韓関係を記録する会 ed. 1979, *Materials of Biological Warfare* 資料細菌戦, Tokyo: Banseisha.

Nishino, Rumiko 西野留美子 1995, A Study of Unit 1855 in Beijing 北京甲一八五五部隊の検証, *Senso sekinin kenkyu [Report on Japan's War Responsibility]*, 9: 46–53.

Nishiyama, Akira 西山明 1984, *Documenting Vivisection: Patients' Human Rights and Medical Ethics* ドキュメント生体実験：患者の人権と医の倫理, Tokyo: Hihyosha, pp. 208, 253–275, 378–379.

Nishizato, Fuyuko 西里扶甬子 1996a, *The Still Unpunished Ishii Unit, Part 1: The Twin Character of the Japanese–American Deal* 裁かれなかった石井部隊 Part 1：日米取引の二重構造, *Senso sekinin kenkyu*, 11: 80–87.

—— 1996b, *The Still Unpunished Ishii Unit, Part 2: How Prisoners of the Allied Forces Were Turned into Maruta* 裁かれなかった石井部隊 Part 2：マルタにされた連合軍捕虜, *Senso sekinin kenkyu*, 12: 80–87.

—— 1996c, The Testimony of Ishii Shiro, No.1: Ishii's Eldest Daughter, Ishii Harumi 証言
石井四郎　その(1)長女石井ハルミ, Akirakani suru kai, Tsushin.

—— 2002, *Biological Army Unit 731: The Japanese Army's War Crimes Exempted from
Prosecution by the United States* 生物戦部隊七三一＿＿アメリカが免罪した日本軍
の戦争犯罪, Tokyo: Kusanone shuppan.

Noda, Masaaki 野田正彰 1998, *War, Crime and Responsibility* 戦争と罪責, Tokyo:
Iwanami shoten.

[Examines the unwillingness of Japanese to bear responsibility for crimes committed
during the Second World War. The author analyzes the process by which Yuasa Ken 湯
浅謙, a member of the Ishii network, gradually acquired a sense of guilt.]

Oga, Kazuo 大賀和男 1989, Unit 731 of the Kwantung Army (Germ Troops) 関東軍第七
三一(細菌戦)部隊, in *What Did the Japanese Army Do in China?* 日本軍は中国で
何をしたのか, Fukuoka: Ashi shobo, pp. 56–71.

Omata, Waichiro 小俣和一郎 2003, *Investigating Human Experimentation: Unit 731 and
Nazi Medical Science* 検証　人体実験＿＿731 部隊・ナチ医学, Tokyo: Daisan
bunmeisha.

[A comparative study of atrocities committed by Unit 731 and Nazi medical researchers.]

Osanai, Hiroshi 小山内宏 1975, *The Department of Epidemic Prevention and Water Supply
of the Kwantung Army – The Mystery behind the Name* "関東軍防疫給水部"のナゾ,
in *An Introduction to the Army's Nakano School* 陸軍中野学校入門, Tokyo: Nihon
bungeisha, pp. 93–100.

Ota, Masakatsu 太田昌克 1999, *Exempting Unit 731 from Prosecution: Germ Troops
and Secret Files* 731 免責の系譜: 細菌戦部隊と秘蔵のファイル, Tokyo: Nihon
hyoron sha.

—— 2001, Unit 731 and the Mystery behind its Exemption from Prosecution for War
Crimes 七三一部隊 "戦犯免責" の謎, *Rekishi tokuhon*, January 733: 158–163.

Ozaki, Kimiko 尾崎祈美子 1997, *Nightmare Heritage: Consequences of Biological
Warfare in Hiroshima, Taiwan and China* 悪夢の遺産,＿＿毒ガス戦の果てに〜ヒロ
シマ〜台湾〜中国 Tokyo: Gakuyo shobon.

Pollitzer, R. 1941, A report dated December 30 by Austrian Doctor R., an epidemiologist
with the National Health Administration, containing a detailed investigation of the
outbreak of plague in Changde, Hunan Province. Available in Kondo 2003.

Powell, John W. 1981, Japan's Biological Weapons: 1930–1945, A Hidden Chapter in
History. *Bulletin of the Atomic Scientists*, 37, 8: 44–52.

[This article, based on declassified top secret reports, reveals that the United States
guaranteed Ishii and his colleagues immunity from war crime prosecution in order to
obtain their research results.]

Qinhua rijun 731 budui zuizheng chenlieguan (Museum of Unit 731 Evidence) 侵华日军
七三一部队罪证陈列馆 ed. 2005, *Unit 731: A Japanese Biological Warfare Unit in
China* 侵华日军关东军七三一细菌部队, Beijing: Wuzhou chuanbo chubanshe.

[A bilingual (Chinese and English) publication including a large number of
photo-graphs.]

Qiu, Mingxuan 邱明轩 1999, *Proof of Crime: Japanese Army's Biological Warfare
Campaign in Quzhou* 罪证: 侵华日军衢州细菌战史实, Beijing: Zhongguo sanxia
chubanshe.

Quzhoushi weishengzhi bangongshi 衢州市卫生志办公室 1991, The Plague Epidemic
and Prevention Efforts 衢州鼠疫流行状况和防治工作, in Zhengxie Zhejiang
Quzhoushi weiyuanhui 政协浙江衢州市委员会, ed., *Historical Documents of
Quzhou No. 9* 衢州文史资料 第九辑.

Ran, Weijun 冉炜君 2005, *The Devil's Tank: Investigating Victims of Japanese Biological Warfare in Inner Mongolia* 魔鬼的战车——内蒙古侵华日军细菌战受害者调查, Beijing: Kunlun chubanshe.

Renmin ribao (People's Daily) 人民日報 1950 年, Huade Hospital Chief of Changde, Hunan, Witnessed Japanese Spreading Plague by Airplane which Caused Many Deaths' 湖南常德華德医院院長證明　日冦曽用飛機散布鼠疫 常 徳地区很多同胞因此死亡, February 5.

Rikugun Guni gakko boekigaku kyoshitu (Department of Epidemics Prevention, Military Medical School) 陸軍軍医学校防疫学教室 ed. 1939–1941, *Research Reports of the Military Medical School* 陸軍軍医学校防疫研究報告, Vols 1, 2, 3, 4, 5, 6, 7, 8, in *Top-secret Documents from the 15-year War* 十五年戦争極秘資料集, Tokyo: Fuji shuppan, Vol. 23, Nos 1–8, 2004–2005.

[These reports document the research work conducted by the Ishii network.]

Rong, Qirong 容啓栄 1942, *Report on the Prevention of Plague in West Hunan Province* (防治湘西鼠疫経過報告書).

[Estimates the number of victims in Changde in Hunan Province affected by the Japanese spreading of plague bacteria. Available in Matsumura 1997a.]

Saito, Mitsunori 斉藤充功 1987, *A Secret War: Documenting the Army's Noborito Research Institute* 謀略戦—ドキュメント陸軍登戸研究所, Tokyo: Jiji tsushinsha, pp. 125, 154–155, 215–219, 227. Revised edn published in 2001 by Gakushu kenkyusha (Tokyo).

Sanders, Murray 1945, Report by Murray Sanders, November 1.

[Details the postwar investigation of Unit 731 by the U.S. Available in Kondo 2003.]

Sass, Hans-Martin 2003, Ambiguities in Judging Cruel Human Experimentation: Arbitrary American Responses to German and Japanese Experiments. *Eubios Journal of Asian and International Bioethics*, 13: 102–104.

Seki, Ryo 関亮1988 (new edn 1998), The Department of Epidemic Prevention and Water Supply 防疫給水部, Cholera and the Expeditionary Force to Shanghai 上海派遣軍とコレラ, Balloon Bombs and Bacteria Bombs 風船爆弾と細菌弾, in *Stories of Medical Surgeons* 軍医サンよもやま物語, Tokyo: Kojinsha.

Seki, Seiwa 関成和 et al. eds 2000, *The Village Destroyed by Unit 731: A Social History of Pingfang* 七三一部隊がやってきた村—平房の社会史, Tokyo: Kochi shobo.

[A historical and anthropological study of the impact of Unit 731 on Pingfang.]

Senba, Yoshikiyo 仙波嘉清 1963, *The Vivisection Incident* 生体解剖事件, Tokyo: Kongo shuppan.

[Describes the vivisection conducted at Kyushu University, including the participants' belief that the American pilots had been sentenced to death.]

Sha, Dongxun 沙东迅 1995, *Exposing Unit 8604: The Biological Warfare Campaign Carried out in Guangdong Province by the Japanese Army in China* 揭开"８６０４"之谜：侵华日军在粤秘密进行细菌战大暴光, Guangzhou: Huacheng chubanshe.

Shen, Mingxian 沈铭贤 2005, Retrospection on Unit 731 after More than Half a Century 731 部队—半个多世紀后的反思. *Yixue yu zhexue*, pp. 32–34.

Shibata, Shingo 芝田進午 1997, People Associated with Unit 731 Prohibited from Entering the US: The Hidden Reason「七三一」関係者入国禁止：その隠された真の意味. *Ronza*, 27: 76–81.

—— 1998, Ethics and Responsibilities of Medical Personnel: Unresolved Medical War Crimes 医学者の倫理と責任：「医学者」の戦争犯罪の未決済と戦後被害, in Kenichiro Yamaguchi 山口研一郎, ed., *Managing Life and Death: From the Beginning of Life to the End* 操られる生と死：生命の誕生から終焉まで, Tokyo: Shogakukan, pp. 205–242.

[Reveals how some key members of Unit 731 took up important positions after the war including senior posts in Japanese medical schools and the National Preventative Hygiene Research Institute.]

Shimamura, Kyo 島村喬 1967 (revised edn 1981), *Human Experiments Carried out on Three Thousand People: The Secret Biological Weapon Research Institute of the Kwantung Army* 三千人の生体実験：関東軍謎の細菌秘密兵器研究所, Tokyo: Hara shobo.

Shimozato, Masaki 下里正樹 1985, *Between Evil and Humanity: Interviews with Former Members of Unit 731* 悪魔と人の間：「七三一部隊」取材紀行, Osaka: Nihon kikanshi shuppan senta.

Shinozuka, Yoshio and Takayanagi, Michiko 篠塚良雄, 高柳美知子, 2004, *There Was Also a War in Japan: Confessions of a Former Junior Member of Unit 731* 日本にも戦争があった：七三一部隊元少年隊員の告白, Tokyo: Shinnihon shuppansha.

Sun, Jinshi and Ni, Weixiong 孫金鈼, 倪維熊, 1963, The Outbreak and Spread of Plague in Ningbo 寧波鼠疫的発生和経過. Reprinted in *Ningbo Historical Record* 寧波文史資料, 2, October 1984.

Takahashi, Masae 高橋正衛 ed. 1982, Documents Relating to Ishii's Unit 731 石井部隊（第七三一部隊）関係文書, *Modern Historical Documents, Supplementary Series (No. 6): The Military Police* 続・現代史資料 (6) 軍事警察, Tokyo: Misuzu shobo, pp. lii–lx, 627–636. Reprinted in 1996 and 2004.

Takahashi, Taketomo 高橋武智 1997, *Acknowledging the Crimes of Unit 731 in Post-war Japan* 七三一部隊の犯罪は戦後日本でどのように認識されるようになったか, Nihon shakai bungaku 日本社会文学, ed., *Modern Japan and Manchuria* 近代日本と「偽満州国」, Tokyo: Fuji shuppan, pp. 161–165.

Takana, Tomi 高名トミ 1982, *The Devil's Gluttony* – A Nurse's Testimony 「悪魔の飽食」看護婦の証言, *Fujin koron*, February.

[Records how 40 members of Unit 731 infected with disease were killed with potassium cyanide during the Unit's withdrawal from Manchuria.]

Takasugi, Ichiro 高杉一郎 1996, Unit 731 and the Wolves 七三一部隊と狼！狼！狼, in *Memories of Returned Soldiers* 征きて還りし兵の記憶, Tokyo: Iwanami shoten, pp. 286–293. Reprinted in 2002.

Takasugi, Shingo 高杉晋吾 1973, How Science Turned to Slaughter 「科学」を「虐殺」にみちびくもの, in *Japan's Human Experiment: Concept and Organization* 日本の人体実験：その思想と構造, Tokyo: Mikasa shobo, pp. 192–194, 201, 205, 272–273, 305, 309.

—— 1974, The War Responsibility of Medical Personnel 医者の戦争責任, in *The State and the Will to Slaughter: the Time of State Security and Mass Killing* 国家と殺意保安処分＝管理と虐殺の時代, Tokyo: Tabata shoten, pp. 282–292.

—— 1982a, *Pursuing the Doctors of Unit 731: the Continuing Horror of Human Experimentation* 七三一部隊細菌戦の医師を追え——今も続く恐怖の人体実験, Tokyo: Tokuma shoten.

—— 1982b, Unit 731: Survivors' Testimonies to the Three Great Outbreaks of Biological Warfare 七三一部隊　三大細菌戦の生き証人, *Shio*, 284: 258–280.

—— 1984, *Investigating the Japanese Auschwitz* 日本のアウシュウィッツを追って, Tokyo: Kyoiku shiryo shuppankai.

Takeda, Eiko 武田英子 1987, Human Experimentation Using Poison Gas 毒ガスの生体実験, *The Island that Disappeared from the Map: Okuno Island as a Poison Gas*

Factory 地図から消された島：大久野島　毒ガス工場, Tokyo: Domesu shuppan, pp. 105–112.

Takehana, Kyoitsu 竹花香逸 1991, *A Young Man's Record of Army Life among Fleas, Rats and Pest Bacteria* ノミと鼠とペスト菌を見てきた話: ある若者の従軍記, Hamamatsu: the author.

[Describes the author's experiences of breeding lice and rats at Unit 9420 in Singapore.]

Takidani Jiro 滝谷二郎 1989, *Confessions by Biological Warfare Troops from the Factory of Death: Unit 731* 殺戮工廠・七三一部隊　発見された細菌部隊兵士の告白調書, Tokyo: Niimori shobo.

[A collection of confessions by members of the Ishii Network which have been widely quoted.]

Tamura, Yoshio 田村良雄 1982, Biological Warfare: Atrocities of Unit 731 細菌戦：七三一部隊の蛮行, ed. Chugoku kikansha renrakukai, new edn, *The Three-All Policy, Volume 1: What the Japanese Did in China* 新編三光　第1集　中国で日本人は何をしたか, Tokyo: Kobunsha, pp. 27–48.

[The author's testimony has been widely quoted. Reprinted in 1985 under the new title 完全版　三光.]

Tan, Xuehua 譚学華 1942, Discovering the Plague in Changde, Hunan: A Summary of Dr. Tan Xuehua's Letter 湖南常徳発見鼠疫経過(譚学華医師来函摘要), *Xiangya yixueyuan yuankan*, March.

Tan, Yuanheng 譚元享 2005, *Japanese Army's Biological Warfare Campaign: The Black Unit 8604* 日军细菌战：黑色 "波字8604," Guangzhou: Nanfang ribao chubanshe.

[Deals with the death of over 100,000 people as a result of biological warfare in Guangzhou.]

Tanaka, Akira and Eda, Izumi 田中明, 江田いづみ 1989, Current Research on Unit 731 by Chinese Scholars 「七三一」部隊の研究における中国人研究者の動向について. *Mita gakkai zasshi*, October, 83, 3.

Tanaka, Akira and Matsumura, Takao 田中明, 松村高夫 eds 1991, *Documents from Unit 731* 七三一部隊作成資料, Tokyo: Fuji shuppan.

[A collection of studies by medical scientists from Unit 731 on human experimentation.]

Tanaka, Toshiyuki 1988, The Story Japan Would Like to Forget: Japan's Secret Poison Gas Complex. *Bulletin of the Atomic Scientists*, 44, 8: 10–19.

Tanaka, Yuki 1996, *Hidden Horrors: Japanese War Crimes in World War II,* Boulder, CO: Westview Press.

Tatsumi, Tomoji 辰巳知司 1993, Okuno Island and Unit 731 大久野島と七三一部隊, in *Evidence from the Secret Island of Poison Gas in Hiroshima Prefecture* 隠されてきた「ヒロシマ」毒ガス島からの告発, Tokyo: Nihon hyoronsha, pp. 102–107.

Thomas, Michael 2003a, Ethical Lessons of the Failure to Bring the Japanese Doctors to Justice. *Eubios Journal of Asian and International Bioethics*, 13: 104–106.

—— 2003b, Let's Deal with the Issue: Commentary on Leavitt. *Eubios Journal of Asian and International Bioethics*, 13: 166–167.

Thompson, Arvo, 1945, Report by Arvo Thompson, May 31.

[Describes postwar investigation of Unit 731 by the U.S. Available in Kondo 2003.]

Tong, Zhenyu 佟振宇 1998, *The Japanese Invasion of China and Japan's Crimes of Biological Warfare* 日本侵华与细菌战罪行录, Harbin: Harbin chubanshe.

Tono, Toshio 東野利夫 1979, *Disgrace: The Truth behind the Vivisection at Kyushu University* 汚名「九大生体解剖事件」の真相, Tokyo: Bungei shunju.

[A participant of the vivisection of eight American pilots describes the incident and the trial.]

Torii, Yasushi 鳥居靖 1999, Thoughts on the Ruling on the Lawsuit regarding Unit 731, Nanjing Massacre and Indiscriminate Bombing 七三一部隊・南京虐殺・無差別空爆事件訴訟の判決に思う, *Senso sekinin*, November, 2, 3: 60–71.

Tsuchiya, Takashi 2000, Why Japanese Doctors Performed Human Experiments in China 1933–1945. *Eubios Journal of Asian and International Bioethics*, 10: 179–280.

—— 2003a, In the Shadow of the Past Atrocities: Research Ethics with Human Subjects in Contemporary Japan. *Eubios Journal of Asian and International Bioethics*, 13: 100–102.

—— 2003b, A Reply to Leavitt's Commentary. *Eubios Journal of Asian and International Bioethics*, 13: 167–168.

—— 2008, The Imperial Japanese Experiments in China. Ezekiel Emanuel, et al. eds. *The Oxford Textbook of Clinical Research Ethics*. Oxford: Oxford University Press. pp. 31–45.

Tsuneishi, Keiichi 常石敬一 1981, *The Germ Warfare Troops that Vanished: Unit 731 of the Kwantung Army* 消えた細菌戦部隊：関東軍第七三一部隊, Tokyo: Kaimeisha.

[This pioneering historical study documents the development of Unit 731, and is based on primary sources and court documents as well as on studies by medical researchers from the Ishii network. A new edition was published in 1989 and reprinted in 1993 by Chikuma shobo (Tokyo).]

—— 1984, *Targeting Ishii: Unit 731 and the American Army's Intelligence Service* 標的・イシイ：七三一部隊と米軍諜報活動, Tokyo: Otsuki shoten.

[A translation of reports by American researchers on Unit 731, including the Sanders report, the Thompson report, and secret documents held by the U.S. Army's GHQ and the Department of Army.]

—— 1985, Scientists and War: Is Clandestine Research Efficient? 科学者と戦争：秘密研究は効率的か. *Sekai*, September, 479: 93–102.

—— 1990, *Japanese Medical Scholarship and Unit 731* 日本医学アカデミズムと七三一部隊, Tokyo: Guni gakko atochi de hakkensareta jinkotsu mondai o kyumeisuru kai. Reprinted in 1993 by Kinohana sha (Tokyo).

—— 1992, *The Dead Bones Speak: Reading Sakura's Report* 骨は告発する：佐倉鑑定を読む, Tokyo: Guni gakko atochi de hakken sareta jinkotsu mondai o kyumeisuru kai.

—— 1994a, *Organized Crimes by Medical Researchers: Unit 731 of the Kwantung Army* 医学者たちの組織犯罪：関東軍第七三一部隊, Tokyo: Asahi shimbunsha.

[Based on historical documents and four reports compiled by American military scientists, this book presents a detailed picture of Unit 731. Underlines the lack of self-reflection by the Japanese medical establishment, and the futility of their experiments.]

—— 1994b, The Researchers of Unit 731 第七三一部隊を利用した研究者たち, Shigeru Nakayama 中山茂 and Yoshioka Hitoshi 吉岡斉, eds, *A Social History of Post-War Science and Technology* 戦後科学技術の社会史, Tokyo: Asahi shimbunsha, pp. 36–39.

—— 1995, *Unit 731: The Truth about Biological Weapons and Crimes* 七三一部隊：生物兵器犯罪の真実, Tokyo: Kodansha.

[17th reprint, 2005. Describes the experiments performed by Unit 731 and the use of the biochemical bombs and recording the voices of victims' families.]

—— 1998, Medical Research and War: Questions to Medical Establishment 医学と戦争いま、医学界に問われていること, in Saito Takao 斉藤孝雄 and Koyama Arifumi 神山有史, eds, *Lectures on Bioethics* 生命倫理学講義, Tokyo: Nihon hyoronsha, pp. 189–216.

[Describes the mentality of military doctors during the war as background to the medical atrocities of the Ishii network.]

—— 2002a, *Crossroads of Conspiracy: An Investigation into the Imperial Bank Incident and Unit 731* 謀略のクロスロード—帝銀事件捜査と731部隊, Tokyo: Nihon hyoronsha.

[An analysis of the investigation documents ("Kai Notes") on the Imperial Bank incident. The author confirms that in 1948 the Japanese police already knew about human experiments performed by the Ishii network and its exemption from prosecution by the U.S.]

—— 2002b, Biological Weapons and Unit 731 of Japanese Army 細菌兵器と日本軍七三一部隊, in Hata Ikuhiko, Sase Masamori and Tsuneishi, Keiichi 秦郁彦, 佐瀬昌盛, 常石敬一, eds, *Encyclopedia of War Crimes in Modern History* 世界戦争犯罪事典, Tokyo: Bungei shunju, pp. 93–106.

—— 2005a, *Epidemiology of the Battlefield* 戦場の疫学, Tokyo: Kaimeisha.

[Examines the outbreak of plague in Shinkyo (today's Changchun) and Unit 731's role. Also describes the U.S.'s exemption of the Ishii network from prosecution in exchange for experimental data. The author discovers that while information about victims was not recorded, details were kept about Japanese who died following medical treatment and were later dissected.]

—— 2005b, New Facts about US Payoff to Japan's Biological Warfare Unit 731. *Japan Focus. The Asian Pacific Journal*, August 15.

—— 2007, Unit 731 and the Human Skulls Discovered in 1989: Physicians Carrying Out Organized Crimes, in William R. LaFleur et al., eds, *Dark Medicine: Rationalizing Unethical Medical Research*, Bloomington: Indiana University Press.

Tsuneishi, Keiichi and Asano, Tomizo 常石敬一, 朝野富三 1982, *Germ Warfare Troops and Two Medical Researchers who Committed Suicide* 細菌戦部隊と自決した二人の医学者, Tokyo: Shinchosha.

[A documentary novel of a former lieutenant general and an associate professor from Tokyo Imperial University who committed suicide because of their consciousness of the atrocities.]

Ura, Naoto 浦直人1981, *The Enemy is in the Bush: The War Record of the Special Water Supply Unit* テキは薮の中に在り—特殊部隊「給水班」モテモテ奮戦記, Tokyo: Sairyusha.

Utsumi, Aiko 内海愛子 et al. eds 1992, Questions about the Human Bones Discovered at the Site of the Military Medical College 軍医学校跡地で発見された人骨問題, in *Handbook of Post-war Reparations* ハンドブック戦後補償, Tokyo: Nashi no ki sha, pp. 108–113.

Wada, Juro 和田十郎 1995, *The First and Last Veterans of the Japanese Army, from the Soviet Invasion to Demobilization: A Record of Unit 731* 日本陸軍最初と最後の復員 ソ連軍侵攻から復員まで: 七三一部隊の記録, Toyoura, Yamaguchi prefecture: self-published.

[Wada shows that the demobilization of Unit 731 was given top priority. Members and their families were the first to return to Japan in the closing stages of the war.]

Wang, Guodong 王国栋 ed. 2005, *Japan's Biological Warfare Criminals: Documents of the Khabarovsk Trials* 日本细菌战战犯 伯力审判实录, Changsha: Hunan renmin chubanshe. A reprint of the Chinese version of the Khabarovsk Trial 1950.

Wang, Shiheng 王詩恒 1942, *Report on the Plague in Changte and Measures for its Control*, July 20. Available in Kondo 2003.

Wang, Zhengyu 汪正宇, 1942, Inspection of Goods Dropped by Enemy Airplanes 敵機於常德首次投擲物品検験経過, in Chongqing yiyao jishu zhuanke xuexiao *Yiji tongxun* 重慶医薬技術専科学校「医技通訊」, December. Available in Matsumura 1997a.

Watanabe, Toshihiko 渡辺利彦 1993, Unit 731 and Nagata Tetsuzan 七三一部隊と永田鉄山, in Chuo daigaku jinbun kagaku kenkyusho 中央大學人文科學研究所, *The Japan-Chinese War* 日中戦争, Tokyo: Chuo daigaku shuppanbu, pp. 275–302.

Williams, Peter and Wallace, David 1985, *Unit 731: Did the Emperor Know?*, London: Television South.

[This television documentary examines the work of Unit 731, includes interviews with former prisoners who were used in experiments, and investigates why the perpetrators remained unprosecuted after the war.]

—— 1989, *Unit 731: The Japanese Army's Secret of Secrets*, London: Hodder & Stoughton.

[Mostly based on research by Tsuneishi Keiichi and Asano Tomizo and materials from the U.S., Britain, Japan, and the Soviet Union. It documents biological weapons developed by the Allied forces and the postwar deals struck between Japan and the U.S. The many interviews include one with Ishii Shiro's daughter. Translated into Japanese by F. Nishizato and published as 七三一部隊の生物兵器とアメリカ—バイオテロの系譜 in 2003 by Kamogawa shuppan (Kyoto). Also translated into Chinese by T. Wu as 七三一部隊 and published by Guoshiguan (Taipei) in 1992. The American edition, published by Free Press in 1989, omitted Chapter 17 on the Korean War which alleged that American forces had used biological weapons.]

Wu, Tianwei, Hu, Hualing, and Sun, Yingzhe 吳天威, 胡華玲, 孫英哲 1995, Special Issue: Unit 731: Japan's Biological Warfare Campaign Against China 侵華日軍七三一細菌部隊專集. *Journal for the Study of Japanese Aggression against China* 日本侵華研究, 21 and 22.

[Includes primary sources and secondary studies in both Chinese and English.]

Wu, Yongming 吳永明 2005, *Crimes under Hinomaru: Exposing Japanese Army's Bacteriological Warfare Campaign in Shangrao* 太阳旗下的罪恶：侵华日军上饶细菌战揭密, Nanchang: Jiangxi renmin chubanshe.

Xie, Zhonghou, Zhang, Ruizhi, and Tian, Susu 谢忠厚, 张瑞智, 田苏苏 ed. 2005, *Archival Materials on Crimes Carried out by the Japanese Army in China, No. 5 – Germ Warfare* 日本侵略华北罪行档案 5, 细菌战, Shijiazhuang: Hebei renmin chubanshe.

Xinhua shishi congkanshe 新華時事叢刊社 ed. 1950, *Justice on Trial: Japanese Biological War Crimes before the Soviet Courts* 正義的審訊：蘇聯審訊日本細菌戰犯案經過, Shanghai: Xinhua shudian.

[Selected documents from the Khabarovsk Trial.]

Xing, Qi and Chen, Daya 邢祁, 陳大雅 eds 1995, 1941, *Calamity: The Bacteriological War in Changde* 辛巳劫難：一九四一年常德細菌戰紀実, Beijing: Zhonggong zhongyang dangxiao chubanshe.

Xu, Jielin 許介鱗 1984, The Japanese Biochemical Unit in China 在中国的日本化学細菌戰部隊, in Zhongyang yanjiuyuan jindaishi yanjiusuo 中央研究院近代史研究所, ed., *A Symposium on Nation-building during the First Ten Years of the Anti-Japanese War*, Vol. 2 抗日前十年国家建設史研討会論文集 (下), Taipei: Zhongyang yanjiuyuan jindashi yanjiusuo.

Xu, Wenfang 徐文芳 1986, The Linkou Branch of Unit 731 of the Japanese Army in China 侵華日軍第七三一部隊・林口支隊, in Zhengxie Heilongjiangsheng weiyuanhui 政協黑竜江省委員会, ed., *Historical Documents of Heilongjiang, Volume 22* 黑龍江文史資料第二十二辑, Harbin: Heilongjiang renmin chubanshe.

Yamada, Seizaburo 山田清三郎 1973, The Final Statement 最終陳述, in *A Record of Internment in the Soviet Union* ソビエト抑留紀行, Tokyo: Toho suppansha, pp. 169–210.

[An account of a Japanese prisoner held in Khabarovsk who confessed to involvement in human experiments.]

—— 1974, *Documentary Novel: Bacteriological Warfare on Trial* 記録小説　細菌戦軍事裁判, Tokyo: Toho shuppansha, 1974.

[Based on Khabarovsk Trial documents and the author's experience as editor for the magazine *Nihon shimbun*, published for the Japanese interned in the Soviet Union after the war.]

Yamaguchi, Kenichiro 山口研一郎 1995, Medical Crimes in History: Unit 731 and Nazi Medical Science 医療の歴史的犯罪　七三一部隊とナチスの医学, in *A Waste of Life – The Destructive Side of Modern Medicine* 生命をもてあそぶ現代の医療, Tokyo: Shakai hyoronsha, pp.178–211.

[Describes the crimes of Unit 731 and shows its mentality remained a part of the medical society after the War.]

Yang, Yulin and Xin, Peilin 杨玉林, 辛培林 eds. 2002, *Biological Warfare* 细菌战, Harbin: Heilongjiang renmin chubanshe.

[Includes studies from China and Japan and testimonies of how the biological warfare was conducted in China.]

Yang, Yulin, Xin, Peilin, and Diao, Naili 杨玉林, 辛培林, 刁乃莉 2004, *Tracking Down the "Special Transportation" used by the Kwantung Army: An Investigation of Human Experimentation in Japanese Bacteriological Warfare* 日军关东宪兵队" 特别输送" 追踪：日军细菌战人体试验罪证调查, Beijing: Shehui kexue wenxian chubanshe.

Yoshifusa, Torao 吉房虎雄 1957, "Special Transportation": Experiments with Biological Weapons 特移扱：細菌実験, in Kanki Haruo 神吉晴夫, ed., *The Three-All Policy: Confessions of Japanese War Criminals in China* 三光　日本人の中国における戦争犯罪の告白, Tokyo: Kobunsha, pp. 27–37.

[Revised and reprinted in 1958, 1982, and 1984 by Shindokushosha (Tokyo) with a new title 侵略—中国における日本戦犯の告白.]

Yoshikai, Natsuko 吉開那津子 1981 (reprinted 1993, 1996), *Memories that Cannot be Erased: A Record of Vivisection by Military Doctor Yuasa* 消せない記憶：湯浅軍医生体解剖の記録, Tokyo: Nicchu shuppan.

Yoshimi, Yoshiaki and Iko, Toshiya 吉見義明, 伊香俊哉 1995, *Links between Unit 731, the Emperor and the Army Command* 七三一部隊と天皇・陸軍中央, Tokyo: Iwanami shoten.

[Based on diaries kept by army chiefs, this booklet reveals that the use of poison gas and biological weapons by Unit 731 would not have been possible without the assent of Emperor Hirohito.]

Yoshimi, Yoshiaki and Matsuno, Seiya 吉見義明, 松野誠也 1997, *Documents on Poison Gas Warfare Vol. 2*, 毒ガス戦関係資料 II, Tokyo: Fuji shuppan.

Yoshimura, Akira 吉村昭 1970, *Bacteria* 細菌, Tokyo: Kodansha.

[A documentary novel of Japanese biological warfare and human experimentation by Unit 731. It was retitled *Fleas and Bombs* 蚤と爆弾 and reprinted in 1975 by Kodansha and in 1989 by Bungei shunju (Tokyo).]

Yoshinaga, Haruko 吉永春子 1976a, Ishii's Germ Troops: Thirty Years after the War 石井細菌戦部隊の戦後三〇年. *Shokun, September 8, 9.*

—— 1976b, *The Bruise – The Terror of Unit 731* ある傷痕・魔の七三一部隊. A documentary programme screened on November 2, 1976 and June 29, 1982 by the Tokyo Broadcasting System.

[Based on her interviews with former Unit 731 members and other relevant individuals in Japan and the U.S.]

—— 1982, Experiments on Human Subjects – Testimonies from Ishii's Germ Troops 「石井細菌戦部隊」被験者の証言. *Shokun*, 14, 9.

[The author describes her interviews with Ishii network members and American investigators.]

—— 2001, *Tracking Down the Leaders of Unit 731* 七三一追撃・そのとき幹部達は, Tokyo: Chikuma shobo.

[Presents interviews with participants in the medical atrocities and also tells the process of making the 1976 documentary.]

Yoshimura, Hisato 吉村寿人 1984, *A Retrospection of his 77 Years* 喜寿回顧, privately published.

[The author is well known for his frostbite experiments on human subjects. He writes: "The experiments I did were not so cruel," although "Ishii's unit was like hell to me, and I was tormented there."]

Zhang, Limei 张丽梅 2006, Research during the Past Decade on Japanese Army's Biological Warfare Campaign in China 近 10 年侵华日军细菌战研究综述. *Beihua daxue xuebao (shehui kexue ban)*, 4.

Zhang, Shixin 張世欣 ed. 1999, *The Japanese Army's Bacteriological Warfare Crimes in Chongshan Village of Zhejiang Province: Demanding Compensation as Victims' Rights* 浙江省崇山村侵华日军细菌战罪行史实—受害索赔, 崇山人的正当权利, Hangzhou: Zhejiang jiaoyu chubanshe.

Zhang, Zhiqiang and Zhao, Yujie 张志强, 赵玉洁 2003, *Research on "Special Transportation": Sourcing Unit 731's Human Subjects* "特别移送" 研究：侵华日军七三一部队人体实验材料之源, Changchun: Jilin renmin chubanshe.

Zhongguo Heilongjiangshen danganguan (Heilongjiang Prefecture Archive) 中国黑龙江省档案馆 et al. eds 2001, *Irrefutable Evidence on Unit 731: Archival Documents Regarding the "Special Transportation" used by Gendarmerie of the Kwantung Army* "七三一"部队罪行铁证——关东宪兵队"特殊输送" 档案, Harbin: Heilongjiang renmin chubanshe.

[Includes two volumes, the first in Chinese and the second in Japanese.]

Zhongguo Jilinshen danganguan (Jilin Prefecture Archive) 中国吉林省档案馆 et al. eds 2003, *Irrefutable Evidence on Unit 731: Selected Archival Documents on "Special Transportation and Epidemic Prevention"* "七三一" 部队罪行铁证–特别移送. 防疫档案选编, Changchun: Jilin renmin chubanshe.

Zhongyang danganguan (China Central Archive) 中央档案馆 et al. eds 1989, *Selected Archival Documents on the Invasion of China by the Japanese Imperialists: Bacteriological and Poison Gas Warfare* 日本帝国主义侵华档案资料选编：细菌战与毒气战, Beijing: Zhonghua shuju.

[This major Chinese publication based on archival documents has been translated into Japanese by K. Eda et al, and published in 1991 to 1992 by Dobunkan (Tokyo). *Witness to Vivisection: War Crimes of the Former Japanese Army* 証言生体解剖：旧日本軍の戦争犯罪; *Witness to Human Experiments: Unit 731 and its Wider Network* 証言人体実験：七三一部隊とその周辺; *Witness to Biological Warfare: The Origins of Biochemical Weapons* 証言細菌作戦：BC 兵器の原点.]

Appendixes

Compiled by Suzy Wang

A The experiments conducted under the Third Reich and Imperial Japan[1] and postwar use of such data

	WARTIME / TOTALITARIAN REGIME (FASCISM)		WARTIME / TOTALITARIAN REGIME (MILITARISM)
	NAZI GERMANY (and conquered territories)		IMPERIAL JAPAN (and conquered territories) 1932–1945
A. Medico-military research			A. Medico-military research
	September 1939–April 1945 (various times between dates)	Lost (mustard) gas experiments, *Sachsenhausen, Natzweiler, and other concentration camps*	Infectious disease experiments – *First at Unit 731, then also at the various subunits that were created as Japan conquered more lands and was faced with more tropical diseases. The subjects were then vivisected and the organs conditions recorded..:*
	December 1941–February 1945	Spotted fever/Typhus (Fleckfieber) experiments, *Buchenwald, Natzweiler and other concentration camps*	Botulism, Brucellosis, Cholera, Dysentry, Gas gangrene, Glanders, Influenza, Meningococcus, Salmonella, Smallpox, Tetanus, Tick encephalitis, Tuberculosis, Tularemia, Typhoid epidemic, Hemorrhagic fever, Tsutsugamushi fever, Plague, Anthrax, Streptococcus bacteria (Navy experiments)
	February 1942–April 1945	Malaria experiments, *Dachau concentration camp*	
	March 1942–August 1942	High-altitude experiments, *Dachau concentration camp*	Freezing experiments
	July 1942–September 1943	Sulfanilamide experiments, *Ravensbrueck concentration camp*	
	August 1942–May 1943	Freezing experiments, *Dachau concentration camp*	High-altitude experiments
	September 1942–December 1943	Bone, muscle, and nerve regeneration and bone transplantation experiments, *Ravensbrueck concentration camp*	Poison experiments

	Dates	Experiment	
	June 1943–January 1945	**Epidemic jaundice experiments,** *Sachsenhausen and Natzweiler concentration camps*	**Fugu (blowfish) toxin, snake poison** **Artificial blood substitutes**
	July 1944–September 1944	**Sea-water experiments,** *Dachau concentration camp*	**Experiments using tourniquets (Navy experiments)**
	Dates unclear	**Tuberculosis experiments,** *Bullenhauser Dam*	**Field tests** – *Most were conducted on civilians in Shanghai, Ninpo, Nanking, Kantong, Hunan, Zhejiang but preliminary testing was conducted at Unit 100 on prisoners tied to a stake to test bomb wounds.*
			Diary entries:
			30 January 1943
	Dates unclear	**Phosgene gas experiments,** *Fort Ney, Strassburg, France*	23 February 1943
			Robert Peaty (senior officer at Muken Camp)
			"Everyone received a 5 cc Typhoid-paratyphoid A inoculation."
			"Funeral service for 142 dead. 186 have died in 5 days, all Americans."
			Sterilization of lepers
			C. Medical Institutions
B. Miscellaneous, ad hoc experiments	November 1943–January 1944	**Incendiary bomb experiments,** *Buchenwald concentration camp*	**Vivisections** – *for training newly employed army surgeons in the various Army hospitals in China to teach them how to treat wounded soldiers in the field (appendectomies, tracheotomies, bullet extraction, amputation, etc.).*
	December 1943–October 1944	**Experiments with poison,** *Buchenwald concentration camp*	
C. Racially motivated	March 1941–January 1945	**Sterilization experiments,** *Auschwitz, Ravensbrueck, and other concentration camps* **experiments**	
	Dates unclear	**Artificial insemination experiments,** *Auschwitz, Block 10*	
	Dates unclear	**Twin experiments,** *Auschwitz*	
	1943	**Jewish skeleton collection,** *Natzweiller-Struhof concentration camp → Strassburg University*	

A The experiments conducted under the Third Reich and Imperial Japan and postwar use of such data (*Continued*)

	WARTIME / TOTALITARIAN REGIME (FASCISM)		WARTIME / TOTALITARIAN REGIME (MILITARISM)	
	NAZI GERMANY (and conquered territories)		*IMPERIAL JAPAN (and conquered territories) 1932–1945*	
			United States	
	Dates	**Material used**	**Material used by**	**Results**
Use of Nazi/ Japan's BW Data	Immediate postwar	Unit 731 data collected as a result of 14 years of human experimentation	U.S. Military (it is believed that information gathered was utilized during the Korean War)	Immunity from prosecution offered to the doctors/researchers
	1980s	Alexander Report on the hypothermia experiments at Dachau	Dr. Robert Pozos, Director of Hypothermia Laboratory at the University of Minnesota of Medicine at Duluth	Publication denied by the *New England Journal of Medicine*
	1986	Collection at the Vogt Institute of the Brain Research in Dusseldorf (collected between 1928 and 1953).	Dr. Berhard Bogerts presented findings of schizophrenic brains at the meeting of the American College of Neuropsychopharmacology.	Warning to Bogerts, 2 questionable specimens to be excluded in research.

B The experiments conducted under the U.S. government[2]

	Dates	Experiments conducted	Award in exchange for experiments	Subjects/facility	Experimentation conducted by
Prison experiments (Pre-WWII)	1906	Plague	Tobacco	**Prisoners who were condemned to death, *Bilibid prison in Manila, The Philippines* (13 deaths)**	**Dr. Richard P. Strong, Director of the Biological Laboratory of the Philippine Bureau of Science, later Professor of Tropical Medicine at Harvard University**
	1910	Beriberi	Tobacco	**Prisoners who were condemned to death, *Bilibid prison in Manila, The Philippines (number of deaths)***	**Dr. Richard P. Strong, Director of the Biological Laboratory of the Philippine Bureau of Science, later Professor of Tropical Medicine at Harvard University**
	1914	Pellagra	"Accordingly rewarded"/promise of Governor's pardon – pardoned plus free medical care until recovery (rejected)	**White male convicts at the Rankin Prison Farm, Mississippi.** *Many begged to be released from experiment, but were not allowed*	**Dr. Goldberger and Wheeler of the U.S. Public Health Service**
	1919–1922	Testicular transplants (some with animal glands)	Unclear	**500 of San Quentin's inmates, California**	**Dr. L. L. Stanley**
	1934	Tuberculosis	Governor's pardon	**Carl Erickson/Mike Schmidt – 2 Colorado prisoners selected to participate in Denver's National Jewish Hospital experiment on TB**	**Doctors at Denver's National Jewish Hospital**
(WWII) *Appeal to patriotism and altruism*	1942	Blood (beef) substitute	Unclear	**64 inmates at a state prison in Norfolk, Massachusetts** *(20 became ill, 1 death)*	**U.S. Navy and Dr. Edward J. Cohn, a distinguished Harvard biochemist**

(Continued)

B The experiments conducted under the U.S. government (*Continued*)

Dates	Experiments conducted	Award in exchange for experiments	Subjects/facility	Experimentation conducted by
during WWII	Malaria, blood plasma substitutes, Dengue fever, Sand-fly fever, Sleeping sickness	Certificates of merit (parole consideration)	New Jersey Prison	U.S. Army (test of diseases found in the field)
1941–1945 ($25 million)				
during WWII	Atabrine and other drugs	Unclear	Sing Sing Prison inmates, New York	U.S. Army (to determine whether, under the drug's influence, soldiers could carry full workloads)
1945 ($700,000) during WWII	Various	$100.00, certificate of merit, and reduction of sentence	Federal Correctional Institution at Seageville, Texas	Unclear
during WWII	Malaria/8 new untested drugs, Atabrine, Quinine, and Plasmochon	$100.00 and certificate of merit	130 inmates at the U.S. Penitentiary at Atlanta, Georgia	The National Research Council, Division of Medical Sciences, and the Committee on Medical Research of the Office of Scientific Research and Development
September 1944–1946	Malaria	Reduction in sentence (317 were granted commutations of sentence or parole)	432 inmates[4] at the Stateville Penitentiary, Illinois	University of Chicago and U.S. Army
(POST NUREMBERG CODE)				
~1955 ($36 million) 1951–1972	Various experiments (shampoo-in-eye, poison ivy, thumb nail	Payments varied from $3.00 to $1500 per test per man	Inmates in the Holmesburg Prison in Pennsylvania. *Most were in prison waiting for a hearing and couldn't afford to post bail or hire an attorney*	Dr. Albert M. Kligman, Director of Ivy Research Laboratories, Inc., Clover Laboratories, Inc., and Betro Laboratories, Inc.

Date	Topic		Subjects	Sponsor
	extraction, various creams and ointments, dioxin, Retin-A, radioactive isotope, LSD, etc.)/			Johnson and Johnson Company; Merck; Sharp and Dohme; Smith, Kline & French Laboratories; Wyeth Laboratories U.S. Army
1950	Viral hepatitis	Unclear	200 female inmates at Clinton Farms, New Jersey	U.S. Army, Dr. Joseph Stokes, Jr., of Children's Hospital of Philadelphia, and the University of Pennsylvania Professor Juko Katsura of Niigata University, funded by U.S. Army
November 1952 – January 1956	Rickettsia Tsutsugamushi	Unclear	118 inmates of a psychiatric hospital (*8 died, 1 committed suicide*)	National Heart Institute
1953	Relationship between chemicals in blood and development of heart disease	Unclear	20,000 inmates at Leavenworth, Atlanta, and Terre Haute	
1953	Amoebic dysentery	Unclear	175 inmates at Seagoville, Texas	Unclear
1953	Athlete's foot	Unclear	U.S. Penitentiary at Atlanta, Georgia	Communicable Disease Center
1953	Common cold	Unclear	The Federal Reformatory in Chillicothe, Ohio	Microbiology Institute

(Continued)

B The experiments conducted under the U.S. government (*Continued*)

Dates	Experiments conducted	Award in exchange for experiments	Subjects/facility	Experimentation conducted by
mid-1950s	Cancer	Unpaid with "no expectation or hope of altering their time of discharge"	about 170 inmates from Ohio prisons	Drs. Chester M. Southam[5] and Alice E. Moore of Manhattan's Sloan Kettering Institute for Cancer Research and Dr. Charles A. Doan, director of medical research at Ohio State University
1950s	Mind-control experiments	Unclear	142 inmates at Iona State Hospital in Michigan	Central Intelligence Agency
? ~ 1957	Tularemia	Army certificates of achievement	31 inmates from Ohio prisons – *treated with streptomycin*	U.S. Army and Ohio State University Research Foundation
early 1960s – early 1970s	Radiation	Unclear	More than 130 inmates in Oregon and Washington prisons – *10-year-long study, estimated ½ died as a result of experimentation*	Atomic Energy Commission, scientists at the National Aeronautics and Space Administration
? ~ 1961	Infectious hepatitis	Unclear	Between 137 and 200 inmates at the Illinois State Penitentiary at Joliet – *5-year-long study*	Dr. Joseph D. Boggs, Director of Laboratories at Children's Memorial Hospital in Chicago and Associate Professor of Pathology at the Northwestern University School of Medicine
1962	Antibiotic designed to treat acne vulgaris	Unclear	50 (either juvenile delinquents or mental defectives)	Unclear

1970 ($1.5 billion to 11,000 grams, 1/3 required human experimentation)[3]				
July 1963	Injection of live cancer cells	None – no informed consent	22 chronically ill and debilitated patients at the Jewish Chronic Disease Hospital of Brooklyn, New York	Dr. Southam and two other doctors. Research funded by United States Public Health Service and the American Cancer Society
1968	Drug that causes temporary paralyses – led to suffocation	None. Prisoners were told to associate agony with misbehavior	Violence-prone inmates at Vacaville, California State Prison	Unclear
1971–1973	Malaria	Additional food, ice cream, fruit juice, improved quarters and $50.00 honorarium	107 inmates of the Jackson County Jail in Kansas City, Missouri	Unclear
June 1975				*Only 12 state prisons systems left hosting medical experiments*
March 1, 1976				*End of medical research on federal prisoners in the U.S.*

Notes

1 Please note that this is not an exhaustive list of experimentations that took place during the periods indicated. Sources compiled for the table may be found in: *Trials of War Criminals before the Nuremberg Military Tribunals under Control Council Law No. 10*. Nuremberg, October 1946 – April 1949. Washington D.C.: U.S. Government Printing Office, 1949–1953; Baruch C. Cohen *The Ethics of Using Medical Data From Nazi Experiments*. Jewish Law. http://jlaw.com/Articles/ NaziMedEx.html (accessed May 18, 2005); Erhard Geissler and John Ellis von Courtland Moon (eds). *Biological and Toxin Weapons: Research, Development and Use from the Middle Ages to 1945*. New York: Oxford University Press, 1999; 20 July 1945. "Japanese Biological Warfare." Intelligence Research Project #2263 of Military Intelligence Service, WDGS. Located in the National Archives: NND857146; 裁かれる細菌戦 : 資料集シリーズ。東京: 7 3 1 部隊細菌戦被 害国家賠償請求訴訟弁護団, *1999*; Peter Williams and David Wallace. *Unit 731: Japan's Secret Biological Warfare in World War II*. New York: Free Press, 1989; David Guyatt. "Unit 731: Human Logs Light Military Research Fires." 1997. http://www.copi.com/articles/guyatt/unit_731.html (accessed May 23, 2005).

2 Please note that this is not an exhaustive list of experimentations that took place during the periods indicated. Sources compiled for the table may be found in: Baruch C. Cohen. *The Ethics of Using Medical Data From Nazi Experiments*. Jewish Law. http://jlaw.com/Articles/NaziMedEx.html (accessed May 18, 2005); Andrew C. Ivy. *The History and Ethics of the Use of Human Subjects in Medical Experiments*. Science, New Series, Vol. 108, No. 2792 (July 2, 1948); *[Testimony presented by Sydney M. Wolfe, M.D. of the Health Research Group in Washington D.C. before the Senate Sub-Committee on Health, Hearings on Human Experimentation, March 7, 1973]* and *[U.S. Congress Senate, Committee on Labor and Public Welfare. Hearings before Sub-Committee on Health, 92nd Congress, 1st Session, 1973 (U.S. Government Printing Office, Washington, D.C.) 1973, pp. 803– 813, 1125]* in Alvis V. Adair. *Human Experimentation: An Ancient Notion in a Modern Technology Occasional Paper*. Institute for Urban Affairs and Research, Vol. 1, No. 3; Len Doyal and Jeffrey S. Tobias (eds). *Informed Consent in Medical Research*. London: BMJ Books, 2001; and the following in Allen M. Hornblum. *Acres of Skin: Human Experimentations at Holmesburg Prison*. London: Routledge, 1998.

   [David J. Rothman, Strangers at the Bedside. New York: Basic Books, 1991]; 1953 experiment information taken from *["Federal Prisons Year End Review," 1953, p. 31–33]; ["Women Prisoners Aid Jaundice Test," New York Times, September 4, 1950]; [Nicholas Horrock, "Records Show CIA Tested LSD on Sex-psychopaths," New York Times, August 5, 1977, p. A10]*, p. 95; *["Prison Volunteers Test Vaccine for Tularemia," Science News Letter, June 22, 1957: 386]*, p. 95; *[Walter Sullivan, "Scientist Reports Isolating 2 Strains of Hepatitis," New York Times, June 29, 1961]* and *["Vaccination Reported for Infectious Hepatitis," New York Times, May 5, 1961] pp. 100–101; [Gary Lee, "The Lifelong Harm to Radiation's Human Guinea Pigs," Washington Post, National Weekly Edition, November 28, 1994, p.33] pp. 107–108; ["Government to Ban Medical Research on Federal Inmates," New York Times, March 2, 1976], p. 113.]*

3 Numbers taken from [David J. Rothman, *Strangers at the Bedside*. New York: Basic Books, 1991, p. 53] in Allen M. Hornblum. *Acres of Skin: Human Experimentations at Holmesburg Prison*. London: Routledge, 1998. p. 85–86.

4 Consent form /waiver form signed by inmates of the Stateville Penitentiary for the malaria experiment:

   I . . . hereby declare that I have read and clearly understood the above notice, as testified by my signature hereon, and I hereby apply to the University of Chicago, which is at present engaged on malarial research at the orders of the Government, for participation in the investigations of the life-cycle of the malarial parasite. I hereby accept all risks connected with the experiment and on behalf of my heirs and my personal and legal representatives I hereby absolve from such liability the University of Chicago and all the technicians and assistants taking part in the above mentioned investigations. I similarly absolve the Government of the State of Illinois, the Director of the Department of Public Security of the State of Illinois, the warden of the State Penitentiary at Joliet-Stateville and all employees of the above institutions and Departments, from all responsibility, as well as from all claims and proceedings or Equity pleas, for any injury or malady, fatal or otherwise, which may ensue from these experiments. I hereby certify that this offer is made voluntarily and without compulsion. I have been instructed that if my offer is accepted I shall be entitled to remuneration amounting to [xx] dollars, payable as provided in the above Notice.

[M. H. Pappworth, Human Guinea Pigs. Boston: Beacon Press, 1967, p. 62] quoted in Allen M. Hornblum. *Acres of Skin: Human Experimentations at Holmesburg Prison*. London: Routledge, 1998, p. 82.

5 When asked in a 1996 interview by Allen M. Hornblum if Dr. Chester M. Southam of Manhattan's Sloan-Kettering Institute was abiding by the Nuremberg Code when conducting experiments on inmates in Ohio, he responded that he was "unaware of the Nuremberg Code and its code of conduct." He also added that "Most of the publicity on the [prison] experiments was favorable during the 1950s." quoted in Allen M. Hornblum. *Acres of Skin: Human Experimentations at Holmesburg Prison*. London: Routledge, 1998. p. 95.

Index